50 Big Debates in Reproductive Medicine

Edited by

Roy Homburg
Homerton University Hospital, London, UK

Adam H Balen
Leeds Fertility, UK

Robert F Casper
TRIO Fertility and University of Toronto, Canada

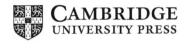
CAMBRIDGE
UNIVERSITY PRESS

CAMBRIDGE
UNIVERSITY PRESS

University Printing House, Cambridge CB2 8BS, United Kingdom

One Liberty Plaza, 20th Floor, New York, NY 10006, USA

477 Williamstown Road, Port Melbourne, VIC 3207, Australia

314–321, 3rd Floor, Plot 3, Splendor Forum, Jasola District Centre,
New Delhi – 110025, India

103 Penang Road, #05–06/07, Visioncrest Commercial, Singapore 238467

Cambridge University Press is part of the University of Cambridge.

It furthers the University's mission by disseminating knowledge in the
pursuit of education, learning, and research at the highest international levels
of excellence.

www.cambridge.org
Information on this title: www.cambridge.org/9781108986601
DOI: 10.1017/9781108986373

© Cambridge University Press 2022

First published 2022

Printed in the United Kingdom by TJ Books Limited, Padstow Cornwall

A catalogue record for this publication is available from the British Library.

ISBN 978-1-108-98660-1 Paperback

•••

Contents

Section III The Best Policy

Section IV Embryology

Contributors

Ashok Agarwal
American Center for Reproductive Research, Glickman Urological Institute, Cleveland Clinic, Cleveland, OH, USA

Megan Allyse
Biomedical Ethics Research Program and Department of Obstetrics and Gynecology, Mayo Clinic, Rochester, MN, USA

Wael Almajed
Division of Urology, Department of Surgery, McGill University, Montreal, QC, Canada; Division of Urology, King Abdullah bin Abdulaziz University Hospital, Riyadh, Saudi Arabia

Claus Yding Andersen
Copenhagen University Hospital and Faculty of Health and Medical Sciences, University of Copenhagen, Copenhagen, Denmark

Ahmed Badawy
Director of Mansoura University Regenerative Medicine Center, Mansoura University, Egypt

Gulam Bahadur
Reproductive Medicine Unit, North Middlesex University Hospital, London UK; Homerton Fertility Centre, Homerton University Hospital, London, UK

Kylie Baldwin
Centre for Reproduction Research, De Montfort University, Leicester, UK

N Ellissa Baskind
Leeds Fertility, Leeds Teaching Hospitals NHS Trust, UK

José Bellver
Instituto Valenciano de Infertilidad, IVI-RMA, Valencia; Department of Pediatrics, Obstetrics and Gynecology, Faculty of Medicine, University of Valencia, Italy

Harish M Bhandari
Leeds Fertility, Leeds Teaching Hospitals NHS Trust, Seacroft Hospital, Leeds, UK

Virginia N Bolton
Formerly of Guy's Assisted Conception Unit, Guy's Hospital, Guy's and St Thomas' NHS Foundation Trust, London, UK

Ernesto Bosch
Instituto Valenciano de Infertilidad, Valencia, Spain

Mark Bowman
Genea Fertility, Sydney Australia; The University of Sydney and Royal Prince Alfred Hospital, Sydney, Australia

Mats Brännström
Department of Obstetrics and Gynecology, University of Gothenburg, Göteborg, Sweden; Stockholm IVF-EUGIN, Stockholm, Sweden

Frank Broekmans
Department of Gynecology and Reproductive Medicine, Division Female and Baby, University Medical Centre, Utrecht, The Netherlands

William Buckett
Division of Reproductive Endocrinology and Infertility, Department of Obstetrics and Gynecology, McGill University, Montreal, Quebec, Canada

Elizabeth Burt
University College London Hospital, London, UK

Ying Cheong
University of Southampton, Southampton, UK

Tim Child
Oxford Fertility and The Fertility Partnership; University of Oxford, UK

Justin Chu
Birmingham Women's and Children's NHS Foundation Trust, University of Birmingham, Birmingham, UK

Helen Clarke
Jessop Fertility, Sheffield, UK

Ana Cobo
IVIRMA, Valencia, Spain

Ben Cohlen
Isala Women's and Children's Hospital, Head of Isala Fertility Center, Isala, The Netherlands

Arri Coomarasamy
Tommy's National Centre for Miscarriage Research, University of Birmingham, Edgbaston, UK

Melanie Davies
Consultant Obstetrician and Gynaecologist, University College London Hospitals, London, UK

Marie-Madeleine Dolmans
Pôle de Recherche en Gynécologie, Institut de Recherche Expérimentale (IREC), Université Catholique de Louvain, Brussels, Belgium; Gynecology Department, Cliniques Universitaires Saint Luc, Brussels, Belgium

Jacques Donnez
Université Catholique de Louvain, Société de Recherche pour l'Infertilité, Brussels, Belgium

Grace Dugdale
Balance Fertility, Leeds, UK

Juan A Garcia-Velasco
IVI RMA Madrid, Spain; Rey Juan Carlos University, Madrid, Spain

Stephan Gordts
Leuven Institute for Fertility and Embryology, Leuven, Belgium

Ingrid Granne
Nuffield Department of Women's and Reproductive Health, University of Oxford, Oxford, UK

Ellen Greenblatt
Department of Obstetrics and Gynaecology, Mount Sinai Hospital, Toronto, Ontario, Canada

Valentina Grisendi
Mother-Infant Department, Institute of Obstetrics and Gynecology, University of Modena and Reggio Emilia, Modena, Italy

Jigal Haas
Infertility and IVF Unit, Chaim Sheba Medical Center, Tel Aviv University, Israel

Lesley Haddock
Research and Development Manager, Examenlab Ltd, Belfast, UK

Mark Hamilton
University of Aberdeen, Aberdeen Fertility Centre, Aberdeen Maternity Hospital, Aberdeen, UK

Roger J Hart
Division of Obstetrics and Gynaecology, Medical School, University of Western Australia, Perth, WA, Australia

Catherine Hayden
Leeds Fertility, Leeds Teaching Hospitals NHS Trust, Leeds, UK

James Hopkisson
NURTURE Fertility, Nottingham, UK

Peter Humaidan
The Fertility Clinic, Skive Regional Hospital and Faculty of Health, Aarhus University, Aarhus, Denmark

Jason Kasraie
Shropshire & Mid-Wales Fertility Centre, Shrewsbury, UK

Louise Kellam
CARE Fertility, Nottingham, UK

Efstratios Kolibianakis
Department of Obstetrics and Gynaecology, Aristotle University of Thessaloniki, Greece

Georgios Lainas
Scientific Director, Eugonia IVF, Athens, Greece; Coordinator, SIG Reproductive Endocrinology, ESHRE, Belgium

Antonio La Marca
Mother-Infant Department, Institute of Obstetrics and Gynecology, University of Modena and Reggio Emilia, Modena, Italy

Cornelis B Lambalk
Department of Reproductive Medicine, Amsterdam UMC, Vrije Universiteit, Amsterdam, The Netherlands

Carl Laskin
TRIO Fertility and University of Toronto, Canada

Joop Laven
Division of Reproductive Endocrinology and Infertility, Division of OBGYN, Erasmus MC University Medical Center, Rotterdam, The Netherlands

Christine Leary
The Women and Children's Hospital, Hull Royal Infirmary, Hull, UK; Hull York Medical School, University of Hull, Hull, UK

William Ledger
School of Women's and Children's Health, Faculty of Medicine, University of New South Wales, Sydney, Australia

Richard S Legro
Department of Obstetrics and Gynecology, Penn State College of Medicine, Hershey, PA, USA

Sarah Lensen
Obstetrics and Gynaecology, University of Melbourne, Royal Women's Hospital, Parkville, Victoria, Australia

Mathew Leonardi
Sydney Medical School Nepean, University of Sydney, Nepean Hospital, Sydney, NSW, Australia; Department of Obstetrics and Gynecology, McMaster University, Hamilton, Canada

Shirley Eve Levitan
Queen's University Law School, Toronto, Ontario, Canada

Sheena EM Lewis
CEO, Examenlab Ltd, Belfast, UK; Queens University Belfast, UK

Gillian Lockwood
Medical Director, CARE Fertility, Tamworth, Staffordshire, UK

Julio Ricardo Loret de Mola
St. John's Hospital, Southern Illinois University, Springfield, IL, USA

Nick Macklon
London Women's Clinic, London, UK and Visiting Professor, University of Copenhagen, Denmark

Arnold M Mahesan
Trio Fertility, Toronto, Ontario, Canada

Kevin Marron
Sims IVF Clinic, Dublin, Ireland

Mariano Mascarenhas
Leeds Fertility, Leeds Teaching Hospitals NHS Trust, Leeds, UK

Raj Mathur
Department of Reproductive Medicine, Saint Mary's Hospital, Manchester Academic Health Sciences Centre, Manchester University NHS Foundation Trust, Manchester, UK

Mostafa Metwally
Consultant in Reproductive Medicine, Sheffield Teaching Hospitals and the University of Sheffield, Sheffield, UK

Mohamed F Mitwally
Odessa Reproductive Medicine Center and San Antonio Reproducive Associates, Helotes, TX, USA

Lewis Nancarrow
The Hewitt Fertility Centre, Liverpool Women's Hospital, Crown St, Liverpool, UK

Jeff Nisker
Department of Obstetrics and Gynaecology, Schulich School of Medicine and Dentistry; Children's Health Research Institute, Western University, London, ON, Canada

Raoul Orvieto
Department of Obstetrics and Gynecology, Chaim Sheba Medical Center (Tel Hashomer), Ramat Gan, Israel; Sackler Faculty of Medicine, Tel-Aviv University, Israel

Allan Pacey
Department of Oncology and Metabolism, University of Sheffield, Sheffield, UK

Stefano Palomba
Unit of Obstetrics and Gynecology, Grande Ospedale Metropolitano of Reggio Calabria, Italy

Guido Pennings
Bioethics Institute Ghent (BIG), Department of Philosophy and Moral Science, Ghent University, Gent, Belgium

Alan Penzias
Boston IVF, Waltham, Massachusetts; Beth Israel Deaconess Medical Center/Harvard Medical School, Boston, MA, USA

Cecilia Petriglia
Departments of Obstetrics and Gynaecology, University of Cagliari, Policlinico Universitario Duilio Casula, Monserrato, Cagliari, Italy

Catherine Pretty
CARE Fertility, Woking, UK

Matt Prior
Newcastle Fertility Centre, Newcastle, UK

Nicholas Raine-Fenning
Queen's Medical Centre, Nottingham, UK

Raj Rai
St Mary's Hospital, London, UK

Claudia Raperport
Homerton University Hospital, London, UK

Kirsten Riggan
Biomedical Ethics Research Program, Mayo Clinic, Rochester, MN, USA

Isla Robertson
University of Southampton, Southampton, UK

Matheus Roque
MATER PRIME – Reproductive Medicine, São Paulo, Brazil

Zev Rosenwaks
Ronald O. Perelman and Claudia Cohen Center for Reproductive Medicine, Weill Cornell Medical College, New York, NY, USA

Hassan N Sallam
Professor in Obstetrics and Gynaecology, the University of Alexandria in Egypt; Alexandria Fertility and IVF Center, Alexandria, Egypt

Ippokratis Sarris
Consultant in Reproductive Medicine, King's College Hospital, London, UK

William D Schlaff
Sidney Kimmel Medical College, Thomas Jefferson University, Philadelphia, PA, USA

Sam Schoenmakers
Division of Obstetrics and Fetal Medicine, Division of OBGYN, Erasmus MC University Medical Center, Rotterdam, The Netherlands

Juan-Enrique Schwarze
Reproductive Medicine Unit at Clinica Las Condes, Santiago, Chile

Amit Shah
Consultant in Reproductive Medicine, Homerton Fertility Centre, London, UK

Hassan Shehata
Epsom and St Helier University Hospitals NHS Trust, Epsom, UK; St George's Hospital Medical School, London, UK; Centre for Reproductive Immunology and Pregnancy, London and Surrey, UK

Francoise Shenfield
Institute for Women's Health, University College London, London, UK

Gon Shoham
Sackler Faculty of Medicine, Tel Aviv University, Ramat Aviv, Tel Aviv, Israel

Zeev Shoham
The Reproductive Medicine and IVF Unit, Kaplan Medical Center, Rehovot, Israel; Hadassah Medical School, Hebrew University, Jerusalem, Israel

Kevin Smith
Division of Health Science, School of Applied Sciences, Abertay University, Dundee, UK

Rachel Smith
Care Fertility Group, UK

Garima Srivastava
Homerton Fertility Centre, Homerton University Hospital, London, UK

Elisabet Stener-Victorin
Karolinska Institutet, Biomedicum B5, Department of Physiology and Pharmacology, Stockholm, Sweden

Jane A Stewart
Newcastle Hospitals NHS Foundation Trust, Gosforth, Newcastle upon Tyne, UK

Tom Gunnar Tanbo
Department of Reproductive Medicine, Oslo University Hospital Rikshospitalet, Oslo, Norway

Karen Thompson
Clinical Lead of Embryology and HFEA, Leeds Fertility, Leeds, UK

Filippo Maria Ubaldi
GENERA Center for Reproductive Medicine, Clinica Valle Giulia, Rome, Italy

Fulco van der Veen
Amsterdam University Medical Center, Amsterdam, The Netherlands

Madelon van Wely
Amsterdam University Medical Center, Amsterdam, The Netherlands

Lisa Webber
Consultant Gynaecologist and Subspecialist in Reproductive Medicine, St Mary's Hospital Imperial College Healthcare NHS Trust, London

Ariel Weissman
Department of Obstetrics and Gynecology, The Edith Wolfson Medical Center, Holon, Tel-Aviv, Israel; Sackler Faculty of Medicine, Tel-Aviv University, Tel-Aviv, Israel

Susan P Willman
Reproductive Endocrinology and Infertility, Contra Costa Regional Medical Center, Martinez, CA, USA

Lucy Wood
Jessop Fertility, Sheffield, UK

Bryan Woodward
X&Y Fertility, Leicester, UK

Ephia Yasmin
University College London Hospitals, NHS Foundation Trust, London, UK

John Yovich
PIVET Medical Centre, Perth, Western Australia; Department of Pharmacy and Biomedical Sciences, Curtin University, Perth, Western Australia, Australia

A Albert Yuzpe
Western University, Ontario, Canada;
University of British Columbia, Canada;
Olive Fertility Centre, Vancouver, BC,
Canada

Armand Zini
Division of Urology, Department of Surgery,
McGill University, Montreal, QC, Canada;
OVO Fertility Clinic, Montreal, QC,
Canada

Foreword

Appearing in what I hope is the wake of the worst pandemic this world has seen in over 100 years, there has never been a more timely appearance of a book that provides the full range of evidence for and against most of the major issues that reproductive medicine specialists face. During this pandemic, we have seen scientific and open debate about how to solve this medical crisis being subjected to political expediency. Dissent by scientists at times has been crushed by autocratic leaders, with honest and open debate the exception and not the rule. We cannot accept the same approach to the many unsolved issues of reproductive medicine. This book has been written by leaders in the field, leaders who I am sure are greatly respected by their patients, in their departments, in their countries and throughout the world, leaders who have strong opinions on how to approach these issues. But on every issue in this book there is a leader who argues for and a leader who argues against. Dear reader, it is up to you to decide who, if either, you will follow.

Renowned physicist and scientist Richard Feynman once noted, 'Religion is a culture of faith; science is a culture of doubt.' We, as practitioners of reproductive medicine, must constantly doubt the current orthodoxy and reassess our practices based on the ever-emerging best evidence. This book provides not only the best evidence but also the ways to assess this evidence. As you read it, you will find even your most cherished practices and beliefs constantly challenged not only by the data cited from key primary sources but also by the eloquence of these thought leaders as they stand by their position and challenge the other. This book is both entertaining and enlightening, and the shortened format of each debate has allowed the authors to distil the essence of their arguments to their purest form.

Those of you like myself who, due to the pandemic restrictions, have been deprived of the intellectual stimulation of our in-person professional meetings and the electricity of a packed hall, and the back and forth of a good debate, complete with a few witty and personal jabs thrust in, look no further for immediate satisfaction than this book. In such spirit, I would be remiss without acknowledging that I have heard the senior editor of this book, Professor Roy Homburg, argue convincingly in his inimitable way both sides of most of these issues in his long and distinguished career. Therefore, I can think of no better person to select presenters for each side of these 50 great debates, assisted, of course, by his accomplished co-editors-in-chief, Professor Adam Balen and Professor Robert Casper. Congratulations to the editors and the authors for this outstanding work.

Richard S Legro, MD, FACOG, FRCOG, ad Eundem
University Professor and Chair, Department of Obstetrics and Gynecology, Penn State College of Medicine, Hershey, PA, USA

Introduction

Human reproduction is the most basic of human functions and is the foundation of our very existence. When considering the bodily mechanisms involved, from the delicacy of the interacting endocrine network to the wonder of the cyclical changes in the ovary and uterus and the mechanism of sperm production, it is a constant source of amazement that the integration needed to produce another human being does not go wrong more often.

The understanding of this process and the possibilities of treating infertility is a rapidly advancing science and there are many variations on a theme, often confusing, and new ideas for improvements, not always scientifically sound, are proffered with startling regularity. It is no surprise then that reproductive medicine constantly provides debate, whether it be scientific, ethical or medical procedural.

This book is a completely unique venture in the field of reproductive medicine. It presents, in the form of debates, two opposing arguments for and against topical, controversial questions. Debates are being utilised increasingly in conferences and have proved to be a wonderful source of information in presenting two sides to an argument which has often been more valuable than a straight frontal lecture. It was with this in mind that we decided to use the same idea in book form and had the enthusiasm and energy of Nick Dunton of Cambridge University Press to encourage us. We thank Nick for all his help and wish him a happy retirement.

Having decided on the most controversial issues in our profession, we approached not only world authorities in the particular fields but also bright young lights to express their opinion in 1000 words. The response was overwhelmingly enthusiastic and we are enormously grateful to the contributors who have done an amazing job. A few of them even admitted that it was not necessarily their opinion that they were expressing but for the sake of debate did their level best to present the other side of the argument.

> Only those afraid of the truth seek to silence debate, intimidate those with whom they disagree, or slander their ideological counterparts. Those who know they are right have no reason to stifle debate because they realize that all opposing arguments will ultimately be overcome by fact.
>
> Glenn Beck, 2009

We hope that this unique form of presentation will be as rewarding for readers as it has been enjoyable for us to put together.

Roy Homburg, Robert Casper and Adam Balen

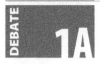

Female Age 42 Years Should Be the Upper Limit for Conventional IVF/ICSI Treatment
For

Jane A Stewart

The premise of this argument is that there is an appropriate age limit for conventional in vitro fertilisation/intracytoplasmic sperm injection (IVF/ICSI) treatment. Why should there be a limit at all? It may be argued that as long as we can squeeze an egg out of an ovary and a woman wishes to proceed, that should be enough for us to proceed.

Good medical practice dictates that doctors advise patients with honesty and integrity and that might include advising no treatment – there is no compulsion to provide a patient with treatment on request or payment. For fertility specialists to fulfil every patient request, whatever the 'cost', would class us alongside commercial surgery. If we are to argue that infertility is a medical diagnosis then we must not accept the definition of 'industry'.

There are a number of reasons why we might not accede to a request for IVF/ICSI in women past their 43rd birthday.

Uncertain Diagnosis

Any woman who continues to ovulate (pre-menopausal) has the potential for natural conception; however, fecundity declines significantly during the fifth decade such that it is rare for a natural conception to occur in a woman over 45.

In practical terms the diagnosis of infertility is based on knowledge of ovulatory function, tubal patency and semen analysis. Whilst more subtle features may be sought, IVF and ICSI are technologies that work around a problem rather than treating an underlying issue. This has become an acceptable way to increase the chance of pregnancy when there is a relative reduction in potential. Very few couples, however, are absolutely infertile and may be better described as subfertile. In women who are older, the margins of benefit of treatment may be very limited, as the effect of age increasingly becomes a major contributory factor to their problem – particularly where it is otherwise unexplained – thus affecting treatment success.

Success Rates

A woman trying to become pregnant in her 40s has a significant risk of failure and a further significant risk of not achieving a live birth even if she does become pregnant. Her chance of success declines year on year and is substantially less at 43 than at 40. She does, however, have an ongoing cumulative pregnancy chance which cannot be matched by a single cycle of treatment. Egg age is the key, and treatment success rates also decline significantly in women in their 40s. This is the result of declining ovarian reserve limiting the number of eggs available, but primarily of egg quality decline. In the United Kingdom the average live birth rate per embryo transferred for women at 40–42 is 11%, whilst at >43 it is 4.5%, demonstrating clearly the effects of these factors [1].

Cost-Effectiveness

Artificial or arbitrary age limits are sometimes applied by commissioners in jurisdictions where state-funded treatment is provided. This is to limit the financial commitment, ensuring that funding helps those most likely to succeed and reducing the number of wasteful cycles. NICE guidance in the United Kingdom recommends a single cycle of treatment for women between 40 and 43 years of age if she has a reasonable ovarian reserve [2]. This was considered a fair approach to address what variability in prognosis may occur at that age point and maintain reasonable cost-effectiveness for state-funded treatment. That same premise may be applied to guide patients who are funding their own treatment where a realistic end point is desired.

Health of Mother and Child

There are a number of challenges in undertaking pregnancy and childbirth in older age:

Pregnancy/fetal health: the risk of miscarriage is significantly raised in older women – over 50% of clinical pregnancies will miscarry in women in their 40s, and the risk increases exponentially each year [3]. The risk of a baby with significant chromosomal abnormality increases with age. Intervention may be required to confirm a diagnosis, which adds risk to the pregnancy and mother even if unaffected, and managing a pregnancy problem incurs physical and mental health risks.

Maternal risk: there is an increased risk of pre-eclampsia and other medical complications with age, which lead to increased intervention and subsequent complications. Whilst only 4% of births in the United Kingdom are to women in their 40s, 11% of maternal deaths are in this age group (24/100,000 maternities; RR 4.34) [4].

Neonatal risk: prematurity risk increases with a woman's age as does perinatal death [5].

Child health and well-being: a woman over 43 will be over 60 when her child reaches adulthood. She is less likely to contribute greatly to their adult years and much less likely to be involved with her grandchildren.

Treatment Burden

IVF/ICSI techniques have become widely accepted as the mainstay treatment of infertility and yet remain a significant challenge to patients. Treatment programmes, although considered relatively safe, may not be without complication. Often described as an emotional rollercoaster, treatment is both physically and mentally demanding, sometimes at significant financial cost.

At what point on this rollercoaster does a woman get off? When she can't cope any more? When she runs out of money? When the medical team get fed up with her? The time to stop must be the concern of the specialist team. They should provide support, advice and counselling to allow patients to come to terms with ending the process before any of those 'breaking' points are reached. One factor for aiding that decision is the ongoing prognosis. If this is sufficiently low, the best advice may be a planned stop rather than to persist indefinitely. If poor prognosis is considered a legitimate guide to ending treatment, then it is a consideration for some as to whether to commence treatment in the first place. It is not uncommon for couples to state that they would 'do anything' or that they need to have 'tried everything' so as to have no later regrets. Specialists providing fertility treatment are not obliged to treat everyone who is prepared to put themselves forward and must manage those for whom treatment is not appropriate (for whatever reason) with both integrity and sensitivity.

Conclusion

IVF/ICSI (assisted reproductive treatment) is a technology that allows us to bypass specific (though sometimes unspecified) fertility problems in order to assist a woman to become pregnant when natural conception may not happen readily. It does not, however, overcome the natural process of fertility decline; success rates decline in parallel with natural conception and with age.

A woman who has a genuine fertility issue necessitating treatment may indeed have a higher pregnancy chance through treatment, but the overall success in a single cycle is limited. So-called unexplained subfertility in an older woman will almost certainly have age as a significant influence, and the cycle of treatment she may contemplate may not better her cumulative chance. To avoid reaching breaking point, appropriate intervention by the specialist may simply be to advise acceptance of continuing to try naturally.

I would advocate this approach for many women for whom age is the most significant factor in their failure to achieve pregnancy. For those women, their cumulative pregnancy rate, through the remainder of their reproductive lives, whilst limited, may yet be better than can be offered through treatment, and if a threshold is to be made, the age of 42 (up to the 43rd birthday) is an appropriate limit.

References

1. HFEA. *Fertility treatment 2018: trends and figures.* 2020; available from: www.hfea.gov .uk/media/3158/fertility-treatment-2018- trends-and-figures.pdf.

2. NICE. *Fertility Problems: assessment and treatment. NICE Clinical Guideline [CG156].* 2013 [updated 2017]; available from: www.nice.org.uk/guidance/cg156/ resources/fertility-problems-assessment- and-treatment-pdf-35109634660549.

3. Magnus MC, Wilcox AJ, Morken N, Weinberg CR, Håberg SE. Role of maternal age and pregnancy history in risk of miscarriage: prospective register based study. *BMJ* 2019;364:l869.

4. MBRRACE-UK. *Saving lives, improving mothers' care.* 2019; available from: www .npeu.ox.ac.uk/assets/downloads/mbrrace- uk/reports/MBRRACE.

5. MBRRACE-UK. *Perinatal mortality surveillance report.* 2019; available from: www.npeu.ox.ac.uk/assets/downloads/ mbrrace-uk/reports/MBRRACE.

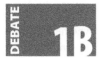

Female Age 42 Years Should Be the Upper Limit for Conventional IVF/ICSI Treatment

Against

Tim Child

I was delighted when asked to write against the proposal to deny women aged 42 years or more the chance of their own genetic motherhood. Indeed, it is challenging to imagine the points that my opposing author will use to try to limit a woman's reproductive choice!

To debate the matter we need to (1) examine the IVF/ICSI live birth rate for women in their 40s; (2) consider the risks to the health of these mothers and their baby(ies) and what can be done to mitigate any concerns; and (3) contemplate the grounds for denying such treatment, and the offered alternatives (childlessness?).

Table 1B.1 reports the live birth rate per cycle started for women in their 40s based on data from the Human Fertilisation and Embryology Authority (HFEA) (2015–17), Oxford Fertility (2009–18) and Cornell IVF [1]. The HFEA and Oxford Fertility data reveal that women aged 43 to 44 years have at least a 5% chance per cycle started of a live birth (with two non-PGT-A embryos most commonly being transferred). Clearly the success rate per oocyte retrieval procedure, and particularly per embryo transfer, will be higher as not all cycles started reach these stages – the figures in the table are therefore a worst-case scenario. For many women aged 43 to 44 years, a live birth rate of 5% per cycle started might not be considered sufficient considering the costs of treatment, both financial and emotional. However, the alternative is childlessness, oocyte donation or adoption, which for some couples may not be acceptable, or at least only acceptable after trying a treatment cycle with their own gametes. For many patients aged 43 to 44 years, a success rate of 5% is absolutely preferable to a chance of zero. On what grounds can treatment, after appropriate counselling, be denied?

The Oxford and Cornell data report a 3% live birth rate per cycle started at the age of 45 years. In my view, even women at the age of 45 years, as long as they have sufficient ovarian

Table 1B.1 Live birth rate per cycle started at specific ages: X% (number of cycles started)

	Age									
	40	41	42	43	44	45	46	47	48	49
HFEA database 2015–17	14%			5%		–	–	–	–	–
Oxford Fertility 2009–18	18% (794)	14% (555)	9% (371)	6% (269)	5% (127)	3% (39)	0% (12)	0% (2)	–	–
Cornell, 2018 [1].	–	–	–	–	–	3% (679)	0.5% (198)	0% (51)	0% (19)	0% (5)

reserve, should be allowed to decide what to do with their body and whether to have treatment. The situation beyond 45 years is different, with success rates of essentially zero.

The primary reason for the reduction in live birth rate with female age is the increasing rate of oocyte embryo aneuploidy. It could be argued that pre-implantation genetic testing for aneuploidy (PGT-A) should be offered to improve outcomes and quicken the time to live birth through earlier identification and transfer of euploid blastocysts (if any exist). Ubaldi et al. [2] reported on the use of 150 PGT-A cycles in women aged 44–47 years. Sixty-eight per cent of cycles resulted in blastocysts suitable for biopsy (though a mean of only 1.0) and only 12% were euploid. Following elective single-embryo transfer (eSET), the live birth rate was 57% per transfer and 8.0% per cycle started. Eleven of the 12 deliveries achieved were in women aged 44 years. My view is that these results are not sufficient to support the routine use of PGT-A in this patient group.

A potential issue with patients in their 40s is the increased prevalence of underlying health conditions such as hypertension, diabetes, obesity, fibroids and other diseases [3]. There is a higher rate of pre-eclampsia, gestational diabetes, pre-term birth and a number of other adverse maternal and perinatal outcomes. We should be screening and counselling all of our patients before offering fertility treatment, regardless of age, and this is particularly so for older women [4]. We can advise and work with our patients to help them improve their pre-treatment health, whether through improved hypertension or diabetic control or through weight loss. For complex cases, the input of an obstetric physician to assist in assessing and modifying risks and to plan for pregnancy care is vital. Where there are risk factors then eSET can be employed to minimise the multiple birth rate, though this can also limit the chance of pregnancy. PGT-A could be useful if eSET is desired.

Oocyte donation is an alternative to conventional IVF with success rates of 40–60% per cycle. However, such pregnancies are independently associated with a higher rate of pre-eclampsia (odds ratio of 3 to 4) and small for gestational age [5]. This could be due to immune tolerance issues between the fetus and mother (since the fetus is considered to be an allogenic graft to the woman). Therefore, if safety issues are a concern for conventional IVF/ICSI beyond the age of 42, the risks with oocyte donation are even higher! Furthermore, the potential for loss of donor anonymity in the future (whether through legal channels such as the HFEA, or through unregulated routes such as home genetic testing, e.g. www.ancestry.com) is a concern, or unacceptable, for some patients.

In conclusion, women can succeed with IVF beyond the age of 42 years using their own eggs. Whilst success rates are low, they are not zero, and it should be the patient's choice. Pre-pregnancy and pre-treatment assessment and mitigation of risk factors can reduce maternal and perinatal risks. Indeed, the pregnancies are safer than those from donor oocyte IVF. Let the woman decide.

References

1. Gunnala V, Irani M, Melnick A, Rosenwaks Z, Spandorfer S. One thousand seventy-eight autologous IVF cycles in women 45 years and older: the largest single-center cohort to date. *J Assist Reprod Genet.* 2018;35(3):435–40.

2. Ubaldi FM, Cimadomo D, Capalbo A, et al. Preimplantation genetic diagnosis for aneuploidy testing in women older than 44 years: a multicenter experience. *Fertil Steril.* 2017;107(5):1173–80.

3. Sydsjö G, Lindell Pettersson M, Bladh M, Skoog Svanberg A, Lampic C, Nedstrand E.

Evaluation of risk factors' importance on adverse pregnancy and neonatal outcomes in women aged 40 years or older. *BMC Pregnancy Childbirth*. 2019;19(1):92.

4. American College of Obstetricians and Gynecologists. Prepregnancy counselling.

ACOG Committee Opinion No. 762. *Obstet Gynecol*. 2019;133:e78–9.

5. Savasi VM, Mandia L, Laoreti A, Cetin I. Maternal and fetal outcomes in oocyte donation pregnancies. *Hum Reprod Update*. 2016;22(5):620–33.

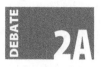

Women with a BMI over 40 Should Be Refused Fertility Treatment

For

José Bellver

The Magnitude of the Problem

The prevalence of overweight individuals has increased in recent decades, reaching epidemic proportions worldwide and affecting about 2 billion people over the age of 18. In some developed countries, such as México, the USA or New Zealand, the prevalence of overweight adults is as high as 70–75%, while obese and morbidly obese (body mass index-BMI $\geq$35 kg/m^2) adults account for 30–35% and 10–15%, respectively. This trend continues to rise, and is reflected in developing countries due to a general shift towards a more western lifestyle. Among women of reproductive age, rates of overweight and obesity are reported to be as high as 64% in some populations, which has made pre-conception weight control a public health priority.

The Negative Effects on General Health

Weight excess leads to high morbidity and mortality rates, and represents significant direct and indirect economic burdens for society. As a systemic disease, obesity affects all the tissues and organs in the body, inducing or exacerbating several comorbidities, including cardiovascular and cerebrovascular diseases, type 2 diabetes, asthma, sleep apnea, gastrointestinal diseases, osteoarthritis and cancer.

The Negative Effects on Conception (Natural or Assisted)

The negative effects of excess weight on male and female fertility are well-documented. Female obesity is associated with an increased risk of subfertility and infertility in both ovulatory and anovulatory women, and with significantly lower implantation, pregnancy and live birth rates after IVF/ICSI, in a BMI-dependent manner, whether own or donated ova are employed, probably through alterations in gamete/embryo quality and endometrial receptivity [1]. In addition, the 'gonadotropic resistance' of obese women reduces ovarian response, increases the dosage of medication required, and leads to more abandoned or cancelled cycles and less oocytes and mature oocytes obtained, thus resulting in higher costs and poorer outcomes than in normal weight women.

The Negative Effects on Pregnancy

Once pregnancy is achieved, whether naturally or by assisted reproductive technology (ART), the risk of complications is higher for the mother – gestational diabetes, pre-eclampsia, gestational hypertension, depression, instrumental and caesarean birth, surgical site infection, and problems related to anaesthesia – and for the fetus – greater risk of preterm birth, large-for-gestational-age babies, congenital anomalies and perinatal death. Additionally, breastfeeding initiation rates are lower and early breastfeeding cessation is more likely. These adverse outcomes can result in longer hospital stays, with the concomitant implications for resources. To counteract all these problems, not only is it necessary for overweight prospective mothers to lose weight before conception, but weight gain during pregnancy should also be minimised.

The Negative Effects on Offspring

Pre-gestational maternal obesity and excessive weight gain during pregnancy have been related to an increased risk of metabolic diseases – obesity, type 2 diabetes, cardiovascular disease, metabolic syndrome – and non-metabolic diseases – cancer, osteoporosis, asthma, neurologic alterations – in the offspring, which all seem to be mediated by epigenetic mechanisms of fetal programming. These diseases can appear during childhood, adolescence or adulthood, thus predisposing subsequent generations to increased rates of chronic disorders.

Policies Adopted to Control the Problem and Related Ethical Issues

In many countries, fertility societies and/or governments have implemented policies to limit the access of obese women to publicly-funded assisted reproduction programmes, an approach that has also been adopted by some private clinics. Cut-off points for denying treatment vary from 32 to 40 kg/m^2, with 35 kg/m^2 representing a standard. This decision has been motivated by economic and health reasons; as stated before, obese women attending a fertility clinic usually require a greater investment than those of normal weight due to their poorer ovarian response and clinical results. In this context, greater cost-effectiveness can be achieved if candidates begin treatment with a more favourable body weight. In fact, some infertile obese women become pregnant spontaneously merely by reducing their weight, especially when polycystic ovary syndrome (PCOS) is associated. The high and increasing prevalence of obesity among women of fertile age multiplies costs in a higher proportion than other less prevalent conditions associated with infertility. Nevertheless, why obesity is considered a factor for denying ART and the aforementioned conditions are not is a matter of ethical controversy.

Approaches to Weight Reduction Tested in Infertile Obese Women

Intervention programmes for weight reduction based on lifestyle modifications prior to IVF have been applied with disparate results. Programmes including close follow-up and monitoring of a reduced group of obese women by a multidisciplinary team have proved to be effective in improving live birth and cumulative live birth rates in randomised studies comparing intervention versus no intervention over a sufficient period of time (12 weeks) before initiation of the IVF cycle [2, 3]. Programmes with larger sample sizes and longer intervention periods, but more heterogeneity among centres and poorer follow-up and monitoring, have not provided evidence of any benefit in terms of live birth rates of weight reduction prior to IVF cycles when compared against no intervention in randomised studies. However, even in the latter randomised trials, a significant proportion of women in the intervention group achieved pregnancy spontaneously while waiting for initiation of the IVF cycle [4, 5]. Therefore, perhaps only strict, multidisciplinary intervention programmes are useful for improving IVF outcome in obese women. Pharmacotherapy to achieve weight reduction for fertility purposes has failed to show any benefit, and bariatric surgery is a risky procedure associated with morbidity and even mortality, as well as long recovery periods before pregnancy can be attempted, and an increased risk of some maternal and fetal complications in comparison to non-operated obese women. In light of this, it should not be considered an initial option for fertility purposes.

Conclusions

In defence of refusing IVF cycles to women with class III obesity, increased economic costs, poor ART outcome, maternal and fetal complications during pregnancy, and an increased risk of diseases in the offspring can be argued, all of which may be minimised or even avoided by reducing weight before conception. However, before denying treatment to any woman, other fertility factors, such as maternal age, also need to be considered, and patients should be assessed on an individual basis, as occurs in other chronic medical conditions. Moreover, a strict multidisciplinary weight-reduction programme should be offered in both public and private settings in an attempt to achieve significant weight reduction in the shortest period of time possible before initiating any IVF procedure.

References

1. Sermondade N, Huberlant S, Bourhis-Lefebvre V, et al. Female obesity is negatively associated with live birth rate following IVF: a systemic review and meta-analysis. *Hum Reprod Update*. 2019;25:439–51.

2. Sim KA, Dezarnaulds, GM, Denyer GS, Skilton MR, Caterson D. Weight loss improves reproductive outcomes in obese women undergoing fertility treatment: a randomized controlled trial. *Clin Obes*. 2014;4:61–8.

3. Espinós JJ, Polo A, Sánchez-Hernández J, et al. Weight decrease improves live birth rates in obese women undergoing IVF: a pilot study. *Reprod Biomed Online*. 2017;35:417–24.

4. Mutsaerts MAQ, van Oers AM, Groen H, et al. Randomized trial of a lifestyle program in obese infertile women. *NEJM*. 2016;374:1942–53.

5. Einarsson S, Bergh C, Friberg B, et al. Weight reduction intervention for obese infertile women prior to IVF: a randomized controlled trial. *Hum Reprod*. 2017;32:1621–30.

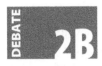

Women with a BMI over 40 Should Be Refused Fertility Treatment

Against

Richard S Legro

Introduction

Obesity in a patient seeking fertility summons many knee-jerk reactions from both providers and health systems alike, who deny access to infertility care on the basis of obesity. These decisions are not evidence-based, in fact they lie in deep-seated conscious biases against women who are obese and the more obese the greater the condemnation. Women with 'morbid' obesity, i.e. a BMI $\geq$ 40 kg/m^2 are the most likely to be denied treatment. Never in the course of human history has there been a more fortuitous time to cast these biases away. They are as follows: (1) Obesity is a personal choice and not an illness and weight loss can be readily obtained with some self-control and dieting and exercise; (2) Weight loss will restore these patients to normal fertility and optimal pregnancy outcomes; (3) 'Morbid' obesity causes unacceptable lower pregnancy rates, as well as an increased rate of pregnancy complications. Let us explore each one of these exaggerated claims and biases.

BIAS: Obesity is a personal choice, easily reversed.

FACT: Obesity is not a personal choice, it is a disease.

The WHO and every major health organisation has acknowledged that obesity is a disease, in the same way that infertility, cancer and COVID-19 are diseases. A disease is a disease and we cannot carve out one disease for exemptions from infertility care and give blanket inclusion to others. It is time to stop blaming the patient for obesity and examine the context within which it originated. Extensive research has shown that the environment shaped by our industries, our institutions and our government has contributed to the epidemic of obesity, not just in the USA (perhaps the most flagrant example) but to varying degrees, in every nation on this earth. Further, weight is much more easily gained than lost. This is not a choice issue, this is a physiological fact that central homeostatic mechanisms reset to the highest weight gained and attempt to maintain or restore it, if lost. Caloric restriction in the context of obesity results in initial steady weight loss but counter-regulatory mechanisms kick in within weeks to (1) slow basal metabolic rate to conserve energy and fat mass; (2) increase orexigenic hormones to restore the lost weight. These latter elevations persist for years, even in those who maintain their weight and these mechanisms contribute to the well-known phenomenon of rebound weight gain often exceeding the basal weight, especially prevalent in fad or extreme diets that over-restrict caloric intake. Additionally to maintain weight loss over time, caloric restriction must be continually reduced to account for the smaller body mass resulting from successful weight loss. Consequently, the amount of weight that can be safely lost through lifestyle changes is relatively modest [1]. At best it ranges from 5–10% over the course of a year. This can be elevated up to 15% through the use of obesity drugs, and the most effective drugs are combination therapies. Thus in the short term, the amount of weight loss will never bring a patient with Class III obesity, i.e. BMI > 40 ever into a normal range, and this becomes extremely unlikely when patients start weight loss with a BMI ≥ 50. They will always be obese to some degree unless they can maintain their lifestyle programme for years. For those at the lower ends of Class III obesity, bariatric surgery is the only treatment that will enable weight loss within a reasonable time; however in the U.S. only 1% of eligible patients ever opt for it AND qualify for it, and this has its own issues when related to fertility as discussed below.

BIAS: Weight loss will restore women with obesity to normal fertility and optimal pregnancy outcomes.

FACT: Weight loss, per se, has not been shown to improve fertility and pregnancy outcomes.

We have seen two recent multicentre studies that shatter the bias that weight loss improves fertility and pregnancy outcomes. The Dutch LIFEstyle study which randomised obese women with a variety of infertility diagnoses to either a six-month weight loss lifestyle based programme followed by standard infertility care or to immediate standard infertility care showed that women who received the intervention were statistically LESS likely to have a live birth over a 2-year period of observation than the immediate group (Figure 2B.1) [2].

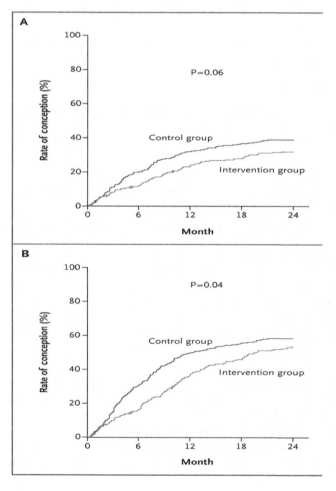

Figure 2.B1 Time to pregnancy (intention-to-treat analysis). Kaplan–Meier curves show the time to pregnancy resulting in the vaginal birth of a healthy singleton at term (panel A) and the time to pregnancy resulting in a live birth (panel B). Crosses indicate women who were lost to follow-up. (From Mutsaerts et al., *NEJM*, 2016 [2].)

Further there were disturbing trends towards more pregnancy loss among those who lost weight. Finally there was no difference in birth weight between the two groups, implying that pregnancy complications were comparable. Some pundits have criticised the study for inadequate weight loss as the mean weight loss in the intervention group was less than the 5% targeted. However in another multicentre study by a Swedish group with a similar design of randomisation to pre-treatment caloric restriction or immediate IVF, the intervention group achieved through the use of liquid diets and extreme caloric restriction an almost 10% weight loss [3]. Again the results were comparable. There was no benefit to weight loss on the live birth rate and again a trend towards pregnancy loss in the intervention group.

There are small single-centre studies and observational studies that can offer opposite and rosily reassuring results about weight loss and fertility. These studies do not enter the hall of evidence-based medicine. However we can resort to well-done observational and case/control studies where there are no RCTs to guide us. Certainly, national registries that have linked the outcomes of pregnancy in women after bariatric surgery should be the crown jewel documenting how weight loss improves pregnancy outcomes. These data are available. Indeed, epidemiologic data from Sweden capturing the women who underwent bariatric surgery (most with Roux-en-Y gastric bypasses that led to on average 40% weight loss after a year) and their pregnancy and the neonatal outcomes of their babies have been published [4]. However, the surprising, even shocking data show that women who had a bariatric surgery compared to obese controls who did not have surgery, were significantly more likely to experience spontaneous preterm delivery and labour, a higher chance of a small for gestational age infant and overall smaller babies than the untreated obese women. So in 'curing' obesity with surgery, the intervention has led to an exacerbation of the number one world-wide perinatal issue contributing to infant mortality: i.e. prematurity and low birth weight. Physician Non Nocere!

BIAS: 'Morbid' obesity causes unacceptable lower pregnancy rates and an increased rate of pregnancy complications.

FACT: Class III obesity is associated with lower pregnancy rates compared to non-obese women and higher complication rates, but not to the degree imagined and less than age and other co-morbidities where caregivers and guidelines cast a blind eye.

Everyone will agree that obesity, from the epidemiologic evidence, is associated with subfertility and increased rates of pregnancy complications, most pronounced in women with a BMI > 40. However these are associations and not causally linked. The evidence of cause, as noted from the discussion above or from the myriad interventions to control gestational weight gain, has shown that none of these have ever improved one significant maternal or fetal morbidity. The primary misconception about the link between obesity and fertility in women is not whether it exists, but how small the effect size truly is. We are making a mountain out of a molehill. The relative risks of IVF failure in women with a BMI of 40–45 are actually smaller than those compared to the adverse effects of increasing maternal age or for instance, maternal smoking. Further obesity as a negative predictor of IVF success appears to be most relevant at younger ages and disappears with advancing maternal age [5]. Similarly obesity *per se*, stripped of co-morbidities such as diabetes or hypertension, appears to only marginally increase risk for maternal complications of pregnancy [6].

In conclusion obesity is a complex disease, recalcitrant to most forms of therapy, which, in and of itself has only a mild impact of subfertility and adverse pregnancy outcomes. There is no Level I evidence that weight loss either pre-conception or post-conception improves live birth rates or maternal health. The possibility remains that weight loss may even cause harm, such as delay in the time to conception. It is time to throw away our biases, conscious and unconscious, and work with women regardless of their obesity status.

References

1. Hall KD, Sacks G, Chandramohan D, et al. Quantification of the effect of energy imbalance on bodyweight. *Lancet*. 2011;378:826–37.

2. Mutsaerts MA, van Oers AM, Groen H, et al. Randomized trial of a lifestyle program in obese infertile women. *New England J Med*. 2016;374:1942–53.

3. Einarsson S, Bergh C, Friberg B, et al. Weight reduction intervention for obese infertile women prior to IVF: a randomized controlled trial. *Hum Reprod*. 2017;32:1621–30.

4. Johansson K, Cnattingius S, Naslund I, et al. Outcomes of pregnancy after bariatric surgery. *New England J Med*. 2015;372:814–24.

5. Sneed ML, Uhler ML, Grotjan HE, Rapisarda JJ, Lederer KJ, Beltsos AN. Body mass index: impact on IVF success appears age-related. *Hum Reprod*. 2008;23:1835–9.

6. Kim SS, Zhu Y, Grantz KL, et al. Obstetric and neonatal risks among obese women without chronic disease. *Obstet Gynecol*. 2016;128:104–12.

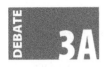

3A Female Age of Menopause Is a Fair Limit for Ovum Donation

For

Melanie Davies

Menopause is a universal experience and widely recognised as the end of female fertility. Review of attitudes to menopause across multiple countries and cultures shows this consistently, and indeed, it is often viewed positively as bringing freedom from further risk of pregnancy. The median age at menopause in industrialised countries is 51 years, but in fact fertility ceases 8–10 years earlier. Studies in both historical and modern populations who do not use birth control show that the last child is typically born at age 42, and only about 10% of women achieve live birth at 45 [1]. There would need to be good reasons for extending fertility treatment beyond these naturally imposed limits.

No doubt menopause made evolutionary sense to ensure that children had parental care when life expectancy was short. Looking back 150 years, female life expectancy for those who survived infancy was 60 years. It could be argued that now '60 is the new 40' and childbearing should be extended accordingly. Unfortunately biology has not changed so quickly! There are strong medical arguments against post-menopausal pregnancy.

Risks of virtually every obstetric complication are increased in older mothers, rising in parallel with maternal age [2]. The maternal death rate in the UK is 24 per 100,000 for women over 40 compared to 7 per 100,000 age 30–34 [3]. Women over 44 have a threefold higher rate of Caesarean delivery compared with women aged 30-34, and only 1 in 4 achieve unassisted vaginal birth. The relative risk of haemorrhage is 1.5, pregnancy hypertension >1.5, and risk of gestational diabetes is more than doubled [2]. For the baby, there is a doubling of the risk of delivery before 32 weeks with the associated complications of prematurity which include cerebral palsy and neonatal death.

Ovum donation is itself an independent risk factor for pregnancy complications, in particular hypertension and postpartum haemorrhage. A systematic review found that women who had IVF with donor eggs were at higher risk of hypertension (odds ratio 3.92, 95% confidence interval 3.21–4.78) with a third of women developing pregnancy hypertension compared with 17% having IVF with their own eggs [4].

In addition, women having assisted conception have a higher rate of multiple pregnancy with donor eggs than using their own eggs. Twins or triplets increase pregnancy risks further. The complications for mothers and babies are significant enough for the Royal College of Obstetricians and Gynaecologists to have commissioned an 'impact paper' on multiple pregnancy after assisted conception [5]. It is 20 years since the first report of maternal death in the UK associated with twin pregnancy after egg donation.

Women over 45–50 are more likely to experience medical conditions such as cancer and heart disease which increase in incidence with age. The latest report into maternal deaths in the UK highlighted that several women have died from ischaemic heart disease after becoming pregnant through assisted reproduction [3]. There was no evidence that their cardiovascular risk had been considered prior to pregnancy and these deaths could be considered avoidable. Disastrous outcomes have been reported following ovum donation;

in Spain twins born to a 66-year-old were left orphaned when she was diagnosed with cancer within a year of giving birth.

From a public health perspective, currently in the UK about 1% of births are to women over 45, but these make disproportionate use of medical resources. The commercialisation of fertility treatment and advertising by clinics worldwide has led to 'medical tourism' or 'cross-border care' with women paying for treatment abroad, often with multiple embryos transferred to boost pregnancy rates, returning to their home country reliant on government-funded health systems for the ensuing complications. This is particularly acute with ovum donation in the UK as the regulatory system, which restricts payment to donors and allows offspring access to donor identity, contrasts with wider availability of treatment and donor anonymity in unregulated markets overseas.

Donor eggs are a scarce resource. Particularly in the UK, where donation is unremunerated, the availability of donor eggs falls short of demand. In this context, priorities need to be set – what are the views of society and the egg donors themselves? Public opinion would surely prioritise young women, and those with medically induced ovarian failure, rather than post-menopausal women with age-related infertility. A study of the motivation and attitudes of anonymous egg donors in the USA found that 'The greatest reservations were in donating to recipients over 50 years of age.'

Social outcomes for the families created after the age of menopause by ovum donation are not yet known. In general, older parents will have greater emotional and economic resources – an exception occurred in Spain where twins born to a 64-year-old woman had to be taken into care. Concerns that children could become carers for their ageing parents or experience bereavement, with potentially devastating psychological effects, have led some countries to impose upper age limits for assisted reproduction. And social acceptance is still a hurdle for these families, with stigmatisation of 'pensioner parents' and hurtful comments at the school gates, a factor taken into account by adoption agencies in setting parental age limits. Becoming parents over 50 has been described as a selfish act. Although societal norms have changed, with 30 now the average age of motherhood in the UK, extending childbearing for another 20 years is a sociological experiment. The female age of menopause remains a fair limit for ovum donation.

References

1. Heffner LJ. Advanced maternal age – how old is too old? *New Engl J Med.* 2004;351:1927–9.

2. Luke B, Brown MB. Elevated risks of pregnancy complications and adverse outcomes with increasing maternal age. *Hum Reprod.* 2007;22(5):1264–72.

3. Knight M, Bunch K, Tuffnell D, et al. (eds.) on behalf of MBRRACE–UK. *Saving Lives, Improving Mothers' Care – Lessons learned to inform maternity care from the UK and Ireland Confidential Enquiries into Maternal Deaths and Morbidity 2015–17.* Oxford: National Perinatal Epidemiology Unit, University of Oxford, 2019.

4. Jeve YB, Potdar N, Opoku A, Khare M. Donor oocyte conception and pregnancy complications: a systematic review and meta-analysis. *BJOG.* 2016;123(9):1471–80.

5. RCOG. *Multiple pregnancies following assisted conception.* Scientific impact paper no. 22. 2018. doi: 10.1111/1471-0528 .14974. https://obgyn.onlinelibrary.wiley .com/doi/full/10.1111/1471-0528.14974.

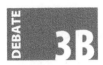

Female Age of Menopause Is a Fair Limit for Ovum Donation

Against

Gillian Lockwood

There is very little that is 'fair' in human reproduction. It is not 'fair' that at the age of 38 a woman has about 2 years to have a reasonable chance of a healthy pregnancy whereas a man has two or three decades.

It is not 'fair' that even in the 'developed' world women risk dying in pregnancy, during delivery or soon after, whereas I have never heard of a man dying as a result of becoming a father! In the 'developing' world the risks for mothers and their babies are truly horrendous with maternal death rates that rival those of medieval Europe.

This situation is all the more 'unfair' because a woman's life expectancy is longer than a man's (a healthy baby girl born today in the UK can expect to live to 86 and be fit and active well into her 70s). Our society has developed so rapidly since the Second World War only because women have been prepared to take on two jobs, worker **and** mother. The 'natural' age of menopause, 51 years, has changed only slightly over the past few decades although we now know that women who live near green parks have a later menopause [1] and women who smoke have an earlier one [2]. Evolutionary biologists tell us that the decades of 'post-reproductive' life that women endure are because being a good grandmother supports Dawkin's 'selfish gene' hypothesis. This may be true for the Minke whale, but is unlikely to prove convincing in London where 10% of births last year were to women over 40.

Today's young women, encouraged to go to university, instructed to train for a 'good' job, denied the prospect of affordable housing and romantically involved with young men who are often 'not ready to settle down yet', have precious little time to also become mothers before the brute biology of sub-fertility, miscarriage and chromosomal abnormality blight their reproductive prospects [3]. And for those that do manage to 'get in under the wire' and have a 'late' baby, those babies are likely to be 'lonely onlys' as the chance of a subsequent sibling is low even with IVF.

The likelihood of divorce for 'graduate' couples is high (>35%) with childless couples more likely to divorce and co-habiting childless couples even more likely to separate. Many women in their 40s therefore find themselves single, with unresolved desires for motherhood. Others may move into second and happier relationships and here the desire for parenthood may be powerful, and yet female age may make this unlikely or impossible.

Ever since the first donor egg baby was born in Australia in 1983, the possibility of achieving (relatively) safe motherhood in a woman's late 40s or even 50s has tantalised and traumatised medical ethicists and obstetricians alike. We recognise that women in their late 40s and early 50s are at a significantly higher risk of pregnancy-induced hypertension (PIH), gestational diabetes, thrombo-embolism and premature or assisted delivery. Yet many much younger women, whose medical histories pre-dispose them to these or even more serious obstetric complications are provided with fertility treatment and specialist support through-out pregnancy. Autonomy, considered the most important of Beauchamp and Childress's 'Four Principles of Medical Ethics' – the others are beneficence, non-maleficence and justice – should surely allow older healthy women with many decades of healthy life as devoted and happy mothers ahead of them to choose to achieve this too having had the risks and costs and benefits outlined.

So why is it that when a 60 something (male) rock star announces the birth of his 9th child with his 5th wife it's 'cigars all round', but a 48-year-old woman choosing to pursue motherhood alone or with a partner, is held up to public scrutiny as 'unnatural' and 'selfish'? Babies don't notice wrinkles, they just thrive in a loving and emotionally and financially stable environment. A whole generation of children were previously brought up by their grandmothers as their natural mothers had either died or, inconveniently pregnant as teenagers, were passed off as ' big sisters' and not their mothers at all.

Age is arbitrary and ageism is unacceptable. Biological age and chronological age, for women, can often differ by 3 or 4 years. A strong family history of early menopause can be a devastating prospect for a woman who, like her peer group, thinks 35 is a good time to start 'hinting' about a baby. Lucky women with grandmothers and great grandmothers who had healthy babies well into their mid-40s can be more sanguine about the passage of time, but a miscarriage rate of 70–80% for conceptions with 45-year-old eggs seems to be a universal constant.

The central tenet of the HFEA Act has always been that 'the welfare of the child' who may be born as a result of treatment offered must be paramount. The philosophical issue of whether it is better to be born to 'an old lady' by dint of ovum donation than not be born at all, is beyond the scope of this debate, but we do need to consider the evidence about the 'welfare of the child'. Women accessing motherhood via donor eggs are better educated, financially more stable and emotionally more secure on average. Often their reasons for 'delaying' motherhood are not explanations but simply the tough stuff that is real life: they had to care for a sick parent, their partner left, they got ill. . . In the same way that there is no rule that states that someone will be a 'good' mother up to midnight the day before her 45th birthday, but mysteriously morph into Cruella de Vil the minute she turns 45, so the biological 'random event' which is menopause does not and should not influence access to treatment with donor eggs. 'Every child a wanted child' would seem to apply to this debate and as long as we are delighted for the woman who achieves a healthy delivery 'against all the odds' if it happened 'naturally', then we should be prepared to be equally welcoming to the baby who arrives courtesy of that most altruistic of women, the egg donor.

References

1. Treibner K, Markevych I, Hustad S, et al. Residential surrounding greenspace and age at menopause: a 20 year European study. *Environ Internat.* 2019;132:105088.

2. Whitcomb B, Purdue-Smith AC, Szegda KL, et al. Cigarette smoking and risk of early menopause. *Am J Epidemiol.* 2017;187 (4):696–704.

3. Magnus M, Wilcox A, Morken N-H, et al. Role of maternal age and pregnancy history in risk of miscarriage: prospective register based study *BMJ.* 2019;364:1–8.

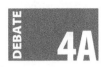

Social Egg Freezing Should Be Available Up To the Age of 40 Years

For

Ana Cobo

In today's society, many women are delaying pregnancy later than the younger years of childbearing. This trend affects mainly the developed countries, most of which are experiencing a significantly reduced birth rate. The motives behind this relate to multiple causes closely linked to current sociological order. Modern women are often forced to choose between their career and the pressure posed by the progression of their biological clock, which is responsible for the well-known decline in fertility in the over 30s. Financial security and lack of a partner are also frequent reasons to delay maternity. In some cases, the decision to remain childless is completely voluntary and simply relates to the particular decision of many women who want to make strides in other facets of their life, other than motherhood. Under such circumstances, if these women ever consider getting pregnant, they will be forced to use assisted reproduction technology (ART), leading to repeated failed cycles due to advanced maternal age or, in many cases, they will ultimately need ovum donation. With an increasing number of women deciding to delay motherhood there is growing interest in the fertility preservation (FP) approaches available, in order to safeguard their options of attaining biological offspring in the future. This choice is commonly known as elective fertility preservation (EFP), or FP for social reasons or anticipated gamete exhaustion [1].

Vitrification has become the most preferred option for FP of the female gamete in post-pubertal women, due to its capacity to circumvent the most significant drawbacks associated with oocyte cryopreservation [2]. This ice-free technology has been routinely available for a little over a decade and its efficiency was initially demonstrated on a large scale using donor oocytes [3]. Later publications showed the success rates achieved after EFP for age-related fertility decline [4]. In this study, the majority of women who chose EFP were highly educated, single and heterosexual. Remarkably, the study showed that women are deciding for EFP at an advanced age, which together with the number of oocytes vitrified were identified as the most powerful variables related to success [4]. A later study including the large series published so far showing EFP outcomes, confirmed these observations and provided detailed analysis of the results achieved by EFP patients compared to women diagnosed with cancer who decided for FP prior to the oncological treatment [5]. The distribution of age showed that the great majority of EFP women (81.1%) had their oocytes vitrified older than 35 years of age and a significant 15.8% were aged 40 years or older. Surprisingly, a minority were younger than 30 years of age [5]. As expected, we witnessed a greater impact of age in older women who used EFP showing impaired outcomes when compared to young women. Hence, the number of oocytes retrieved and the number of metaphase II (MII) oocytes finally vitrified, oocyte survival, pregnancy and live birth rates were affected by the age at vitrification. The most noticeable consequence of advanced age is the natural depletion of the ovarian reserve and increased chromosomal abnormalities. Therefore, in our study, a larger number of oocytes were retrieved and vitrified in patients aged 35 y or younger when compared with patients older than 35 y and the lowest figures

Table 4A.1. Cumulative live birth rate (CLBR) according to age at retrieval and number of oocytes used [5].

Age ≤35		Age >35	
No. oocytes	CLBR(95% CI)	No. oocytes	CLBR(95% CI)
5	15.8 (8.4–23.1)	5	5.9 (3.6–8.3)*
8	32.0 (22.1–41.9)	8	17.3 (13.3–21.3)*
10	42.8 (31.7–53.90)	10	25.2 (20.2–30.1)*
15	69.8 (57.4–82.2)	15	38.8 (32.0–45.6)*
20	77.6 (64.4–90.9)	20	49.6 (40.7–58.4)*
24	94.4 (84.3–100.4)		

* $P<0.05$.
CLBR is expressed in percentage and 95% confidence interval.

were observed in patients aged 40 y or older (5.1 (95% CI = 4.2–6.0) mean retrieved and 3.9 (95% CI = 2.6–5.0) mean MII vitrified) [4]. This reveals that most women over 40 will need more than one ovarian stimulation cycle to increase the number of oocytes available and thus the chance of future success [5]. Additionally, a number of embryo transfers in patients who had their oocytes vitrified at advanced aged are cancelled due to absence of chromosomally normal embryos [5].

Age is also related to oocyte survival. Significantly lower survival rates are observed in older patients (85.3% for women ≤ 40 years old) compared with women younger than 30 years of age (94.5%) [4]. As expected, the cumulative probability of having a child according to the number oocytes used is significantly lower in older women [4, 5]. Accordingly, with eight oocytes the probability of having a child is around 17% in patients older than 35, while it is almost double if the patient is younger (≤35 years). Additionally the gain in yield per additional oocyte is much lower in older patients and, also a time comes when no matter what the increase in the number of oocytes, the results do not improve from that point onward (Table 4A.1) [5]. In other words, older patients need more oocytes to approximate the results seen in young women, but they will never reach the highest outcomes of the younger patients. However, despite the evidence of substantially scarcer chances for patients who had their oocytes vitrified in their 40s, the probability of having a child is not 0%. In light of this, our obligation as care-givers is to provide appropriate counsel in order to avoid false expectations. Individualised treatment for older women is mandatory. Needless to say, women who wish to preserve fertility should be encouraged to do so at early ages when the chances of success are significantly higher.

References

1. Stoop D, van der Veen F, Deneyer M, Nekkebroeck J, Tournaye H. Oocyte banking for anticipated gamete exhaustion (AGE) is a preventive intervention, neither social nor nonmedical. *Reprod. Biomed.* 2014;28:548–51.

2. Martinez F. Update on fertility preservation from the Barcelona International Society for Fertility Preservation-ESHRE-ASRM 2015 expert meeting: indications, results and future perspectives. *Hum Reprod.* 2017;32:1802–11.

3. Cobo A, Meseguer M, Remohi J, Pellicer A. Use of cryo-banked oocytes in an ovum

donation programme: a prospective, randomized, controlled, clinical trial. *Hum Reprod.* 2010;25:2239–46.

4. Cobo A, Garcia-Velasco JA, Coello A, Domingo J, Pellicer A, Remohi J. Oocyte vitrification as an efficient option for elective fertility preservation. *Fertil Steril.* 2016;105:755–64.e8.

5. Cobo A, Garcia-Velasco J, Domingo J, Pellicer A, Remohi J. Elective and Onco-fertility preservation: factors related to IVF outcomes. *Hum Reprod.* 2018;33.2222–31.

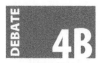

4B Social Egg Freezing Should Be Available Up To the Age of 40 Years

Against

Kylie Baldwin

The last decade has seen a significant increase in the number of egg freezing cycles performed across the world. Often described as a fertility preservation or fertility extension technology, social egg freezing (henceforth SEF) has the potential to allow women to defer childbearing to later in their reproductive lives which can benefit users in a multitude of different ways [1]. However, there are several reasons we should think twice before recommending such an elective procedure to otherwise healthy women.

The chance of a live birth with frozen eggs depends on the age of the woman at the time of undergoing the procedure; the number of eggs frozen; and the expertise and experience of the clinic providing the technology. However, as SEF remains somewhat novel, only small numbers of women have returned to use their eggs in fertility treatment. It is therefore difficult to provide potential users with accurate, individualised information about their chance of achieving a live birth in the future. Indeed, the evidence emerging from fertility clinics, at least in the UK, is showing egg freezing to have low levels of efficacy and is resulting in live births in only a small number of women [2]. Many clinics providing the technology have yet to achieve a live birth with previously frozen eggs and thus may rely on published studies from other centres to provide indications of possible success rates which they may or may not be able to replicate [3]. The absence of high quality, individualised, clinic-specific success rates available to potential users thus poses problems for informed consent and may lead women to overestimate the efficacy of the technology [4].

Cobo argues in the previous chapter that SEF should be made accessible to women until the age of 40. However, this may give the false impression that eggs taken from a woman in her late 30s can be used to achieve a live birth with relative ease. The typical user of SEF tends to be in her late 30s or early 40s and is thus often drawing on the technology after her fertility (her egg quality and quantity) has significantly declined. In most cases women need to be making use of the technology at a younger age to increase their chance of a live birth. Since egg quality declines as women age, older women often need to bank more eggs than their younger counterparts to increase their chance of a live birth in the future [4]. As such they may need to undergo multiple rounds of stimulation and retrieval with the associated costs, yet it can be difficult to predict the number of cycles required to bank enough eggs at the outset. Users may also need to undergo multiple rounds of IVF in the future with their frozen eggs in an attempt to achieve a live birth, which remains far from guaranteed. This is significant as the process of freezing eggs for future use, and using them to try and conceive, is not risk free and is often significantly emotionally challenging for its users [5]. It is indeed also important to also note that unlike other fertility patients, at the time of undergoing egg freezing, users of SEF are assumedly healthy with no known reproductive pathology and who could therefore conceive naturally without the risks and costs associated with medicalised fertility treatment.

Social egg freezing is not funded by the NHS in the UK and the cost of one cycle of egg freezing can exceed £3350, not including the costs of medication [2]. As a result, the procedure remains the preserve of middle-class, privileged women and excludes those from more insecure or precarious financial backgrounds. Most women who freeze their eggs pay for the procedure themselves; however a smaller number of women are able to access the technology though their employer who 'sponsors' the procedure on their behalf. Whilst company sponsored egg freezing may open up the technology to a greater number of women, it is important to recognise that that this 'benefit' is unlikely to ever be extended to women in insecure employment or in low-wage, low-status jobs and is unlikely to become widely covered by public health systems [4]. Indeed, widespread use of the technology may instead further re-entrench and aggravate racial and class inequalities exacerbating the chasm between highly educated and privileged groups and those with less economic and social power. Therefore it is important to remember that whilst SEF grants some of its users greater reproductive choice and control, it remains beyond the reach of most women and is perhaps one of the latest examples of what is often referred to by social scientists as stratified reproduction.

To conclude, only small numbers of women are seeing success, in the form of a live birth, with frozen eggs and few clinics are highly experienced at performing the procedure. In the absence of age and clinic-specific success rates potential users of the technology may have to rely on published data, often from specialist centres, when deciding whether to engage with the technology. Many women who undergo the procedure do so at an older than desirable age such as in their late 30s and early 40s at which point their egg quality and quantity will have significantly declined. As a result, these women may be advised to undergo multiple rounds of stimulation and retrieval to bank enough eggs; this can be significantly expensive and requires women to undergo medical procedures which carry risks on multiple occasions even before they actively try to conceive. These women then face further risks when trying to conceive a pregnancy later in life as, whilst they are using younger genetic material, they remain at an elevated risk for some obstetric complications due to their advanced reproductive age. Finally, whilst egg freezing offers some women greater reproductive choice about the timing of motherhood, the technology remains out of reach for most women due to the high cost of the procedure further exacerbating social class inequalities. Thus, whilst SEF may be a beacon of hope for some women it offers no guarantee of a live birth, it carries risk, is costly and is highly exclusionary.

References

1. Baldwin K. *Egg Freezing, Fertility and Reproductive Choice: Negotiating Hope, Responsibility and Modern Motherhood.* Emerald: Bingley, 2019.

2. HFEA. *Egg Freezing in Fertility Treatment: Trends and Figures 2010–2016.* HFEA, 2018.

3. Daar J, Benward J, Collins L, et al. Planned oocyte cryopreservation for women seeking to preserve future reproductive potential: An ethics committee opinion. *Fertil Steril.* 2018;110(6):1022–8.

4. Jackson E. The ambiguities of 'social' egg freezing and the challenges of informed consent. *BioSocieties.* 2018;13(1):21–40.

5. Baldwin K, Culley, L. Women's experience of social egg freezing: Perceptions of success, risks, and 'going it alone'. *Hum Fertil.* 2018;1:1–7.

DEBATE 5A

DHEA Is an Effective Treatment for Poor Responders

For

Catherine Hayden and Mariano Mascarenhas

Dehydroepiandrosterone (DHEA) is produced primarily from the adrenal gland (85%) under the influence of adrenocorticotropic hormone (ACTH) and to a lesser extent by the ovaries. DHEA is an intermediate in the sex steroid pathway and is converted to testosterone and estradiol within the ovaries. The anti-ageing properties of DHEA were first described in 1996, together with the decline in DHEA with advancing age. In reproductive medicine, DHEA has been hypothesised to play a role in improving folliculogenesis through multiple mechanisms:

1. Acting as a precursor for increased testosterone levels which, in conjunction with increased expression of androgen receptors appear to increase the sensitivity of ovarian follicles to exogenous ovarian stimulation.

2. Increased insulin like growth factor 1 (IGF-1) levels which also potentiates gonadotrophin-stimulated folliculogenesis.

3. Improving oocyte ploidy and reducing atresia: maternal ageing is associated with an increase in embryo aneuploidy and DHEA supplementation is purported to improve meiotic spindle stability. This mechanism has also been hypothesised to explain the negative correlation of DHEA with cellular ageing and cancer and forms the explanation behind it being marketed as an anti-ageing supplement.

4. Influencing follicular growth at the stage of pre-antral and antral follicles thus increasing the antral follicle count and augmenting the number of gonadotrophin-sensitive follicles leading to an improved ovarian response to stimulation.

The first report of a possible benefit from DHEA in an IVF setting was in a case report published in 2005. A 42-year-old woman with an initial diagnosis of reduced ovarian reserve and who had one oocyte retrieved in her first IVF cycle self-medicated concomitantly with over-the-counter DHEA supplements and acupuncture. Her oocyte yield was noted to be steadily increasing with each ovarian stimulation, with 17 oocytes being retrieved after her ninth stimulation attempt.

This study was followed by case–control studies and randomised control trials (RCTs), and the update of the Cochrane review in 2015 [1] concluded that there was moderate quality evidence for an improvement in live birth rate with the use of DHEA (OR 1.88, 95% CI 1.30–2.71; eight RCTs, n = 878).

A recent network meta-analysis [2] comparing ten different adjuvant therapies for poor responders (testosterone (DHEA), letrozole, recombinant LH, recombinant hCG, oestradiol, clomiphene citrate, progesterone, growth hormone (GH) and coenzyme Q10 (CoQ10), concluded that only DHEA and CoQ10 showed improvement in clinical pregnancy rates (OR 2.46, 95% CI 1.16–5.23).

Despite the non-availability of high quality evidence, considering that DHEA is available as an over-the-counter supplement with minimal side effects [3] and is only one of two adjuvant therapies that have indicated an improvement in pregnancy rates for poor responders, an argument can certainly be made for DHEA supplementation to be offered for the woman undergoing IVF with a predicted poor ovarian response, after clear counselling about the limited nature of the evidence. Indeed, when surveyed, one quarter of respondents to a survey from IVF Worldwide representing 124,700 cycles in 196 centres and 45 countries claimed to be using it [4]. Whether the definitive answer will ever be known is doubtful given the insurmountable difficulties of setting up a well-designed double-blind, placebo-controlled randomised trial investigating a product which is available over-the-counter and which patients with diminished ovarian reserve perceive to be very low risk [5]. The dose and duration varies in the literature with a consensus of 25 mg tds for 12 weeks before IVF stimulation begins [4].

References

1. Nagels HE, Rishworth JR, Siristatidis CS, Kroon B. Androgens (dehydroepiandrosterone or testosterone) for women undergoing assisted reproduction. *Cochrane Database Syst Rev.* 2015 Nov 26.

2. Zhang Y, Zhang C, Shu J, et al. Adjuvant treatment strategies in ovarian stimulation for poor responders undergoing IVF: a systematic review and network meta-analysis. *Hum Reprod Update.* 2020 Feb 28;26(2):247–63.

3. Gleicher N, Weghofer A, Barad DH. Antimullerian hormone (AMH) defines, independent of age, low versus good live birth chances in women with severely reduced ovarian reserve. *Fertil Steril.* 2010;94:2824–7.

4. IVF Worldwide Survey. www.ivf-worldwide.com/survey/poor-responders/ersults-poor-responders.html, 2013.

5. Homburg R, Opoku A. Battle-worn: setting up a multi-centre randomised controlled trial in the UK. *BioNews* 2018;967.

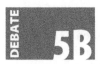

DHEA Is an Effective Treatment for Poor Responders

Against

Mostafa Metwally

DHEA is a pro-hormone produced by the adrenal gland and is a precursor to testosterone and consequently oestrogen production by the ovary. Its use in women with anticipated poor response to IVF has been suggested for some time. The concept behind its use is the potential improvement in follicle sensitivity to FSH through an increase in local androgen production within the ovary. There is also a suggestion that DHEA can improve abnormal mitochondrial dynamics within the cumulus cells in women with poor ovarian response [1].

As attractive as these concepts may be, the use of DHEA in women with potential poor response is supported by very little clinical evidence and consequently its usage seems to stem from a desperation within the clinical community, given the very few options available in this group of women. The majority of studies in the literature are either retrospective or involve a small group of participants. They are also underpowered and associated with significant heterogeneity, with different definitions of poor ovarian reserve used amongst studies. This is despite the introduction by the European Society of Human Reproduction and Embryology (ESHRE) in 2011 of the Bologna criteria for defining poor responders. Since then only some published articles have used these criteria in their designs. Consequently, heterogeneity in study populations casts doubt regarding the validity of the results of these studies. Furthermore, some studies have reported conclusions that are not supported by their statistical findings. For example, a recent paper despite reporting no significant difference in pregnancy rates between those who received DHEA and those who did not, concluded that DHEA supplementation could improve IVF outcomes [2]. There is significant danger in reporting trends that are not supported by robust statistical findings, particularly when busy clinicians are superficially reading the conclusions of such research and implementing the findings in their clinical practices without having the time to critically analyse the findings in detail.

Leaving such an in-depth analysis of the quality of existing research to meta-analyses is also potentially dangerous. Unfortunately, current meta-analyses have done little to shed more light on the situation. Sadly, despite the lack of good quality adequately powered clinical studies, there have been several meta-analyses over the last 5–6 years and whilst meta-analyses offer a useful insight into the evidence they are also potentially dangerous tools which can camouflage deficiencies in the primary studies and portray an overall conclusion which is not befitting the quality of the original research. For example, one meta-analysis in 2018 [3] concluded from five included studies that DHEA led to a significant improvement in clinical pregnancy rates. However, on closer examination of the results, these studies were a mixture of case–controlled studies, randomised controlled trials and retrospective studies. Such a mixture of trial methodologies is not justified in a meta-analysis which should aim to minimise heterogeneity by including only studies of similar design. Such a conclusion, therefore, would have very little validity in clinical practice.

Other studies have suggested that DHEA may lead to a reduction in embryo aneuploidy as evidenced by results obtained from pre-implantation genetic screening for aneuploidy [4].

However, it is now known that pre-implantation genetic screening for aneuploidy has little benefit in improving clinical pregnancy rates in women undergoing IVF, therefore rendering this concept invalid.

Furthermore, most of the preliminary evidence that led to the adoption of DHEA in clinical practice, comes from animal studies and the findings have not then been validated to the same degree in human studies. The data comes mainly from androgen knockout model in mice granulosa cells and although the results did show the indispensable role of androgens in promoting pre-antral follicle growth, this does not lend any justification to the use of DHEA in humans. Rushing an intervention into clinical practice based mainly on concepts developed in the animal model and without a substantial body of evidence to inform human clinical trials is unacceptable and reminiscent of the way that other so-called adjuvant IVF therapies such as endometrial scratch, were quickly adopted into clinical practice without waiting for the results of the necessary studies only to be later proven ineffective in many cases.

There are however other studies that have indeed demonstrated the ineffectiveness of DHEA at a conceptual level. One particular study showed that the concentration of follicular testosterone was completely independent of serum testosterone levels and therefore the concept of manipulating the follicular androgen environment through systemic androgen supplementation is flawed at the very basic level [5]. Other clinical studies have also failed to demonstrate any potential benefit for DHEA on pregnancy rates with IVF.

Proponents of DHEA, however, will however argue where is the harm in prescribing it in a group of women where very little else can be done? This argument is easily refuted by several counter arguments. First of all, the main role of a doctor is to do no harm, and in giving patients false hope regarding a treatment without sound clinical evidence is in a sense causing harm in an already vulnerable group of women, encouraging them to undergo a potentially risky procedure associated with significant physical, mental and financial effects under false pretence. Furthermore, the safety of many so-called IVF add-on treatments such as DHEA and other androgens is not entirely established and in the absence of sound clinical data, any unproven treatment with potential harm should not be given.

Poor ovarian response to ovarian stimulation is a consequence of a diminished ovarian reserve. So far there is no scientific way for replenishing a diminished reserve. It seems completely illogical that an agent such as DHEA could overcome this innate physiological deterioration in ovarian function and lead to some sort of rejuvenation of the ovary. Similar to other adjuvant treatments which have yet to be proven of benefit, DHEA usage should be confined to the research context, using well-powered randomised control studies. Until then, there is no justification for prescribing a drug that is completely unproven and may have potential safety concerns for women with predicted poor response.

References

1. Li CJ, Chen SN, Lin LT., et al. Dehydroepiandrosterone ameliorates abnormal mitochondrial dynamics and mitophagy of cumulus cells in poor ovarian responders. *J Clin Med.* 2018;7(10):293.

2. Mostajeran F, Tehrani H, Ghoreishi E. Effects of dehydroepiandrosterone on in vitro fertilization among women aging over 35 years and normal ovarian reserve. *J Family Reprod Health.* 2018;12:129–33.

3. Schwarze JE, Canales J, Crosby J, Ortega-Hrepich C, Villa S, Pommer R. DHEA use to improve likelihood of IVF/ICSI success in patients with diminished ovarian reserve: a systematic review and meta-

analysis. *JBRA Assist Reprod.* 2018;22:369–74.

4. Gleicher N, Weghofer A, Barad DH. Dehydroepiandrosterone (DHEA) reduces embryo aneuploidy: direct evidence from preimplantation genetic screening (PGS). *Reprod Biol Endocrinol.* 2010;8:140.

5. von Wolff M, Stute P, Eisenhut M, Marti U, Bitterlich N, Bersinger NA. Serum and follicular fluid testosterone concentrations do not correlate, questioning the impact of androgen supplementation on the follicular endocrine milieu. *Reprod Biomed Online.* 2017;35:616–23.

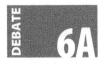

The Addition of LH/hCG to FSH Improves IVF Outcome

For

Claus Yding Andersen

During the natural menstrual cycle both follicle-stimulating hormone (FSH) and luteinising hormone (LH) play important roles in the follicular phase securing follicular growth and development resulting in competent oocytes capable of sustaining further development. It is well-known that after an initial FSH rise in the early follicular phase, FSH becomes down-regulated in the middle of the follicular phase, while the concentration of LH remains relatively constant throughout the follicular phase. Selection of the dominant follicle takes place around the mid-follicular phase at a diameter of 8–10 millimetres. The selected follicle starts to develop LH receptors on the granulosa cells, while FSH receptor expression continues to decline until ovulation [1, 2]. Thus, in the second half of the follicular phase both gonadotropins advance follicular growth with a key contribution from LH. In connection with ovarian stimulation (OS) and assisted reproductive technology (ART) treatment, most protocols use either a gonadotropin releasing hormone- (GnRH)-agonist or a GnRH-antagonist to secure low pituitary output of gonadotropins, especially LH. Therefore, OS protocols don't mimic normal physiology and usually provide supraphysiological concentrations of FSH, while LH/human chorionic gonadotropin (hCG) typically is considerably lower than physiological concentrations. Thus, what are the requirements of LH/hCG and should a lower threshold concentration be surpassed or preferentially be in the physiological range to improve IVF outcome? Many different meta-analyses have compared the use of human menopausal gonadotropin (hMG) and FSH for OS to answer this question, but depending on inclusion criteria, different results have been obtained one favouring one conclusion over the other while the opposite conclusion remains a valid option.

A well-known characteristic of OS with exogenous gonadotropins is the augmented concentrations of oestradiol when LH/hCG is present as compared to a pure FSH preparation, especially in connection with the standard long-agonist down-regulation protocol. The oestradiol levels *per se* do not predict successful IVF outcome, but do suggest that stimulation of both FSH and LH receptors result in additive effects on the reproductive outcome also. This is illustrated by the following two well-conducted studies.

A potential effect of LH/hCG was nicely documented in an RCT comparing administration of HMG and r-FSH in normo-gonadotropic patients undergoing IVF/ICSI treatment following the standard long protocol [3]. The clinical and endocrinological effects of giving either intranasal (IN) or subcutaneous (SC) GnRHa was also compared. The IN administration in the doses given resulted in a less pronounced pituitary down-regulation of LH as compared to SC administration – allowing an assessment of the effect of the endogenous LH. A total of 400 women received either (1) IN/hMG; (2) IN/r-FSH; (3) SC/hMG; or (4) SC/r-FSH with approximately 100 women in each arm, who were similar in baseline characteristics. Number of days used for OS, number of oocytes retrieved and of transferable and transferred embryos were similar in the four groups. Endocrinologically, the four groups differed on stimulation day 8 and on the day of oocyte pick-up (OPU) with significantly higher LH concentrations in those who received IN GnRHa as compared to SC administration. This was also reflected in the concentrations of oestradiol, which were significantly higher following IN GnRHa as compared to SC irrespective of type of gonadotropin preparation administered. Furthermore, hMG resulted in significantly higher oestradiol concentrations as compared to those who received r-FSH. Equally interesting was the clinical pregnancy rate in each of the four groups (1) IN/HMG; (2) IN/r-FSH; (3) SC/ hMG; or (4) SC/r-FSH was 44, 38, 31, 27%, respectively, being significantly higher in the IN/hMG group as compared to the SC/r-FSH group.

The implications of these results are that LH/hCG activity resulting from both endogenous release (i.e. type of down-regulation) and exogenous administration (i.e. either hMG or r-FSH) augment clinical and endocrinological outcome in IVF/ICSI-treated normo-gonadotropic women. However, this study does not demonstrate a causal link between the improved clinical outcome in the IN/hMG group and the augmented output of oestradiol. This may reflect different mechanisms of action, which, however, both appear to be linked to the addition of LH/hCG.

The second study was an RCT performed in women undergoing IVF/ICSI with r-FSH treatment following an antagonist protocol including a total of 333 women. This was a phase II, multicentre, double-blind, randomised dose-finding study of the GnRH antagonix 'Ganirelix' to establish the minimal effective dose preventing premature LH surges during OS [4]. Ovarian stimulation included fixed daily dose of 150 IU for 5 days after which the dose was individualised. From cycle day 7 and until final maturation of follicles Ganirelix was administered once daily by s.c. injection in six increasing doses (i.e. 0.0625, 0.125, 0.25, 0.5, 1.0 and 2.0 mg/0.5 ml).

On the day of ovulation induction, the number of follicles exceeding 11, or 15 or 17 mm was comparable in the six dose groups, similar to the concentration of FSH and progesterone. Furthermore, the number oocytes retrieved, the number of embryos and the good quality embryos were similar in all groups. In contrast, the concentration of LH steadily decreased from 3.6 IU/L in the group with the lowest dose of Ganirelix to 0.4 IU/L in the highest. Interestingly, the concentration of oestradiol followed a similar pattern being three times higher in the lowest Ganirelix group as compared to highest – again demonstrating that the concentration of LH/hCG exerted a pronounced effect on the synthesis of oestradiol. The implantation and ongoing pregnancy rates were highest in the lowest dose group, which effectively eliminated a premature LH rise (i.e. 0.25 mg). Increasing the dose of Ganirelix beyond the 0.25 mg dose more than halved the ongoing pregnancy rate. Taken together, these results may be interpreted as sufficient antagonist dose is required to block for a premature release of LH. Once this is achieved the highest possible LH/hCG activity will enhance chances of an ongoing pregnancy.

These six groups of women were comparable with regard to a number of key clinical parameters differing only in the dose of antagonist administered and thereby in the concentration of endogenous LH. If it is assumed that an increase in the dose of Ganirelix (f.i. going from 0.25 to 0.5 mg per injection) doesn't exert a markedly different direct effect on the ovary itself, these results also appear to support a specific beneficial effect of LH/hCG on the pregnancy potential.

In conclusion, the above two studies demonstrate that when circulating levels of LH/ hCG, either from endogenous or exogenous stores, approach physiological concentrations, the clinical pregnancy rate appears to be positively affected.

References

1. Jeppesen JV, Kristensen SG, Nielsen ME, et al. LH-receptor gene expression in human granulosa and cumulus cells from antral and preovulatory follicles. *J Clin Endocrinol Metab*. 2012;97:1524–31.

2. Kristensen SG, Mamsen LS, Jeppesen JV, et al. Hallmarks of human small antral follicle development: implications for regulation of ovarian steroidogenesis and selection of the dominant follicle. *Front Endocrinol (Lausanne)*. 2018;8:376.

3. Westergaard LG, Erb K, Laursen SB, Rex S, Rasmussen PE. Human menopausal gonadotropin versus recombinant follicle-stimulating hormone in normogonadotropic women down-regulated with a gonadotropin-releasing hormone agonist who were undergoing in vitro fertilization and intracytoplasmic sperm injection: a prospective randomized study. *Fertil Steril*. 2001;76:543 9.

4. Mannaerts B. A double-blind, randomized, dose-finding study to assess the efficacy of the gonadotrophin-releasing hormone antagonist ganirelix (Org 37462) to prevent premature luteinizing hormone surges in women undergoing ovarian stimulation with recombinant follicle stimulating hormone (Puregon). The ganirelix dose-finding study group. *Hum Reprod*. 1998;13:3023–31.

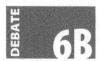

The Addition of LH/hCG to FSH Improves IVF Outcome

Against

Juan-Enrique Schwarze

Our clinical practice, according to evidence-based medicine, should integrate clinical experience and patient values with the best available research information. The latest research revealed that both granulosa cells and theca cells express receptors for LH, thus implying a role in folliculogenesis, and theoretically, in controlled ovarian hyperstimulation (COS) [1]. Several RCTs and systematic reviews have explored whether the addition of LH, either as hCG or rLH, would improve the outcome of IVF cycles. The results are, at least, conflicting [2, 3]. Furthermore, the majority of RCTs include only 'ideal' patients, that is those with normal ovarian reserve, under 37 years, normal semen analysis etc., rendering the results of little use in a regular clinical setting. An alternative source of information to RCT is real-world data, that is observational studies using national registries. If confusion is adequately corrected for, the interpretation of the analysis should be reliable.

Two sources of such real-world data are the Deutsches IVF Register (DIR) [4] and the Latin American Registry of ART (RLA) [5]. Most COS cycles correspond to antagonist cycles (66.8% and 86.3%, respectively), hence I will focus my analysis on the outcome of antagonist cycles.

Probably, the most important outcome of IVF cycles is the clinical pregnancy rate or delivery rate per initiated cycle. Table 6B.1 shows an analysis comparing this outcome according to COS protocols reported to DIR and RLA. Chi-square analysis shows that there is an association between clinical pregnancy rate per initiated cycle and the addition of LH, with a better outcome if rFSH is used alone. Using logistic regression analysis (rFSH as reference), DIR reports an OR of 0.67 (CI 0.62–0.73, $p < 0.001$) for rFSH/hMG, and 0.77 (95% 0.70–0.83, $p < 0.001$) for rFH/rLH; and RLA reports an OR of 0.83 (95% CI 0.77–0.90, $p < 0.001$) for rFSH/hMG and an OR of 0.80 (95% CI 0.73–0.90, $p < 0.001$) for rFSH/rLH.

Such a simple analysis is disposed to different sources of bias, mostly selection bias. For example, older patients or those with a poor ovarian response, are prescribed LH more frequently than younger patients with an adequate ovarian reserve, or are transferred more embryos. A more thorough analysis should include age, the number of embryos transferred, and stage of embryonic development at transfer. We performed such an analysis, and examined 21,212 initiated cycles registered to the RLA [8]. Again, considering rFSH as

Table 6B.1. Comparison of clinical pregnancy rate per initiated cycles as a function of the stimulation protocol in antagonist cycles, DIR (2016) [6] RLA [7] (2017)

	rFSH	rFSH/hMG	rFSH/rLH	p-value
	n/N (%)	n/N (%)	n/N (%)	
DIR (2016)	4632/12940 (26.2%)	1017/3426 (21.4%)	876/4515 (19.4%)	<0.001
RLA (2017)	1165/3548 (32.8%)	3053/10567 (28.9%)	880/3107 (28.3%)	<0.001

reference and correcting for age of the female partner, BMI, number of embryos transferred, and blastocyst-stage transfer, we found that the use of rFSH/hMG had an OR of delivery rate per ET of 1.02 (95% CI 0.91–1.10, p = 0.622), and rFSH/rLH had an OR of 0.96 (95% CI 0.85–1.09, p = 0.569). That is, no clinically significant difference between COS protocols.

Another outcome of interest is the number of mature oocytes recovered. We performed multiple regression analysis and corrected for confusion, compared to rFSH alone, rFSH/hMG had a beta coefficient of –0.59 (95CI –0.84 to –0.35, p < 0.0001), and rFSH/rLH had a beta coefficient of –1.03 (95% CI 1.41 to –0.66, p < 0.001). The difference is not clinically significant.

A possible surrogate for the quality of the oocyte is the natural miscarriage rate. We performed logistic regression analysis, and found that compared to rFSH, rFSH/hMG had an OR of 0.99 (95% CI 0.83–1.32, p = 0.877) and rFSH/rLH of 1.04 (95% CI 0.85–01.42, p = 0.721). Again, of no clinical significance.

Finally, another outcome is the morphology and number of blastocysts according to COS. We analysed 2112 cases of autologous ART performed in our unit [9]; 20% received rFSH, 48% HMG/rFSH, and 32% rFSH/rLH. Blastocyst rate formation was 38%, 35% and 33%, respectively (Chi square p = 0.444). Blastocyst morphology was classified as expanded, cavitated and initial. We found that compared to rFSH alone, the addition of neither hMG or rLH was associated with: (a) an increase in the number of expanded blastocysts, multilevel Poisson regression, rFSH alone [10]; hMG/rFSH IRR 1.08 (95% CI 0.93–1.26, p = 0.301); rFSH/rLH IRR 0.86 (95% CI 0.73–1.92, p = 0.092); (b) number of expanded blastocysts, multilevel mixed logistic regression, rFSH alone [11]; hMG/rFSH OR 1.09 (95% CI 0.76–1.40, p = 0.847); rFSH/rLH OR 1.03 (95% 0.74–5.60, p = 0.162); (c) odds of a blastocyst being expanded over cavitated/initial, rFSH alone [12]; hMG/rFSH OR 1.11 (95% CI 0.87–2.25, p = 0.281); rFSH/rLH OR 1.02 (95% CI 0.93–2.00, p = 0.839). Again, the addition of LH was not associated with a positive effect.

In summary, real-world data does not provide any support to the notion that the addition of LH/hCG to FSH improves the number of mature oocytes recovered, the morphology of the blastocyst, livebirth rate or reduces the natural miscarriage rate.

References

1. Jeppesen JV, Kristensen SG, Nielsen ME, et al. LH-receptor gene expression in human granulosa and cumulus cells from antral and preovulatory follicles. *J Clin Endocrinol Metab.* 2012;97:E1524–31.

2. Mochtar MH, Danhof NA, Ayeleke RO, van der Veen F, van Wely M. Recombinant luteinizing hormone (rLH) and recombinant follicle stimulating hormone (rFSH) for ovarian stimulation in IVF/ICSI cycles. In: Cochrane Gynaecology and Fertility Group, ed. *Cochrane Database Syst Rev.* 2017;18:250–105.

3. van Wely M, Kwan I, Burt AL, et al. Recombinant versus urinary gonadotrophin for ovarian stimulation in assisted reproductive technology cycles. In: van Wely M, ed. *Cochrane Database Syst Rev.* 2011;CD005354. John Wiley & Sons: Chichester.

4 www.deutsches-ivf-register.de/ivf-international.php.

5. https://redlara.com/registro.asp?

6. www.kup.at/kup/pdf/14120.pdf.

7. Unpublished data.

8. Schwarze JE, Crosby J, Zegers-Hochschild F. Addition of neither recombinant nor urinary luteinizing hormone was associated with an improvement in the outcome of autologous in vitro fertilization/

intracytoplasmatic sperm injection cycles under regular clinical settings: a multicenter observational analysis. *Fertil Steril*. 2016;106:1–5.

9. Unpublished data from my clinic.

10. Unpublished data from my clinic.

11. Unpublished data from my clinic.

12. Unpublished data from my clinic.

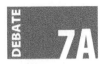

Acupuncture Is a Useful Adjuvant for Fertility Treatment

For

Elisabet Stener-Victorin

Since the beginning of the twenty-first century, acupuncture has been used as an adjunctive treatment before and/or during in vitro fertilisation (IVF). Couples frequently search for information on non-pharmacological treatments with the aim to reduce stress and anxiety linked to IVF treatment and with the hope to increase the success rate and chances of achieving pregnancy and live birth. Between 30 to 50% of all women undergoing IVF in USA are treated with acupuncture before or during IVF treatment [1].

Acupuncture is an ancient method where thin needles are inserted into specific acupuncture points located subcutaneously and preferably in skeletal muscle in the same innervation area as the uterus and ovaries, as well as in the hands and legs to enhance the effect. When inserted, needles are stimulated by manual rotation to evoke a needle sensation reflecting activation of afferent nerve fibres which process information to the central nervous system. In addition, needles can be stimulated with electricity, so called electro-acupuncture. Needle sensation and electrical stimulation of the needles cause afferent activity in the peripheral nerves with local release of neuropeptides resulting in increased microcirculation. Furthermore, depending on the intensity of stimulation, activation of afferent nerve fibres can modulate the transmission of signals in the spinal cord and in the central nervous system, and thus modulate sympathetic reflexes, in this case, to the uterus and ovaries. Thus, hypothetically acupuncture acts via several mechanisms including modulation of neuroendocrine function, namely the hypothalamus-pituitary-adrenal axis, i.e. the stress, anxiety and depression axis; modulation of sympathetic reflexes which results in increased uterine artery blood flow; and modulation of immune factors.

The first published studies between 2002 and 2006 demonstrated that acupuncture given immediately before and after embryo transfer improves the reproductive outcome although no data on live births were provided [2]. Even though these trials were underpowered, most of them showed a benefit of acupuncture over control, and acupuncture before and after embryo transfer quickly became standard clinical practice at many hospitals [3].

Many randomised controlled trials (RCTs) with adequate sample size calculations and of high scientific quality, including blinding and sham/placebo groups, have been published since then. With increasing quality, the evidence of an actual effect of acupuncture on live births has become less clear [4]. Most high-quality, double-blind trials using non-penetrating sham needles, which have been shown to evoke needle sensation (i.e. activation of afferent nerve fibres), find no benefit of acupuncture over sham, or even favouring sham over true acupuncture in pregnancy outcomes [4]. The largest sham-controlled trial of acupuncture within IVF treatment included 824 women who had already failed two or more IVF cycles [5], and they found no beneficial effect of acupuncture over sham acupuncture.

Despite this, the most recent meta-analysis found increased live births and reduced miscarriage rate when acupuncture was compared with no adjunctive control [4]. Furthermore, acupuncture during embryo transfer in women who have had multiple IVF attempts, had a significant effect on the outcome, independent of the comparator group (sham acupuncture or no adjunctive control) [4]. These findings suggest that the major problem in sham-controlled acupuncture trials is the sham procedure *per se*, as it is not an inert control. In addition, meta-analyses indicate that acupuncture treatment for women with poor IVF outcomes might be beneficial, but further studies are warranted. These data imply that there is a need for studies in which acupuncture treatment is optimised with an inert comparator and performed in specific patient groups. This is further supported by a study demonstrating that acupuncture improves IVF outcome and decreases the risk of ovarian hyperstimulation syndrome in women with polycystic ovary syndrome [6].

Finally, true acupuncture has been shown in several studies to give significant benefit in terms of anxiolysis and depression. To get a long-lasting effect on psychiatric variables as anxiety and depression, a course of regular acupuncture treatments is required to mediate measurable clinical effects. The same holds for increase in uterine artery blood flow which has been shown to be increased first after eight acupuncture treatments given twice a week prior to IVF. Therefore, given the physiological reasoning above, it is likely that a course of acupuncture treatments for 1–2 months prior to IVF treatment must be given to improve the IVF outcome. Furthermore, acupuncture intervention must be optimised, and reasonable controls must be used in future studies.

The ultimate question is whether acupuncture can be recommended as an adjuvant treatment during embryo transfer with the aim of increasing the chance of successful IVF treatment. Currently the answer is no, but there are clear indications that a course of acupuncture treatments given prior to IVF with optimised acupuncture protocols has the potential to improve the success rate, but it remains to be further investigated.

Therefore, don't throw out the baby with the bath water!

References

1. Domar AD, Conboy L, Denardo-Roney J, Rooney KL. Lifestyle behaviors in women undergoing in vitro fertilization: a prospective study. *Fertil Steril*. 2012;97:697–701.e691.

2. Domar AD. Acupuncture and infertility: we need to stick to good science. *Fertil Steril*. 2006;85:1359–61; discussion 1368–70.

3. Smith CA, Armour M, Betts D. Treatment of women's reproductive health conditions by Australian and New Zealand acupuncturists. *Complement Ther Med*. 2014;22:710–18.

4. Smith CA, Armour M, Shewamene Z, Tan HY, Norman RJ, Johnson NP. Acupuncture performed around the time of embryo transfer: a systematic review and meta-analysis. *Reprod Biomed Online*. 2019;38:364–79.

5. Smith CA, de Lacey S, Chapman M, et al. Effect of acupuncture vs. sham acupuncture on live births among women undergoing in vitro fertilization: a randomized clinical trial. *JAMA*. 2018;319:1990–8.

6. Jo J, Lee YJ. Effectiveness of acupuncture in women with polycystic ovarian syndrome undergoing in vitro fertilisation or intracytoplasmic sperm injection: a systematic review and meta-analysis. *Acupunct Med*. 2017;35:162–70.

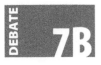

Acupuncture Is a Useful Adjuvant for Fertility Treatment

Against

Isla Robertson and Ying Cheong

Extensive evidence to date makes clear that there is no significant benefit for acupuncture alongside IVF on live birth outcomes, the agreed primary outcome measure in infertility trials, and that acupuncture has no influence beyond placebo on any measures of the success of IVF. However, acupuncture is increasingly used by patients during fertility treatment. We advocate that acupuncture should not be used as an adjuvant for fertility treatment, for the following reasons.

The Regulatory Authority Do Not Recommend the Use of Acupuncture As an Adjuvant to IVF

In the UK 2018 HFEA national patient survey, 26% of those receiving fertility treatments in the last two years reported having received acupuncture. This uptake had increased from 18% in the preceding 3 years. The HFEA chair recently stated, 'From acupuncture to bee pollen, there are many supplements and treatments that claim to work but are simply not supported by evidence.' However, direct-to-patient websites make claims such as, 'A recent trial demonstrated a doubling of IVF success rates when acupuncture was used' [1]. We are concerned that co-location of acupuncture practices within HFEA-licensed clinics and advertising of these services on clinic websites suggests clinical endorsement of these therapies.

Sufficient RCTs Have Been Performed

A Cochrane review in 2013 showed no evidence of improvement in pregnancy or live birth after acupuncture at the time of oocyte retrieval or embryo transfer [2]. In addition, a large 2018 RCT, including 848 women undergoing IVF, showed no difference in live births between those given acupuncture vs. those given sham acupuncture at the time of ovarian stimulation and embryo transfer. A review of seven meta-analyses, published in early 2019, showed acupuncture had no positive effect on clinical outcomes in IVF, whether the procedure was performed around the time of oocyte aspiration, embryo transfer, or when controlled ovarian hyperstimulation was performed [3]. A March 2019 updated meta-analysis, including the 2018 RCT, showed there was no statistical difference between acupuncture and sham control for live birth rate, clinical pregnancy, ongoing pregnancy or miscarriage [4]. The relative risk (RR) of live birth with acupuncture compared with sham control was 1.01 (95% CI 0.80, 1.28), p = 0.93. In this analysis, when acupuncture was compared with no adjunctive treatment, a marginal difference was demonstrated (RR 1.30 (95% CI 1.00, 1.68), p = 0.05). Crucially, the primary outcome showed no evidence of benefit for live birth in 12 studies. Given the number of studies already conducted, are any more studies needed to evaluate the impact of acupuncture on reproductive outcomes?

Are Small Differences Clinically Valuable?

The small differences in outcome demonstrated in some studies when acupuncture is compared with no adjunctive treatment, rather than with a placebo/sham therapy, require consideration. It may be that sham acupuncture devices are not inert, and that some effect may arise when applied, including sensory and psycho-social cues. For this reason, sham acupuncture cannot be defined as an inert placebo and trials require careful interpretation. Acupuncture involves needling, non-needling components (palpation, education, self-care and diagnosis), and non-specific components including time, attention, credibility and expectation. Even if acupuncture needling is not an effective treatment modality, there may be psychological benefit derived from the time, attention and hope associated with treatment, whether sham or traditional. A large RCT study found acupuncture may be associated with reduced anxiety following embryo transfer but with no overall difference in quality-of-life measures [5].

Acupuncture Is Expensive

As there is no evidence of treatment effectiveness, acupuncture should not be included as part of publicly funded fertility care. However, currently most IVF and all acupuncture adjuvant therapies are self-funded, therefore, the patient as consumer makes their own choice regarding treatment. To inform this choice, they assess personal value, defined as improving the outcomes that matter to them for a given amount of resource (e.g. money, time), with their experience of care a critical element. The individual weighs up potential benefits and harms and determines whether greater value could be derived from a different use of resources. As there is minimal risk of harm, other than cost (typically, £55/session), it is a personal decision as to whether to use acupuncture alongside fertility treatment.

Honest Marketing

If acupuncture for fertility patients was marketed in a balanced way, focusing on experience, reduction in anxiety and possible placebo benefit, it would not be incumbent on fertility clinicians to discuss this therapy. However, perusal of relevant consumer marketing and related media reports shows this is not the case. Hence, it is vital to discuss the effectiveness of such add-on therapies, so patients can make informed choices about whether to fund treatments additional to their primary fertility treatment. This is a focus of the HFEA traffic light system; with a red rating being 'there is no evidence that this add-on is effective and safe.' The stated HFEA aim relating to add-on therapies is to prevent patients from being misled (in terms of potentially exploiting unfounded expectations) by ensuring that patients are provided with clear, reliable information. As a quarter of IVF patients are accessing acupuncture, clinicians should be ready to establish dialogue and present up-to-date evidence on this topic, so that patients are not vulnerable to misleading or exploitative marketing.

'First Do No Harm'

Primum non nocere dictates that clinicians be honest with patients. Since acupuncture remains of unproven clinical benefit this should be clearly explained to ensure that patients are fully informed when consenting to treatment. Clinicians should be clear that acupuncture for IVF may have personal value to couples, justifying the associated expense in psychological benefits such as reduction of short-term treatment-related anxiety. However, patients should not be led to believe that this complementary treatment will have any effect on their likelihood of a successful outcome from the IVF process. We should focus research endeavour on other ways to support our patients, establishing evidence of benefit before routine availability and use.

In conclusion, there is currently no evidence on the benefit of acupuncture as an adjuvant for fertility treatment.

References

1. www.emmacannon.co.uk/fertility/acupuncture.

2. Cheong YC, Dix S, Ng EHY, Ledger WL, Farquhar C. Acupuncture and assisted reproductive technology. *Cochrane Database of Systematic Reviews*, 2013.

3. Peng JT, Li TT, Zhang XL, Li JJ, Liang XY. Acupuncture has no significantly positive effect on in vitro fertilization: a review of systematic reviews. *J Reproduct Med.* 2019;64:51–60.

4. Smith CA, Armour M, Shewamene Z, Tan HY, Norman RJ, Johnson NP. Acupuncture performed around the time of embryo transfer: a systematic review and meta-analysis. *Reproduct Biomed.* Online 2019;38:364–79.

5. Smith CA, de Lacey S, Chapman M, et al. The effects of acupuncture on the secondary outcomes of anxiety and quality of life for women undergoing IVF: a randomized controlled trial. *Acta Obstet Gynecol Scand.* 2019;98:460–69.

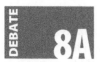

There Is a Role for Pre-conceptional Treatment with CoQ10

For

Grace Dugdale

Making evidence-based decisions with a common primary outcome measure is a key tenet of ethical and effective clinical practice in assisted reproduction technology (ART) in a rapidly evolving scientific landscape. However, interpretation of the evidence must be underpinned by sound biological reasoning and this is especially true when it comes to adjunct antioxidant supplementation in IVF. Furthermore, study design for assessing natural compounds is typically based on protocols established to assess drug-based therapies, that often fail to effectively evaluate efficacy of individual nutrients that occur naturally in vivo, and often groups study patients together with many differing aetiologies. Finally, the gold standard in terms of IVF outcome measure is live birth rate (LBR) but it is vital that we move beyond this narrow perspective and consider obstetric and child health outcomes. With this in mind I will describe the role for pre-conceptional treatment with co-enzyme Q10 (CoQ10).

In order for a human oocyte to achieve optimal developmental competence, cooperative signalling and effective nutrient exchange between cumulus, granulosa and theca cells and the oocyte are needed for the oocyte to grow and mature within the follicular microenvironment. As it leaves the primordial resting pool, the oocyte is sensitive to changes in various aspects of this microenvironment including toxic exposures and fluctuations in nutrient availability [1]. Such environmental changes have the potential to adversely affect the oocyte throughout the follicular growth phase, with impairments to reproductive function mediated predominantly via impact on mitochondrial function. At the same time, adequate levels of CoQ10 are required for optimal mitochondrial function and yet levels within the oocyte microenvironment are known to decline with age along with expression of the enzymes responsible for endogenous production within the oocyte, Pdss2 and Coq6, and in line with mitochondrial function, thus exacerbating the effects of other environmental stressors.

Crucially, therefore, CoQ10 is one component of multiple environmental exposures that can impact oocyte developmental competence but not the only one. Despite this, studies assessing treatment with CoQ10 alone demonstrate significant benefit including improved ART outcomes, up-regulation of mitochondrial biogenesis and delay of cellular senescence [2]. In terms of age-related decline in fertility, animal studies support the case for CoQ10 treatment, with research in an aged mouse model showing that long-term supplementation can slow decline in ovarian reserve, restore gene expression in the oocyte mitochondria, reverse age-induced deterioration of oocyte quality and enhance mitochondrial function [3]. These studies provide mechanistic evidence in the absence of other complexities experienced by human beings in terms of varying diet, lifestyle, nutrient levels, underlying health and other environmental exposures.

In terms of human studies, research also indicates benefit, with studies assessing the follicular fluid (FF) of older patients (>35) undergoing IVF demonstrating that supplementation of CoQ10 improves FF oxidative metabolism and therefore has the potential to improve oocyte quality. An RCT looking at the impact of CoQ10 treatment on IVF outcomes found an aneuploidy rate of 46.5% in the CoQ10 group compared with 62.8% in the control. Clinical pregnancy rate (CPR) was 33% for the CoQ10 group and 26.7% for the control group, though the trial was halted prematurely and therefore was underpowered to draw firm conclusions [4]. Indications are, however, that there was a benefit in the treatment group.

In terms of research into patients with poor ovarian reserve (POR) as defined by the Bologna criteria, in a recent meta-analysis of 19 trials comparing 2677 women with controls [5], CoQ10 supplementation combined with DHEA significantly increased CPR compared to controls [odds ratio (OR) 2.46, 95% CI 1.16–5.23; 2.22, 1.08–4.58, respectively] and other clinical outcomes including reduced requirements for gonadotrophin needed for stimulation. One study that assessed pre-treatment with CoQ10 alone demonstrated improved ovarian response to stimulation and embryological parameters in young women with poor ovarian reserve in IVF-ICSI cycles [6]. A more recent meta-analysis of five RCTs assessing outcomes in general patient cohorts concluded that oral supplementation of CoQ10 alone may increase CPR when compared with placebo or no-treatment, in women undergoing ART procedures, although this did not extend to improvements in overall LBR and miscarriage rates [7].

Although the data suggest benefit in the general patient population, a personalised medicine approach informed by evidence as to which categories of patients particularly likely to respond can help refine more targeted treatment. In vitro maturation research has been informed by the discovery of CoQ10 in FF and experiments have shown particular benefit of CoQ10 supplemented media for oocytes of obese women, for instance. Animal research has demonstrated similar potential for the oocytes of old overweight mice, indicating specific sub-groups of patients may benefit from exposure to CoQ10. Aside from direct effects on the oocyte microenvironment, separate studies in mice show enhanced lipid metabolism in overweight animals, which may confer indirect improvements in terms oocyte quality and reproductive outcomes, further indicating potential advantages of CoQ10 for obese patients.

Other research has explored the impact of CoQ10 on inflammatory markers [8], with a recent meta-analysis [9] demonstrating reduced plasma levels of C-reactive protein, interleukin 6 (IL-6) and tumour necrosis factor alpha (TNF-α) in patients suffering from inflammatory-linked conditions and treated with doses ranging from 60 to 500 mg/day for a 1-week to 4-month intervention period. These inflammatory cytokines are known to be involved in the development of endometriosis and contribute to a sub-optimal oocyte microenvironment in affected patients. Women with underlying inflammatory-linked conditions including PCOS and endometriosis may therefore particularly benefit from treatment with CoQ10. Further, infertile women with endometriosis exhibit excessive consumption of the antioxidants needed to scavenge the excess ROS associated with the condition and achieving greater antioxidant capacity in these patients has been shown to improve outcomes including increased number of oocytes retrieved, number of mature oocytes, and the number of fertilised oocytes. Separate studies have shown that CoQ10 supplementation significantly decreases AMH levels in PCOS patients, one contributor to the sub-optimal oocyte microenvironment in women with PCOS.

Together these studies demonstrate a significant impact for a single antioxidant and therefore recommending stand-alone supplementation of 300–600 mg daily in the suitable patient groups outlined above is more than justified, given this is a low-cost and risk-free intervention. However, the potential to improve outcomes further could be achieved via a systems biology approach where CoQ10 treatment is provided alongside optimisation of other environmental exposures within the follicular microenvironment including micronutrient status. There is increasing evidence to demonstrate the role of zinc in both triggering oocytes from developmental arrest, and supporting transcription and improving meiotic competence in the developing oocyte, for instance. A number of other micronutrients have been implicated in oocyte developmental competence and/or ART success, including vitamins A and D, folate, and iodine. Given the significance of nutrient deficiencies as potential environment stressors in the follicular microenvironment, assessing and optimising overall nutrient status alongside CoQ10 treatment is clinically sound not only in terms of oocyte competence and conception but also for obstetric and long-term child health outcomes. Many women enter pregnancy with low levels of key nutrients needed for conception and pregnancy including zinc, folate, iron, iodine and vitamin A [10] and there is a growing recognition of the importance of pre-conception care, not only for maternal–fetal health but in addressing preventable causes of miscarriage. Since mitochondrial impairments are heritable, age-related decline in mitochondrial function has implications beyond simple conception and live birth. Similarly, given CoQ10 levels decline with age and that the oocyte contains all the nutrients and cellular machinery needed by the pre-implantation embryo, including antioxidants to counter the oxidative stress generated by early development, restoring levels through supplementation is important for this crucial stage of embryonic development that has profound implications for the lifelong health of the child. Therefore a three-month pre-conception care period to address the multiple modifiable factors that can impact both ART and long-term outcomes via a personalised approach, including CoQ10 treatment, is essential if fertility services are to progress in an ethical and patient-centred manner, especially given this is unlikely to have a significantly negative impact on success rates. Indeed, a recent study found that a delay in IVF treatment of 180 days for practical reasons did not affect pregnancy outcomes in women with diminished ovarian reserve and this was without interventions to improve results in the intervening period. Whilst a delay may be specifically contraindicated in some, this approach should be possible and reasonable for most patients.

Overall, the scientific evidence demonstrates that evaluating natural compounds, or indeed any drug, as an individual silver bullet to correct reproductive ageing in a complex biological system represents a failure to effectively direct future research. Furthermore, individual nutrients are not usually able to replicate the effects of a drug on a biological system and a single compound is unlikely to solve the multiple significant combined consequences of infertility and ageing on conception and pregnancy by itself. Despite this, CoQ10 has been shown to have a significant impact on numerous parameters and can help optimise the microenvironment for oocyte development and maturation. Any rationale that eliminates a compound that shows such promise, because by itself it has not yet been shown to increase LBR, will hinder progress in IVF research and clinical outcomes. A shift in perspective is needed away from a narrow focus on a single intervention to increase LBR towards an approach of marginal gains targeting LBR and maternal and child health. If clinicians are able to modify aspects of biological function such that outcomes including clinical pregnancy are improved, a personalised approach can then optimise other parameters that have the potential to increase the chances of a live birth in an individual patient via a systems biology approach.

References

1. Ramalho-Santos R, Varum S, Amaral S, et al. Mitochondrial functionality in reproduction: from gonads and gametes to embryos and embryonic stem cells. *Hum Reprod. Update* 2009;15(5):553–72.

2. Díaz-Casado ME, Quiles JL, Barriocanal-Casado E, et al. The paradox of coenzyme Q10 in aging. *Nutrients.* 2019;11(9):2221.

3. Ben-Meir A, Yahalomi S, Moshe B, Shufaro Y, Reubinoff B, Saada A. Coenzyme Q-dependent mitochondrial respiratory chain activity in granulosa cells is reduced with aging. *Fertil Steril.* 2015;104(3):724–7.

4. Bentov Y, Hannam T, Jurisicova A, Esfandiari N, Casper RF. Coenzyme Q10 supplementation and oocyte aneuploidy in women undergoing IVF-ICSI treatment. *Clin Med Insights Reprod Health.* 2014;8:31–6.

5. Zhang Y, Zhang C, Shu J, et al. Adjuvant treatment strategies in ovarian stimulation for poor responders undergoing IVF: a systematic review and network meta-analysis. *Hum Reprod Update.* 2020;26 (2):247–63.

6. Xu Y, Nisenblat V, Lu C, et al. Pretreatment with coenzyme Q10 improves ovarian response and embryo quality in low-prognosis young women with decreased ovarian reserve: a randomized controlled trial. *Reprod Biol Endocrinol.* 2018;16(1):29.

7. Florou P, Anagnostis P, Theocharis P, Chourdakis M, Goulis D. Does coenzyme Q10 supplementation improve fertility outcomes in women undergoing assisted reproductive technology procedures? A systematic review and meta-analysis of randomized-controlled trials. *J Assist Reprod Genet.* 2020;37(10):2377–87.

8. Hernández-Camacho JD, Bernier M, López-Lluch G, Navas P. Coenzyme Q10 supplementation in aging and disease. *Front Physiol.* 2018;9.

9. Fan L, Feng Y, Chen GC, Qin LQ, Fu CL, Chen LH. Effects of coenzyme Q10 supplementation on inflammatory markers: a systematic review and meta-analysis of randomized controlled trials. *Pharmacol Res.* 2017;119:128–36.

10. Stephenson J, Heslehurst N, Hall J, et al. Before the beginning: nutrition and lifestyle in the preconception period and its importance for future health. *The Lancet.* 2018;391:10132.

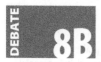

8B There Is a Role for Pre-conceptional Treatment with CoQ10

Against

Roger J Hart

Co-enzyme Q10 (CoQ10), transported in the blood by lipoproteins, is an essential component of the inner mitochondrial membrane and is responsible for electron transport in the mitochondrial respiratory chain for oxidative phosphorylation to generate the energy substrate adenosine triphosphate (ATP), and acts as an antioxidant within the oocyte. Observational studies suggest that the follicular fluid concentration of CoQ10 diminishes with age [1], and low CoQ10 antioxidant status may indeed correlate with oocyte aneuploidy [2]. Consequently it would appear there is a sound rationale for the use of CoQ10 during infertility treatment, perhaps for women with perceived 'poor oocyte quality'. Furthermore the scientific rationale is supported by several animal studies which demonstrate a beneficial effect of CoQ10 supplementation on embryonic development. However, before all clinicians are encouraged to prescribe CoQ10 as the eternal elixir of reproductive youth, evidence for a benefit of supplementation in the IVF clinical setting is required.

The largest study to date using CoQ10 for women undergoing IVF treatment with an expected poor prognosis was performed in China over 14 months in 2015–2016. This was a non-blinded randomised controlled trial of the use of CoQ10 (200 mg three times per day for two months pre-IVF), or no treatment, in women under 35 years of age with an expected poor response to ovarian stimulation, on the basis of their serum anti-Mullerian hormone concentration, or their antral follicle count. The hypothesis for their study was that increased oxidative stress was responsible for a premature decline in ovarian function, which may improve in response to treatment with a course of CoQ10. The power calculation for this study was based on the recruitment of at least 76 women to each arm of the study, and the primary outcome measure was the number of embryos that reached 6–8 cells on the 3rd day of culture. 76 women completed the CoQ10 arm, and 93 women were recruited to the control arm. Most women were treatment naïve with primary infertility. Despite favourable outcomes with respect to the duration of stimulation required, dose of gonadotrophin required, number of oocytes collected, fertilisation rate and an improvement in embryo quality, no benefit of use on clinical pregnancy rate or livebirth was demonstrated [3]. It is acknowledged that the study was not powered for this outcome variable, but it is widely accepted that all studies performed in the infertility setting should have livebirth as the primary outcome for the study. However, it is recognised that studies performed on patients with an expected poor response to treatment have incredible difficulty in recruiting patients [4], but this group only took 14 months to enroll 94 patients to each arm, and hence it is a shame the study was not powered for the primary outcome of livebirth at the outset. Furthermore it is possible that this intervention study investigated the wrong study population, as it is possible that a more appropriate group for analysis is women with 'poor egg' or 'poor embryo' quality.

A retrospective comparative study that looked at the use of a longer duration of treatment with CoQ for 10 8.8 ± 6.2 months with a previous poor response to ovarian stimulation,

RJH is part of the NHMRC Centre of Research Excellence for Polycystic Ovarian Syndrome, Grant number 1078444.

undergoing either intrauterine insemination treatment (IUI) or IVF. The study group (330 patients) were also prescribed dehydroepiandrosterone (DHEA), with the addition of CoQ10, and were treated between the years 2009–2014. This study group was compared to a control group (467 patients) derived from a prior time period, 2006–2014, who were similarly poor responders, who were just prescribed DHEA prior to their treatment cycle. The study group recorded an increase in antral follicles within the ovary, and more dominant follicles at the time of trigger injection prior to IUI or IVF, although there were no differences in pregnancy rates, and no differences in oocytes retrieved in the IVF group [5].

The only other randomised controlled trial of the use of the medication CoQ10, administered to women undergoing IVF treatment, studied its effect on the rate of oocyte aneuploidy, but was unfortunately prematurely terminated due to the safety concerns over the use of polar body biopsy, when only 39 patients had undergone randomisation [2]. It was unfortunate that the study was terminated early as it was a double blind study powered for the primary outcome of oocyte aneuploidy rate. The authors' conclusions were: 'The results show a lower rate of aneuploidy in the CoQ10 group, although the results do not reach statistical significance... More research is needed to study the effects of a longer duration of intake of CoQ10 on female function of various ages.'

Conclusion

Consequently on the basis of this very limited evidence provided, there is no sound basis to advise a woman with limited ovarian reserve, or perceived poor oocyte quality, to postpone the commencement of an IVF cycle for 2–3 months to commence a course of CoQ10 to derive a potentially improved IVF outcome.

The abundant animal work performed demonstrates a rationale for the use of CoQ10 in an IVF cycle, and is therefore very encouraging, however there is limited human clinical work to verify any benefit in the clinical setting. More studies of the use of CoQ10 prior to an IVF cycle are required, and the patient population where any perceived benefit may lie needs further exploration. It is unclear whether a place for treatment may lie within a group of patients with perceived 'poor egg quality' (young, or just the older patient cohort), or in a group of women with a perceived poor ovarian reserve; furthermore it is also unclear how long should any treatment course last, and at what dose.

References

1. Ben-Meir A, Yahalomi S, Moshe B, Shufaro Y, Reubinoff B, Saada A. Coenzyme Q-dependent mitochondrial respiratory chain activity in granulosa cells is reduced with aging. *Fertil Steril*. 2015;104(3):724–7.

2. Bentov Y, Hannam T, Jurisicova A, Esfandiari N, Casper RF. Coenzyme Q10 supplementation and oocyte aneuploidy in women undergoing IVF-ICSI treatment. *Clin Med Insights Reproduct Health*. 2014;8:31–6.

3. Xu Y, Nisenblat V, Lu C, et al. Pretreatment with coenzyme Q10 improves ovarian response and embryo quality in low-prognosis young women with decreased ovarian reserve: a randomized controlled trial. *Reprod Biol Endocrinol*. 2018;16(1):29.

4. Norman RJ, Alvino H, Hull LM, et al. Human growth hormone for poor responders: a randomized placebo-controlled trial provides no evidence for improved live birth rate. *Reprod Biomed. Online*. 2019.

5. Gat I, Blanco Mejia S, Balakier H, Librach CL, Claessens A, Ryan EA. The use of coenzyme Q10 and DHEA during IUI and IVF cycles in patients with decreased ovarian reserve. *Gynecol Endocrinol*. 2016;32(7):534–7.

DEBATE 9A There Is a Role for Pre-conceptional Treatment with Vitamin D

For

Justin Chu

The prevalence of infertility is increasing. Women are choosing to have their families later in life with more couples relying on IVF treatment to achieve pregnancy. Each year, the number of IVF treatment cycles performed around the World is rising, and there is a need to optimise the success rates of treatment. We already know a great deal about how to select the embryo with the highest pregnancy potential. The rate limiting step in improving treatment outcomes seems to be in improving our understanding of endometrial receptivity. There is a need to significantly improve our ability to optimise the implantation environment.

Vitamin D is a fat-soluble pro-hormone. Our main source of vitamin D is through photochemical synthesis in the skin with a small source from dietary intake. Its levels are measured easily by assay of serum 25-hydroxy vitamin D_3. Vitamin D deficiency has been found to be highly prevalent in the infertile population. It has also been found to be of great importance in female reproductive health. Vitamin D plays critical roles in oocyte development, ovarian steroidogenesis and importantly endometrial receptivity [1]. Vitamin D enzymes and receptors are found in the endometrium and deficiency in vitamin D has been shown to lead to poor implantation and placentation due to its immunomodulatory role.

People are at risk of the detrimental effects of vitamin D deficiency at serum 25-hydroxy vitamin D_3 concentrations of less than 50 nmol/L. A level of 50 to 75 nmol/L is considered insufficient and greater than 75 nmol/L is considered vitamin D replete (Table 9A.1). Serum concentrations greater than 374 nmol/L are associated with toxicity [2].

There is some conflicting evidence from clinical research investigating the association between vitamin D levels and IVF treatment outcomes. Some observational studies investigating the link between vitamin D and IVF treatment outcomes have previously shown no association. However, it should be noted that these studies have been small and usually include a low proportion of women who are vitamin D replete. A more recently published cohort study, which included larger numbers with more women replete in vitamin D, showed a dose–response relationship between vitamin D and IVF treatment outcomes. This cohort study showed that women who are deficient in vitamin D have the poorest IVF live birth rates (23.2% [57/246]); those who have insufficient vitamin D levels have intermediate IVF live birth rates (27.0% [38/141]); whereas women who are replete in vitamin D have the best live birth rate (37.7% [29/77]). [3].

A systematic review and meta-analysis of 11 published cohort studies showed that women were more likely to achieve a positive pregnancy test (OR 1.34 ([1.04–1.73]); a clinical pregnancy (OR 1.46 [1.05–2.02]); and a live birth 1.33 [1.08–1.65]) if they had replete vitamin D levels when compared with women with deficient or insufficient vitamin D levels [4].

Table 9A.1. Vitamin D categories

Vitamin D category	Serum 25-hydroxy vitamin D$_3$ (nmol/L)
Deficient	<50
Insufficient	50–75
Replete	>75

So why is it not routine clinical practice to treat women with vitamin D in the pre-conceptional period? Unfortunately, the reason why vitamin D deficiency is not treated more commonly is because there is no available published trial evidence. No published trial has investigated the merit of pre-conceptional treatment of vitamin D deficiency. The reason behind the lack of trial evidence is an ethical one. It would be unethical to perform a placebo-controlled trial in women undergoing IVF treatment who are found to be vitamin D deficient due to the myriad of health benefits associated with treating vitamin D deficiency and reaching replete vitamin D levels. Participants randomised to receive placebo treatment would undergo IVF treatment remaining deficient in vitamin D. These vitamin D deficient patients would be at higher risk of a variety of obstetric complications such as fetal growth restriction, pre-eclampsia and gestational diabetes. In the UK, the associations between vitamin D deficiency and poor obstetric outcome have been recognised. The National Institute for Health and Care Excellence (NICE) has provided guidance to prescribe vitamin D supplementation to all pregnant and breastfeeding women due to the presumed benefit of treating vitamin D deficiency in this 'at risk' group [5].

For the purpose of this debate, the more pertinent question that should be asked is, 'Are there any good reasons why we should NOT treat vitamin D deficiency in the pre-conceptional period?' There are no logical reasons to not screen and treat for vitamin D deficiency. Vitamin D deficiency is well-defined and can be easily identified. The blood test is simple, widely available and cheap, costing roughly £10 per serum assay. Once vitamin D deficiency is diagnosed, there is already clear guidance as to how it should be treated [2]. Importantly, the treatment is simple, safe and cost-effective.

Perhaps, the most important reason to screen for and treat vitamin D deficiency is to optimise reproductive treatment outcomes. The physical, emotional and financial burdens of women undergoing fertility treatments mean that everything should be done to improve the chances of pregnancy. In reproductive medicine, our aim should be to go further than just achieving pregnancy for our patients. Instead, we should provide the best possible start to any pregnancy. The identification and treatment of vitamin D deficiency achieves this. Maternal health can be optimised so that the risks of adverse obstetric outcomes complications may be reduced to achieve the best pregnancy outcomes along with the best start to motherhood.

References

1. Lerchbaum E, Obermayer-Pioetsch B. Mechanisms in endocrinology: Vitamin D and fertility: a systematic review. *Eur J Endocrinol*. 2012;166(5):765–78.

2. Holick M, Binkley NC, Bischoff-Ferrari HA, et al. Full guideline: evaluation, treatment, and prevention of vitamin D deficiency: an Endocrine Society clinical practice guideline. *J Clin Endocrinol Metab*. 2011;96(7):1911–30.

3. Chu J, Gallos I, Tobias A, Tan B, Eapen A, Coomarasamy A. Vitamin D and assisted reproductive treatment outcome: a systematic review and meta-analysis, *Hum Reprod*. 2018;33(1):65–80.

4. Chu J, Gallos I, Tobias A, et al. Vitamin D and assisted reproductive treatment outcome: a prospective cohort study. *Reprod Health*. 2019;16(1):106.

5. NICE. Vitamin D: supplement use in specific population groups. *NICE Public Health Guideline*. 2014; www.nice.org.uk/guidance/ph56.

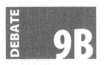

9B
There Is a Role for Pre-conception Treatment with Vitamin D

Against

Amit Shah

Recently, we have been hearing a lot about the potential role of vitamin D supplementation in the pre-conception period. Vitamin D is thought to play a possible role in improving implantation. This is because vitamin D deficiency in animal studies has been shown to reduce fertility capacity. Human data has also pointed towards the positive role that vitamin D may play in improving placental function and thus lowering the risk of pre-eclampsia, gestational diabetes and growth restriction in the fetus [1]. Data has been published supporting vitamin D supplementation in PCOS, IVF and even reducing the risk of caesarean section deliveries [2]. This has then led some to postulate a link with problems in embryo implantation leading to poor placentation and its consequences [3].

Vitamin D deficiency seems quite common in women of reproductive age. This clearly has prompted research to explore vitamin D supplementation and its role. Since, assessing and treating vitamin D deficiency is relatively easy and low cost, clinicians have adopted this strategy based on evidence that is not robust.

Pre-conception vitamin D supplementation in assisted conception treatment has been assessed in a prospective cohort study which showed that once important prognostic factors were adjusted for, the statistical significance of any benefits for vitamin D use was lost [4].

The role that vitamin D may play in improving egg and sperm quality, endometrial receptivity and embryo implantation remains questionable. Studies supporting vitamin D supplementation in preconception care for both IVF and PCOS are usually retrospective, lack solid study designs and are often based on single centre observational data.

Similarly, studies have not supported the beneficial effects of vitamin D in the prevention of pre-eclampsia, gestational diabetes and low birth weight. Often, the associations between its usage and positive outcomes are by chance and not statistically significant. There are no randomised controlled trials available showing that vitamin D supplementation alters these pregnancy specific pathologies.

Even though we have established that maternal vitamin D is important in fetal bone development and also potentially associated with healthy fetal lung function and neonatal immune conditions, such as asthma, it is not clear if pre-conception supplementation of vitamin D would prevent these sequelae. Beneficial effects of vitamin D on neonatal lung development, childhood immune disorders and skeletal development and growth remains to be proved in randomised control trials [5].

Even though vitamin D supplementation appears safe and cheap, and seems to be routinely recommended in clinical practice, there is not enough evidence to support its routine usage. As clinicians and scientists, we should follow good evidence-based practice and unfortunately there just is not enough data supporting vitamin D use at the moment.

Further research is warranted focusing on potential benefits proven by adequately powered randomised controlled studies. Until then, I do not advocate routine vitamin D pre-conceptionally in my clinical practice, and I suggest you do the same and not offer false hope to intending parents.

References

1. Bodnar LM, Catov JM, Simhan HN, et al. Maternal vitamin D deficiency increases the risk of pre-eclampsia. *J Clin Endocrinol Metab*. 2007;92:3517–22.

2. Kosta K, Yavropoulou MP, Anastasiou O, Yovos JG. Role of vitamin D treatment in glucose metabolism in polycystic ovary syndrome. *Fertil Steril*. 2009;92:1053–8.

3. Robinson CJ, Wagner CL, Hollis BW, et al. Maternal vitamin D and fetal growth in early-onset severe pre-eclampsia. *Am J Obstet Gynecol*. 2011;204:566.

4. Chu J, Gallo I, Tobias A, et al. Vitamin D and assisted reproductive treatment outcome: a prospective cohort study. *Reprod Health*. 2019;16:106.

5. RCOG. *Vitamin D in pregnancy*. Scientific Impact Paper No 43. June 2014. RCOG.

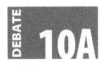

Natural Killer Cell Assay in the Blood Is a Useless Investigation

For

Ingrid Granne

Undertake a web search for 'natural killer (NK) cell testing' or 'reproductive immunology' and the unwary fertility patient or woman with a history of recurrent pregnancy loss will find dozens of clinics offering a bewildering variety of different tests measuring blood NK cells and their 'killing' potential, or measuring 'baby friendly' blood cytokines (presumably in contrast to 'baby unfriendly' cytokines). Depending on the clinic, 'abnormal' percentages or numbers of NK cells, elevated NK cell cytotoxicity, or apparent evidence of NK cell activation, lead to the offer of costly treatment options to 'dampen down' or suppress NK cells. Treatments offered include steroids, intravenous immunoglobulins, intralipids and even biologic agents such as anti-TNFα; all medications with significant side effect profiles.

Blood natural killer cells are part of the innate immune system, where they serve as a first line of host defence to both tumours and virally infected cells; killing by both direct cytotoxicity and by the release of cytokines. NK cells were named because of their ability to kill some leukaemia cell lines. It is perhaps unfortunate that they were ever given this name; one wonders had a different nomenclature been used, the attractive (but incorrect) theory that NK cells were capable of killing trophoblast cells would never been posed.

That blood NK cells were ever thought to influence reproductive outcomes is almost certainly a result of the emerging evidence regarding the important role of uterine NK (uNK) cells in pregnancy. uNK cells were first identified in the human endometrium more than 30 years ago, as cells that expressed CD45 and CD56 but not CD3; thus, demonstrating that these cells were from an NK cell lineage. In the late-secretory phase of the menstrual cycle uNK cells are the dominant immune cell, accounting for more than 30% of the cells in the endometrial stroma. In the early pregnancy decidua, NK cells continue to predominate, particularly around the site of placentation. Considerable progress has been made in understanding the function of these cells in the decidua, where they have a direct influence on the development of a healthy placenta. In pregnancy, NK cells produce growth factors, angiogenic factors and cytokines that promote trophoblast invasion and aid the remodelling of the decidua and the spiral arteries [1].

Uterine NK cells have receptors called killer immunoglobulin-like receptors (KIRs) that interact with HLA-C molecules on fetal extravillous trophoblast cells. Both HLA-C and KIR genes are highly polymorphic; resulting in different combinations of HLA-C/KIR receptors in different pregnancies. Of note, particular heritable HLA-C/KIR combinations that result in strong inhibitory signals are associated with recurrent pregnancy loss. In direct contradiction to the theory that NK cells require suppression for successful pregnancy, NK activation may in fact be required [2].

To understand why blood NK measurements are no surrogate for uterine NK cells, one simply has to note their differing phenotype and function. There are two major types of blood NK cells. The majority (more than 90%) are CD56^{dim} (expressing low levels of this marker) and are CD16 positive, and the rest are CD56^{bright} (expressing high levels of CD56) but are CD16 negative. In contrast, uNK cells are CD56^{superbright} and do not express CD16.

Recent single cell RNA sequencing of first trimester decidua has in fact confirmed the presence of three NK populations, all distinct from blood NK cells [3].

Despite the lack of data implicating blood NK cells in the pathogenesis of recurrent implantation failure or recurrent pregnancy loss, many research groups have looked at the association of blood NK phenotype or function with these conditions, with contradictory findings. Although a meta-analysis has demonstrated that women with subfertility or recurrent pregnancy loss have higher numbers of blood NK cells compared to controls [3], meta-analyses have not shown that blood NK cells reflect subsequent pregnancy outcome after either miscarriage [4] or IVF [3]. This is surely the relevant outcome for patients. Despite this uncertain data and the lack of biological plausibility, many clinics still advise patients to have these tests and go on to offer immunotherapy that is not backed by high quality clinical trial data.

In summary, there is no evidence that altered blood NK parameters lead to implantation or pregnancy failure; but women and couples desperate for pregnancy success will understandably often try any option offered to them, when that they are advised by a clinician they trust that it may give them a better chance of a baby. The reality is that blood NK testing is in fact worse than a useless investigation; it is an investigation that offers patients false hope based on poor science.

References

1. Ander SE, Diamond MS, Coyne CB. Immune responses at the maternal-fetal interface. *Sci Immunol*. 2019 Jan 11;4(31): eaat6114.

2. Colucci F. The role of KIR and HLA interactions in pregnancy complications. *Immunogenetics*. 2017 Aug;69 (8–9):557–65.

3. Vento-Tormo R, Efremova M, Botting RA, et al. Single-cell reconstruction of the early maternal-fetal interface in humans. *Nature*. 2018;563(7731):347–53.

4. Seshadri S, Sunkara SK. Natural killer cells in female infertility and recurrent miscarriage: a systematic review and meta-analysis. *Hum Reprod Update*. 2014 May–June;20(3):429–38.

5. Tang AW, Alfirevic Z, Quenby S. Natural killer cells and pregnancy outcomes in women with recurrent miscarriage and infertility: a systematic review. *Hum Reprod*. 2011;26(8):1971–80.

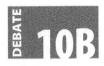

Natural Killer Cell Assay in the Blood Is a Useless Investigation

Against

Kevin Marron

Laboratory testing is one of the cornerstones of modern medical science. Any diagnostic test used inappropriately may have little or no merit. The right test, at the right time, for the right patient, can legitimately add value to the understanding and management of the disease process involved/suspected. The treatment of infertility is peppered with numerous 'add-ons' of varying quality, which have often become part of the landscape, but sometimes without detailed evaluation. One of these, the natural killer (NK) cell assay is poorly understood and perhaps misnamed as it is in fact a reproductive immunophenotype, where many cells are evaluated. The hypothesis that NK cells may be involved in fetal demise stems from their ability to directly lyse target cells in a non-MHC dependent way, and conflation of the nomenclature to include peripheral blood (pNK) and tissue resident uterine forms (uNK) as similar. The immune system and its modulation has, since the time of Peter Medawar been considered integral to successful pregnancy, balancing regulation of inflammation and establishment of maternal immunotolerance. In this context, it's no surprise that deviations from a normal immunophenotype could be involved in abnormal pregnancy development, or 'unexplained' ART failures. Recent advances have led to the possibility of examining immune cell heterogeneity in greater detail; cell populations, transcription factors, activating/inhibitory receptors, cytokines and chemokine expression patterns, all utilise sophisticated crosstalk mechanisms to initiate tissue remodelling and angiogenesis. Cell number/ratio and function of these can now be reasonably evaluated in the laboratory. Importantly, genetic and environmental determinants shape the diversity and function of the NK receptors in particular. Apart from confusing pNK and uNK subtypes, much of the controversy surrounding NK analysis may be traced back to poor study design, excessive bias, and overzealous interpretation of results. Additionally, in many published studies, the patient groups tend to be heterogeneous, often combining diverse groups such as recurrent miscarriage and repeated implantation failure, neither of which have yet achieved definition consensus. In the absence of numerous large prospective randomised trials, few, if any, laboratory tests will meet 'grade A' evidence criteria, and so will not gain mainstream support for their use [1]. There is unfortunately a paucity of such well-designed trials in the world of assisted reproduction.

Identification of the type and relative concentrations of functionally significant white blood cell populations in peripheral blood, however, has actually been shown to be valuable in several studies determining risk factors for pregnancy loss [2]. Placental evaluation post miscarriage, often presents with inflammatory cell infiltration and thromboembolism. Lymphocytes uniquely acquire a more tolerant phenotype during pregnancy [3], while uNKs, in fact facilitate implantation and spiral artery formation, all the while maintaining their innate ability to directly lyse target cells. The evidence for immune dysfunction on some level, in certain patient populations mounts, so full immunological assessment can be a meritorious option. Elevated proportions, and also activation, of NK cells, contributes to spontaneous abortion and recurrent pregnancy loss [4]. It should be stated, however, that meta-analysis of trials do not show statistical significance, but again we must be cautious as this is probably due to the heterogeneity of the patient populations described above as well as the technical methods employed [2]. Focusing on the NK cell alone, however, is like believing the whole iceberg is floating on top of the ocean. Further value appears when peripheral blood examination is not just limited to NKs, but a wider profile of leucocytes. An elevated ratio of CD4+/CD8+ cells is seen in a number of autoimmune disorders including reproductive autoimmune failure syndrome. The mechanism of action is unclear, but it has been hypothesised that during pregnancy the expansion of more anti-inflammatory immune cell subsets predominates over those with a more pro-inflammatory phenotype [4]. Increased pro-inflammatory cytokines, the origin of which is considered most likely to be CD4+ lymphocytes, could potentially play a major role here by direct or indirect mechanisms. Women with recurrent pregnancy loss/recurrent implantation failure (RPL/RIF) demonstrate increased peripheral blood Th1 cells relative to normal fertile women [5] while Th2 cytokines, are known to be essential to prevent rejection of the embryo. It is crucial that the correct balance between these subsets is maintained in order to fight off possible infections whilst also allowing tolerance towards the developing fetus. There are several more players in this game, populations that are said to contribute to a normal pregnancy and when dysregulated contribute to infertility and recurrent miscarriage; NK-T cells and regulatory T-cells (Tregs) are more akin to conductors than foot soldiers, being intricately involved in immunosuppression and induction of tolerance towards the fetal allograft, but perhaps also influenced by NKs. B-lymphocyte numbers and function also exhibit increasing evidence of a profound influence on reproductive outcome, particularly around implantation.

Given the number and possible relevance of these immune cell subsets in particular patients, it has become necessary in recent years to identify and characterise these cells in the peripheral blood and/or endometrium of patients with subfertility in order to establish the normal ranges, to determine when an imbalance exists, and identify patients that could benefit from pharmaceutical intervention [4]. It is argued that endometrial assessment is superior to that of peripheral blood; however blood evaluation has advantages of being non-invasive, not subject to timing pressures, can be assessed during pregnancy, and allows addition of in vitro cytotoxicity/inhibition analysis where appropriate.

To conclude, the finely balanced immunological mechanisms described above must, if logic prevails, be capable of being involved, at some level, in obstetric complications. Cellular conflict is being recognised as important for optimal survival, fitter cells win out over less fit neighbours. Perhaps the embryo is embroiled in this conflict from day one? Given their highly involved interactions, these cells are erroneously looked at, if looked at in isolation. Like any tool this type of test is indeed potentially useless if used in the wrong context. Physicians must, by a process of elimination, systematically remove all the most likely probable causes of pregnancy failure and, rather like Sherlock Holmes found, what is left is likely to be the truth, however fantastical.

References

1. ESHRE Guideline Group on RPL. ESHRE guideline: recurrent pregnancy loss. *Human Reproduction Open*, 2018;2018(2). doi: 10.1093/hropen/hoy004.

2. Seshadri S, Sunkara SK. Natural killer cells in female infertility and recurrent miscarriage: a systematic review and meta-analysis. *Hum Reprod Update*. 2014;20 (3):429–38.

3. Feyaerts D, Benner M, van Craenbroek B, et al. Human uterine lymphocytes acquire a more experienced and tolerogenic phenotype during pregnancy. *Sci Rep.* 2017;7(1):2884.

4. Marron K, Walsh D, Harrity C. Detailed endometrial immune assessment of both normal and adverse reproductive outcome populations. *J Assist Reprod Genet.* 2019;36(2):199–210.

5. Kwak-Kim JYH, Chung-Bang HS, Ng SC, et al. Increased T helper 1 cytokine responses by circulating T cells are present in women with recurrent pregnancy losses and in infertile women with multiple implantation failures after IVF. *Hum Reprod.* 2003;18(4):767–73.

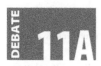

Intralipid Therapy Has a Place in Infertility Treatment

For

Hassan Shehata

Successful implantation depends on balanced a immunological network. This fact is widely recognised, but the exact mechanism and the interaction between maternal and fetal components of this complex system is not entirely understood and ongoing research brings constant development in this area. A number of immune components have been implicated in outcomes of early pregnancy, including lymphocytes, Th 1 and 2, regulatory T-cells (Tregs), natural killer (NK) cells and autoantibodies. Balance between pro- and anti-inflammatory cytokines is required for embryo implantation and early placental development. In normal pregnancy, the survival of the fetus is dependent on the initiation of maternal immune tolerance, with regulatory T-cells and Th 2 anti-inflammatory profile. Any imbalance to this system may lead to recurrent miscarriage and implantation failure.

Th1 and Th2 lymphocytes are lymphocyte T subpopulations with distinctive cytokine profiles. Th1 lymphocytes mediate the pro-inflammatory response and secrete Th1 cytokines which increase significantly fetal loss in animal studies. Several studies showed that increased Th1 cytokine blood levels result in an increased TNF a/IL-10 ratio in recurrent miscarriage and implantation failures.

Regulatory T-cells (Tregs) are potent suppressive cells of Th1- and Th17-mediated immunity. In normal pregnancy, there is an expansion of Tregs within 2 days of conception. Several studies reported a decrease of Tregs in the peripheral blood and the decidua of patients with recurrent miscarriage.

Increased numbers and cytotoxic activity of NK cells have been reported in women with reproductive failures [1] and recurrent miscarriage. Natural killer cells have also been shown to express nuclear receptors known as peroxisome proliferator-activated receptors (PPARs). Activation of these receptors by their fatty acid ligands have been shown to regulate inflammation. Deleting the PPAR gene in mice has been shown to be associated with reduced implantation and decreased litter size.

A number of studies reported that Intralipid infusion may modulate immune function with suppression of NK cytotoxicity and pro-inflammatory cytokine generation. It is hypothesised that administration of Intralipid infusion may engage PPAR receptors in NK cells and decrease their cytotoxic response enhancing implantation and maintenance of pregnancy.

Intralipid® is a fat emulsion containing 20% soybean oil, 1.2% egg yolk phospholipids, 2.25% glycerin, and water. It has been traditionally used as a parenteral source of calories and essential fatty acids. Intralipid fat infusion is also considered as a standard component of total parenteral nutrition in trauma and severely burned patients. Parenteral fat emulsions are known to accumulate in macrophages impairing some of their various functions and those of the reticuloendothelial system. It has been reported that intravenous fat emulsion infusions during the early post-injury period increased susceptibility to infection, prolonged pulmonary failure, and delayed recovery in critically injured patients suggesting that one possible way of acting is by suppression of NK activity. It has been shown in animal studies that the administration of Intralipid 20% could suppress genetic resistance to bone marrow grafts and NK cell activity likely through the impairment of the macrophage function. Intralipids have been shown to stimulate the reticuloendothelial system and remove 'danger signals' that can lead to pregnancy loss.

Data analysing the use of Intralipid in fertility is sparse, with lack of large RCT and good quality meta-analysis; however the existent data is encouraging. Studies have demonstrated improvement in endometrial receptivity and better successful pregnancy rates. This positive effect has been demonstrated both in vitro and in vivo.

A systematic review and meta-analysis to evaluate the effects of Intralipid infusion on pregnancy outcomes in women with previous implantation failure has recently been published [2]. Four studies with 544 participants were included. Live birth rate was statistically higher among the groups of women who received intravenous Intralipid (RR 1.98, 95% CI 1.39–2.80) with significant improvement in clinical pregnancy rate (RR 1.74, 95% CI 1.27–2.40).

Fifty non-pregnant women with recurrent implantation failure with abnormal NK cell activity received one or more Intralipids 20% intravenously. Among them 78% normalised their NK cell activity above 10% after the first infusion and all after more infusions. The duration of NK cell activity suppression lasted for 6–9 weeks in 94% [3].

In another study, 275 women with recurrent implantation failure and miscarriage, Intralipid reduced NK cytotoxicity by nearly 40%, similarly to intravenous immunoglobulins, as well as in patients with normal and elevated NK killing activity [4]. Intralipid infusion markedly inhibited pro-inflammatory cytokine generation, in particular TNF-a, IL-6, IL-8 cytokines by monocytes, and endothelial adhesion and trans-endothelial migration were also significantly reduced.

A single blinded randomised placebo-controlled trial, including 105 women undergoing IVF/ICSI compared Intralipid and placebos. The study demonstrated higher biochemical pregnancy and clinical pregnancy, implantation and baby birth rates in the Intralipid arm [5].

In another study by Mekinian et al. [6] published in 2016, 200 women with recurrent miscarriages (n = 38) and implantation failure (n = 162) and elevated NK cell activity which were treated with intra-lipids, the pregnancy rate was 52%, with pregnancy ongoing/live birth rate of 91%. In 2011, Ndukwe et al. showed evidence of improved outcome following Intralipid infusion in women with recurrent embryo implantation failure after in vitro fertilisation [7].

There are no data to assess the safety of Intralipid during pregnancy, however, although our and other users' experience is reassuring, adequate measures should be taken to prevent the risks (such as infection), of intravenous infusions as usually recommended.

References

1. Thum MY, Bhaskaran S, Abdalla HI., et al. An increase in the absolute count of CD56dimCD16+CD69+ NK cells in the peripheral blood is associated with a poorer IVF treatment and pregnancy outcome. *Hum Reprod.* 2004 Oct;19(10):2395–400.

2. Zhou P, Wu H, Lin X, Wang S, Zhang S. The effect of intralipid on pregnancy outcomes in women with previous implantation failure in in vitro fertilization/intracytoplasmic sperm injection cycles: A systematic review and meta-analysis. *Eur J Obstet Gynecol Reprod Biol.* 2020 Sept;252:187–92.

3. Roussev RG, Acacio B, Ng SC, Coulam CB. Duration of intralipid's suppressive effect on NK cell's functional activity. *Am J Reprod Immunol*. 2008 Sept;60(3):258–63.

4. Roussev RG, Ng SC, Coulam CB. Natural killer cell functional activity suppression by intravenous immunoglobulin, intralipid and soluble human leukocyte antigen-G. *Am J Reprod Immunol*. 2007 April;57 (4):262–9.

5. Singh N, Davis AA, Kumar S, Kriplani A. The effect of administration of intravenous intralipid on pregnancy outcomes in women with implantation failure after IVF/ ICSI with non-donor oocytes: A randomised controlled trial. *Eur J Obstet Gynecol Reprod Biol*. 2019 Sept;240:45–51.

6. Mekinian A, Cohen J, Alijotas-Reig J, et al. Unexplained recurrent miscarriage and recurrent implantation failure: is there a place for immunomodulation? *Am J Reprod Immunol*. 2016 July;76(1):8–28.

7. Ndukwe G. Recurrent embryo implantation failure after in vitro fertilisation: improved outcome following intralipid infusion in women with elevated T helper 1 response. *Hum Fertil*. 2011;14:21–2.

Intralipid Therapy Has a Place in Infertility Treatment

Against

Ephia Yasmin

Intralipid® is a therapy that has no place in evidence-based delivery of fertility treatment. It is one of an ever-increasing list of adjuvants, or add-on therapies. The hype surrounding Intralipid preceded scientific validity. The immunological relationship between the endometrium and the embryo remains an enigma. However, our understanding of the cross-talk between the embryo and endometrium during implantation is increasing. There is an acceptance that the cross-talk involves the stromal decidual cells, trophoblast and immune tolerance. During implantation, maternal immunoactivation and tolerance are not only limited to the decidua but are also observed in the periphery, predominantly affecting the immune system. Whilst several theories exist as to how the immune response is modulated to allow the fetal allograft, none of them are sufficiently established to allow a clear explanation.

The scrutiny of the immune system led to the study of:

- natural killer (NK) cell levels and elevated NK activity in peripheral blood or in the intra-uterine environment;
- dysregulated cytokines;
- presence of antiphospholipid antibodies or other autoantibodies;
- imbalance of T helper (Th) 1 and Th2 cell reaction and elevated Th1/Th2 cell ratio;
- the sharing of human leukocyte antigen alleles between the male and female partners.

In practice when immunological studies are carried out to investigate implantation failure, there is no consensus or standardisation among them. Investigations range from the study of NK cells in venous blood to uterine NK cells to addition of a range of antibody tests. Comparisons are also difficult in studies investigating immunity, where a similar lack of standardisation exists. For the purpose of the debate, we can limit ourselves to NK cells or Th1 and Th2 ratios but even here, the published studies (mostly retrospective data) and clinical practice do not display any consensus of what the measures should be – peripheral, uterine or a combination of both.

Kuroda, along with Quenby's group, detected that elevated levels of uterine NK cells (uNK) in the stroma underlying the surface epithelium are associated with inadequate cortisol biosynthesis by resident decidualising cells in their mid-luteal endometrial biopsies [1]. This suggests that elevated NK cells reduce immune tolerance. As NK cell testing became more popular, the hunt for immunotherapy began to target NK cells. The use of steroids, intravenous immunoglobulins and Intralipid crept in. The reports of apparent success with Intralipid in small cohorts, widely publicised in the media, made it an attractive proposition for patients and clinicians.

Intralipid® is a sterile, non-pyrogenic fat emulsion prepared for intravenous administration as a source of calories and essential fatty acids. It is made up of 10% soybean oil, 1.2% egg yolk phospholipids, 2.25% glycerin, and water for injection. Intralipid is used as parenteral nutrition to replenish calories and essential fatty acids. The product contains aluminium with potential for toxicity and product information states that studies with Intralipid have not been performed to evaluate carcinogenic potential, mutagenic potential, or effects on fertility. Intralipid should not be used in the background of abnormalities of fat metabolism, liver and renal problems and coagulation disorders. Fat embolism is a risk. Therefore, the essential question that should be asked is whether benefits outweigh the risks. However, the use of Intralipid is often justified by the perception that it is just a nutritional product with no significant risk.

Whilst the exact immunomodulatory action of Intralipid is unknown, it has been demonstrated to be effective in decreasing NK cell activation and production of proinflammatory cytokines (Granato et al. 2012) [2]. The proponents of Intralipid therapy claim it has a place in the management of recurrent implantation failure (RIF) and recurrent pregnancy loss (RPL) with a background of elevated NK cells and absence of other identified causes. This indication has a problem, as there is no unanimous definition of RIF. However, absence of implantation after two cycles of embryo transfer with no less than four for cleavage-stage embryos and no less than two for blastocysts is generally accepted in clinical practice to define RIF.

Understanding of implantation failure is the holy grail of assisted reproduction and therefore it was not surprising to see the excitement that greeted the presentation of the non-randomised studies demonstrating significant increase in pregnancy rates after Intralipid therapy in RIF. Whilst there is no consensus that elevated NK cells are responsible for absence of implantation, to target therapies to reduce NK cells is fraught with problems.

Achilli and colleagues carried out a systematic review and meta-analysis, examining the efficacy of immunotherapies [3]. This included Intralipid in IVF and recurrent pregnancy loss. Only randomised controlled trials (RCTs) were included. Their analysis identified only one RCT (published as a conference abstract) evaluating the efficacy of Intralipid in ICSI. The overall outcome of the meta-analysis did not reveal benefit of different immune modulating therapies in RIF. Two RCTs are currently registered with no published outcomes. The paucity of RCTs to evaluate what is considered a cheap and low risk intervention is worth questioning.

An RCT [4] was carried out to investigate the efficacy of Intralipid in recurrent miscarriage with elevated NK cells. This study, performed on 296 women with history of recurrent miscarriage, had a positive hCG as its primary outcome. It showed no difference between the therapy and control group. Live birthrate was their secondary outcome measure and did demonstrate a difference.

Multiple non-randomised, retrospective, cohort studies are available, some demonstrating positive outcomes. However, these studies are heterogeneous with varied study cohorts, different regimens of intravenous Intralipid infusions, different outcome measures and small groups. It is also noteworthy that these studies, including those showing benefit, come with the caveat that well-powered RCTs are necessary before Intralipid can be recommended for use.

Martini et al. 2018 [5] are one such group performing retrospective review of their cohort and conclude that there is no benefit of Intralipid in improving live birth outcome.

The content of this debate highlights that poorly understood conditions like recurrent implantation failure and recurrent miscarriage are often investigated in a differential manner, which makes reading of studies difficult. The popularity of Intralipid is not difficult to fathom. As clinicians we are propelled by our desire to treat and fix problems. However we also have a duty to uphold science. The rationale (or lack of) for using unproven therapies to treat conditions with no agreed definition or standardised investigation seems to defy the very ethos of evidence-based management.

References

1. Kuroda K, Venkatakrishnan R, James S, et al. Elevated peri-implantation uterine natural killer cell density in human endometrium is associated with impaired corticosteroid signalling in decidualizing stromal cells. *J Clin Endocrinol Metab.* 2013;98(11):4429–37.

2. Granato D, Blum S, Rössle C, et al. Effects of parenteral lipid emulsions with different fatty acid composition on immune cell functions *in vitro. JPEN J Parenter Enteral Nutr.* 2000;24:113–8.

3. Achilli C, Duran-Retamal M, Saab W, Serhal P, Seshadri S. The role of immunotherapy in in vitro fertilization and recurrent pregnancy loss: a systematic review and meta-analysis. *Fertil Steril.* 2018;110(6):1089–1100.

4. Dakhly DM, Bayoumi YA, Sharkawy M, et al Intralipid supplementation in women with recurrent spontaneous abortion and elevated levels of natural killer cells. *Int J Gynaecol Obstet.* 2016 Dec; 135(3):324–7.

5. Martini AE, Jasulaitis S, Fogg LF, Uhler ML, Hirshfeld-Cytron JE. Evaluating the utility of Intralipid infusion to improve live birth rates in patients with recurrent pregnancy loss or recurrent implantation failure. *J Hum Reprod Sci.* 2018;11 (3):261–8.

The Endometrial Scratch Has Had Its Day

For

Sarah Lensen

Many couples seek IVF to help them conceive, only to be faced with the reality of probable failure: only 30–40% of IVF cycles result in a live birth. This modest success rate has driven the innovation of numerous IVF add-ons: drugs, procedures, or techniques which can be added to standard IVF methods, and which claim to boost the chance of a successful outcome. These add-ons are rarely subject to robust assessment in randomised controlled trials (RCTs) and have not been confirmed as effective or safe. Yet, these extras can cost patients hundreds, even thousands, of dollars. Endometrial scratching, also known as endometrial injury or trauma, is one such add-on. The procedure is essentially a routine endometrial biopsy, usually performed by a pipelle catheter as an out-patient appointment. The mechanical action of obtaining the biopsy has been suggested to elicit a favourable inflammatory and immune response within the endometrium, thereby increasing the probability of embryo implantation and pregnancy.

The History of Endometrial Scratching

In 2000, an observational study reported an unusually high number of pregnancies among women undergoing multiple endometrial biopsies prior to their IVF cycle. Surprised by their observation, the same research group then undertook a study in 134 women, reporting a twofold increase in the pregnancy rate among women undergoing endometrial biopsy compared with control women [1]. Although this was not an RCT, the study sparked interest among IVF clinicians worldwide, understandably keen to apply new interventions in their practice in the hopes of helping their patients to conceive. A Cochrane review including 14 trials reported moderate-quality evidence of possible benefit from endometrial scratching [2]. However, subgroup analysis suggested this benefit may be restricted to women with recurrent implantation failure, and the authors concluded that further evidence from well-designed trials was needed. Today, over 30 randomised controlled trials have been conducted. Despite the wealth of available data from RCTs, it is difficult to interpret. Reported effects range from implausible benefit to significant harm. This substantial heterogeneity does not appear to be explained by differences between trial populations or variations in intervention, such as the timing or severity of the scratching. Instead, it is suggested to arise from the poor-quality of the contributing trials, and consequent bias in the observed results.

Quality of the Evidence

Although it is well-established that RCTs present the gold standard in evaluating healthcare interventions, not all RCTs are created equal. Indeed, most trials evaluating endometrial scratching display red flags or outright methodologic flaws [3]. Many of the trial reports failed to describe the randomisation process, and may not in fact have been truly randomised. Most of the trials lack adequate trial registration, and many were not registered at all, introducing potential for post-hoc protocol changes and selective outcome reporting, that we remain unable to detect. A number stopped recruitment early after observing a positive effect, which is known to be associated with exaggerated and biased effect estimates. Other methodological issues include planned post-randomisation exclusions and improbable pregnancy rates and effect estimates. For example, one trial reports an impressive live birth rate of 67% after endometrial scratching (compared to 28% in the control arm) yielding an implausible odds ratio of 4.61 in favour of endometrial scratching (95% confidence interval 3.05–6.96) [4]. Such large odds ratios are rare in healthcare and unlikely to represent true treatment effects. Additionally, most trials are available only as conference abstracts, with minimal methodological detail or results, and lack of sufficient peer review. Further, most trials recruited too few women to have enough statistical power to detect clinically relevant effect sizes. Two-thirds of trials reporting live birth recruited 200 women or fewer. A trial of 200 women would only be powered to detect an impressive and unrealistic improvement of 20 percentage points, e.g. from 25% to 45% (at 80% power and 5% significance level). Indeed, an analysis of methodological flaws in this cohort of trials has suggested that much of the data is not consistent with arising from RCTs, and may have resulted from poor study conduct, errors in data management or analysis, or possibly scientific misconduct.

The procedure is also painful, with patients reporting pain scores between 3–7 out of 10. It often causes bleeding and carries a risk of infection. Endometrial scratching often entails the inconvenience of attending for an additional clinic visit, and patients can be charged up to £400 (more than US$500) for an endometrial scratch. Despite a lack of high-quality evidence, endometrial scratching quickly became one of the most commonly used IVF add-ons. In the UK in 2018, it was offered by over 80% of fertility clinicians and used in 27% of all IVF cycles.

In 2019 the results of a large randomised trial were published, which demonstrating no benefit from endometrial scratching; 26.1% of women in both arms achieved a live birth (adjusted odds ratio [OR] 1.00, 95% confidence interval [CI] 0.78–1.27) [5]. This was a large international trial with robust randomisation procedures, pragmatic methodology, and minimal attrition. Pre-specified subgroup analysis did not reveal any population of women who may benefit. In women with at least two previous implantations, the probability of live birth was *lower* among women in the endometrial scratch arm (adjusted OR 0.68, 95% CI 0.39–1.17). This confidence interval leaves very little room for potential benefit in this subgroup. Subgroup analysis also found no trend for any benefit depending on characteristics such as cause of subfertility, timing of scratch, or pain experienced during the procedure.

The End of Endometrial Scratching

We now have high-quality evidence demonstrating no benefit from this painful add-on. Yet, some continue to support the use of this procedure, arguing that endometrial scratching may still benefit specific subsets of women. For this to be true, this argument would most likely require a qualitative interaction – that endometrial scratching somehow helps some women and harms others; an uncommon medical phenomenon. Further, it remains to be hypothesised, let alone established, which defined subsets of patients might benefit. Therefore, such an argument cannot be used to rationalise the ongoing application of this procedure based only on the hope that it might help some subset of women among our clinic cohorts. Indeed, to continue to offer, market and charge for an unnecessary procedure, proven to offer no benefit and confirmed to cause pain, cannot be considered ethical or in the interests of our patients.

Conclusion

Against the background of heterogeneity and poor-quality trials, the available evidence now suggests that an initially promising procedure probably offers no benefit for patients. While it's possible that specific subgroups of patients may benefit, we should wait for evidence of this from robust RCTs, before using this procedure in practice.

Conflict of Interest

I am the lead author of the cited RCT, and a co-author on the cited Cochrane review.

References

1. Barash A, Dekel N, Fieldust S, Segal I, Schechtman E, Granot I. Local injury to the endometrium doubles the incidence of successful pregnancies in patients undergoing in vitro fertilization. *Fertil Steril.* 2003;79(6):1317–22.

2. Nastri CO, Lensen SF, Gibreel A, et al. Endometrial injury in women undergoing assisted reproductive techniques. Cochrane Database of Systematic Reviews 2015, Issue 3.

3. Li W, Suke S, Wertaschnigg D, et al. Randomised controlled trials evaluating endometrial scratching: assessment of methodological issues. *Hum Reprod.* 2019;34(12):2372–80.

4. Mahran A, Ibrahim M, Bahaa H. The effect of endometrial injury on first cycle IVF/ICSI outcome: a randomized controlled trial. *Int J Reprod Biomed.* 2016;14 (3):193–8.

5. Lensen S, Osavlyuk D, Armstrong S, et al. A randomized trial of endometrial scratching before in vitro fertilization. *N Engl J Med.* 2019;24;380(4):325–34.

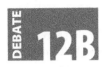

The Endometrial Scratch Has Had Its Day

Against

Nick Macklon

Taking this side of what would appear to be an open and shut case against the further use of the endometrial scratch as a therapeutic intervention would appear to be a lost cause. My opponent in this debate carefully reviews the recent literature relating to randomised trials of the endometrial scratch as a means of improving the chance of successful embryo implantation and ongoing pregnancy after fertility treatments. Normally, arguing the opposite conclusion from the same dataset would rely on challenging the minutiae of interpretation of the presented data or criticising the quality of the data being used to shore up the position much as my opponent has done in her justified criticism of the early studies.

I don't intend to do either. Indeed, like Dr Lensen I believe that the published data which now includes large randomised controlled trials has shown convincingly that the routine use of endometrial scratching should no longer be part of clinical practice. But does this mean it should be completely eliminated as a candidate intervention? Has it indeed had its day? Not yet.

We both agree that, as is often the case with medical 'breakthroughs', the endometrial scratch initially offered considerable promise. The serendipitous observation made by workers investigating tight junctions in endometrial tissue, that women who had undergone biopsy reported high success rates in the immediately following IVF cycle was initially reported with excitement [1]. Planting such a seed of hope into the fertile soil provided by patients and clinicians seeking new treatments to aid implantation resulted in a rapid growth of interest. Initial small and uncontrolled studies appeared to support the counter-intuitive proposition that harming the endometrium might improve its function, and very quickly the endometrial scratch took a firm root in clinical practice.

However, to justify a form of intentional injury as a therapy required some notion of how it might work. A number of plausible theories ranging from altering the immune response to the implanting embryo by means of an injury healing response to improving the quality of decidualisation by stimulating NK cell activity and hence reducing decidual cell senescence [2] can be proposed, but essentially, the scratch remains an intervention devoid of a clear rationale.

The rapid adoption of an intervention without a clear underlying biological mechanism of action bears the hallmarks of a 'bubble', akin to those that have gripped us in the past and which we came to rue. And under the scrutiny of a series of well-powered randomised controlled trials, it might seem that the bubble has now burst.

However, our tendency to over-invest our hopes in a seemingly exciting innovation is only matched by a keenness to rapidly and wholly disinvest if initial, unrealistic hopes and claims are not satisfied.

The case for not dropping the scratch as quickly as we picked it up rests on the simple observation that we have not yet properly researched its value. Most, if not all the studies reporting its lack of efficacy have been based on two false premises. The first is that embryos implant for a single consistent reason that could be ameliorated by a single intervention. The second is that all endometria respond to specific interventions in the same way.

As recently argued in two debate articles [3, 4], testing the effectiveness of a single intervention to treat a condition that has many (as yet poorly defined) causes, is a recipe for negative trial results. It also challenges one of the basic tenants of medicine, that treatment should where possible be directed at the cause rather than the symptom. Implantation failure is simply the manifestation of a complex and variable range of causative factors, not a diagnosis. As such it can be considered as similar to any other symptom with different aetiologies. We do not treat abdominal pain empirically and would not entertain an RCT of an intervention to treat it without diagnosing the cause first. Moreover, the notion that interventions that help some will not harm in others is counter to medical orthodoxy as illustrated by the need for judicious use of therapeutics such as glucocorticoids.

These arguments may be borne in mind when considering the conclusions from subgroup analysis of the large international trial referred to on the other side of this debate [5]. The authors report that no pre-specified subgroup analysis revealed any population of women who may benefit. For illustration, a subgroup of women with at least two previous implantation failures is described. While this defines a cohort with more severe symptoms, it does not describe it in terms of a single likely aetiology, so again, we should not be surprised that no effect is seen.

The concept of diagnosing the endometrium is only now emerging as we begin to understand its many and complex roles in implantation. Unfortunately, clinically useful tests of many of these various functions still elude us. If we are to make real progress in understanding implantation and designing interventions that can treat the causes of failure, we first need to identify the individual causes, and then test interventions designed to treat them. This may require similar resources to those required to perform the large empirical trials that currently seek to shape clinical practice, but it can be argued that such an investment may represent a more productive way forward.

Finally, it should be recognised that requests from medical care do not come from a symptom or pathology but from an individual who brings their values, needs and expectations into the consultation room [6]. The need to interpret the clinical evidence base in the sometimes complex individual context of the patient risks making pronouncements on the value of a specific treatment purely on the basis of RCTs in poorly representative populations simplistic and possibly harmful. The evidence base is there to serve the doctor and patient and not the reverse.

To summarise, at present it is indeed reasonable to conclude that there is no good evidence to support the use of the endometrial scratch in unselected populations. However, the current evidence base remains too crude to completely write-off a treatment from clinical practice. Moreover, simply calling for larger RCTs without any understanding or targeting of a specific aetiology risks wasting significant research resources.

Declaring that the endometrial scratch has 'had its day' is therefore premature and represents an over-interpretation of the available evidence. The empirical use of the scratch should be discouraged. But more evidence is required before we can state that it has no value.

Disclosures

During the last 4 years NS Macklon has received salary/fees or grant support from the following organisations: Abbott, Anecova, ArtPRED, Clearblue, IBSA, Merck Serono, Ferring, Gedeon Richter, London Women's Clinic, Vivoplex, University of Copenhagen, Zealand University Hospital and Zealand Health Region, Denmark.

References

1. Barash A, Dekel N, Fieldust S, Segal I, Schechtman E, Granot I. Local injury to the endometrium doubles the incidence of successful pregnancies in patients undergoing in vitro fertilization. *Fertil Steril.* 2003 June;79(6):1317–22.

2. Brighton PJ, Maruyama Y, Fishwick K, et al. Clearance of senescent decidual cells by uterine natural killer cells in cycling human endometrium. *Elife.* 2017 Dec 11;6. pii: e31274.

3. Lensen S, Venetis C, Ng EHY, et al. Should we stop offering endometrial scratching prior to in vitro fertilization? *Fertil Steril.* 2019 June;111(6):1094–101.

4. Odendaal J, Quenby S, Sammaritano L, Macklon N, Branch DW, Rosenwaks Z. Immunologic and rheumatologic causes and treatment of recurrent pregnancy loss: what is the evidence? *Fertil Steril.* 2019 Dec;112(6):1002–12.

5. Lensen S, Osavlyuk D, Armstrong S, et al. A randomized trial of endometrial scratching before in vitro fertilization. *N Engl J Med.* 2019 Jan 24;380(4):325–34.

6. Macklon NS, Fauser BCJM. Context-based infertility care. *Reprod Biomed Online.* 2020;40(1):2–5.

Corticosteroid Therapy Is Useful in Assisting Implantation

For

Harish M Bhandari

Introduction

Implantation is a complex molecular interaction between a developmentally competent blastocyst and an appropriately primed endometrium. Over half of human conceptions fail to implant into the endometrium. Controlled inflammation and activation of the immune response in the peri-implantation period are vital for the maternal tolerance of an antigenically different fetus. Any perturbation to immune adaptation at implantation is likely to have negative influence on a successful reproductive outcome. Synthetic corticosteroids serve an important role in anti-inflammatory and immunosuppressive therapies. This review provides an overview of the current knowledge about the physiological steroid regulation required for implantation and an argument supporting the use of corticosteroid therapy to women with no overt maternal immunological conditions, with a view to aid establishment of pregnancy.

Role of Glucocorticoids in Ovarian Function

In the ovary, glucocorticoid activity is regulated mainly by the 11β-hydroxysteroid dehydrogenase (11βHSD) enzyme expressed in the granulosa-lutein cells. The interconversion of active cortisol and inert cortisone is mediated by the two 11βHSD isoforms (I and II). It has been shown that exposure of the follicular fluid to higher cortisol concentration is important for follicular development, oocyte maturation and successful implantation. A study [1] found significant improvement with fertilisation and implantation from the oocytes retrieved from unstimulated ovarian follicles with higher cortisol:cortisone ratio. Furthermore, it was found that a higher cortisone level in the follicular fluid was more likely to yield oocytes with reduced fertilisation and implantation potential and is due to predominance of 11β-HSD-II in immature follicles. Even in gonadotropin-stimulated IVF cycles – higher intra-follicular cortisol:cortisone ratios were found in women who conceived compared to non-conception cycles.

21 hydroxylase, the enzyme involved in the biosynthesis of cortisol, is not present within the human ovary and any glucocorticoid present in the follicular fluid must come from the systemic circulation. Hence the potentially important strategy of steroid therapy was subjected to few clinical studies, with a view to improve follicular fluid cortisol:cortisone ratio and implantation. A recent Cochrane review [2] demonstrated that glucocorticoid administration (commenced with ovarian stimulation and continued until oocyte retrieval) possibly increased clinical pregnancy rate in women having gonadotropin-stimulated IVF/ICSI cycles. There was little or no impact on live birth rate. However, the included number of studies in this review was small and the event rates were low.

Role of Glucocorticoids in Peri-implantation Endometrium

The remarkable prevalence of human embryo aneuploidy is the likely reason for reproductive disorders such as infertility, implantation failure and miscarriage. However, the emerging evidence suggests that spontaneous, functional and morphological changes occurring in the endometrium, – a process known as decidualisation – which is independent of the presence of an embryo, is a key determinant to successful implantation. Under the influence of elevated circulating progesterone, decidualising endometrial stromal cells proliferate and secrete cytokines (responsible for recruitment of immune cells) and angiogenic factors (which induce spiral artery remodelling). Any perturbations in this process may contribute more to the reproductive disorder.

Local cortisol biosynthesis plays an integral role in the preparation of the endometrium for implantation. Progesterone enhances the expression and activity of 11βHSD-I in decidualising endometrial stromal cells which has been shown to promote the formation of a corticosteroid gradient at the feto-maternal interface and its inhibition practically eliminates the induction of *HSD11B1*, the gene that encodes 11βHSD-I.

Uterine receptivity and embryo implantation are determined by immune system regulated cells to include uterine natural killer (uNK) cells, cytokines, dendritic cells, and macrophages. uNK cells are the most abundant immune cells in the decidualising endometrium. Studies have shown that an imbalance in the density and temporo-spatial distribution of uNK cells is associated with an increased risk of miscarriage/recurrent miscarriage. Relative corticosteroid deficiency is the likely mechanism as there is a strong inverse correlation between high uNK cell density and expression of 11βHSD-I in the decidualising endometrium. In addition, elevated uNk cells blunt the induction of decidual marker genes *PRL* and *IGFBP1* and cytokines IL-11 and IL-15, connecting steroid deficiency to impaired decidualisation.

The uNK cells express glucocorticoid receptors but lack progesterone receptors, making them directly responsive to cortisol but not to progesterone. Animal studies indicate the pregnancy-promoting potential of glucocorticoids. Prednisolone administration has been shown to effectively reduce elevated uNK density [3] and improve altered endometrial angiogenic growth factor expression and increased endometrial blood vessel maturation associated with RM. In a pilot, double-blind, RCT [4], the administration of prednisolone to women with RM and high uNK density showed a trend towards improving live-birth, but this was not significant – probably due to the small sample size. No further studies have attempted to demonstrate efficacy and safety of this plausible strategy.

Conclusions

Despite extensive research, our understanding of human implantation remains limited. Various factors govern the process of successful implantation and pregnancy health is determined even before the embryo is created. Corticosteroid deficiency in the developing ovarian follicles and peri-implantation endometrium appears to negatively impact embryo implantation and hence it is possible that corticosteroid therapy would benefit in improving this situation, especially in the sub-group of women with previous unexplained reproductive failure, when there are questions about appropriate follicular development or endometrial preparation.

Placental 11βHSD-II plays an important role in safeguarding the fetus from elevated levels of maternal glucocorticoids. Prednisolone is continued to be used in first trimester of pregnancy for women with certain pre-existing medical conditions and studies with good quality postnatal follow-up have not shown any major detrimental effects.

Finally, researchers must be encouraged and supported to conduct large RCTs reporting live birth to validate scientific and clinical observations of potential benefits of corticosteroid therapy. Until further evidence is available, it is advisable to limit the use of corticosteroids to research context and clinicians must resist any temptation to use them routinely for all women with reproductive disorders. This is especially relevant in the context of assisted conception as currently the reproductive immunology tests and treatment are given a 'red light' by the Human Fertilisation and Embryology Authority in the UK.

References

1. Keay SD, Harlow CR, Wood PJ, Jenkins JM, Cahill DJ. Higher cortisol:cortisone ratios in the preovulatory follicle of completely unstimulated IVF cycles indicate oocytes with increased pregnancy potential. *Hum Reprod.* 2002;17 (9):2410–14.

2. Kalampokas T, Pandian Z, Keay SD, Bhattacharya S. Glucocorticoid supplementation during ovarian stimulation for IVF or ICSI. 2017 3(3), CD004752. *The Cochrane Database of Systematic Reviews.*

3. Quenby S, Nik H, Innes B, et al. Uterine natural killer cells and angiogenesis in recurrent reproductive failure. *Hum Reprod.* 2009;24:45–54.

4. Tang AW, Alfirevic Z, Turner MA, Drury JA, Small R, Quenby S. A feasibility trial of screening women with idiopathic recurrent miscarriage for high uterine natural killer cell density and randomizing to prednisolone or placebo when pregnant. *Hum Reprod.* 2013;28(7):1743–52.

Corticosteroid Therapy Is Useful in Assisting Implantation
Against

Cecilia Petriglia and Filippo Maria Ubaldi

Introduction

The main goal in reproductive medicine is to increase the cumulative live birth rate using the safest and most cost-effective treatment. Embryo implantation is the most critical step of the reproductive process requiring synchronised dialogue between maternal and embryonic tissues. Nevertheless, the main features to consider are a receptive endometrium and a competent embryo [1].

A competent embryo is an embryo with a high implantation potential that may be identified by extending the culture in vitro up to the blastocyst stage and adding chromosomal testing. Although there is no conclusive evidence stating that cumulative success rates depend on the stage of embryo transfer (ET), the live birth rate per ET increases from 29% after cleavage stage transfer to 37% after blastocyst stage transfer [2]. Furthermore, aneuploidy rate in blastocysts increase from a 20–30% baseline in women <35 years, up to 70% in advanced maternal age women [3]. Therefore, pre-implantation genetic testing was introduced to detect chromosomal abnormalities in the embryo prior to ET. In fact, transferring embryos with a normal chromosomal composition leads to a lower risk for implantation failures, miscarriages and abnormal pregnancies [4]. Still, a competent embryo requires an optimal endometrial environment to implant successfully, and endometrial selectivity and receptivity must be equally balanced to allow for the implantation of a competent embryo [5].

Corticosteroids and Endometrial Receptivity

The endometrium is a dynamic tissue that can undergo physiological changes in response to steroid hormones assuming a receptive status during the window of implantation. The absence or suppression of molecules essential for the correct endometrial receptivity would result in a decreased implantation rate. The mechanisms are different and complex, including abnormal cytokine and hormonal signalling, as well as epigenetic alterations. However, their individual function and role within the network of endometrial development is still not clear. Even though most of these molecules are involved in the inflammatory response, many still remain unknown. To date, an effective treatment to improve the endometrial receptivity is missing. Corticosteroids were proposed to enhance embryo implantation rate after IVF and prevent miscarriage. It is known that glucocorticoids influence the intrauterine environment by reducing aberrant populations of uterine natural killer (NK) cells, normalising cytokine expression in the endometrium and suppressing endometrial inflammation. Thus, different types of corticosteroids with their corresponding dose, schedule and duration of treatment were suggested to further investigate potential benefits in implantation.

Body of Evidence

In the first studies analysing the effectiveness of corticosteroids in implantation, infertile women positive to autoantibodies (antinuclear antibodies, anti-thyroid antibodies, lupus anticoagulant, anti-cardiolipin antibodies) were enrolled; the results highlighted an enhanced pregnancy rate after IVF. Corticosteroids were also subsequently tested in patients not presenting with immune disorders, however positive results such as increased pregnancy rates occurred only in women who experienced several previous miscarriages. Nevertheless, no other studies identified differences in the implantation rate of IVF patients receiving corticosteroid treatment with either high or low doses [6]. Moreover, a Cochrane review and meta-analysis encompassing 14 trials, concluded that no evidence exists to support the use of peri-implantation corticosteroids administration in routine IVF [7], also underlining the fact that the impact of exogenous glucocorticoids on the physiological immune activation and inflammatory events in early pregnancy remains unexplained.

Against the Administration of Corticosteroids

There is strong evidence to support that a beneficial effect in enhancing embryo implantation in IVF patients derives from the administration of glucocorticoids. Immune activation with controlled inflammation is extremely important for embryo implantation and the correct development of a pregnancy. Nevertheless, there is contrasting evidence of the usefulness of corticosteroids, suggesting that suppression of immune function may interfere with implantation consequently compromising placental development in many patients. The endometrium has a specialised competence to attenuate local cortisol bioavailability. In fact, the gestational tissues in pregnancy are maintained in a low glucocorticoid environment by placental expression of 11β-hydroxysteroid dehydrogenase type 2 which inactivates the glucocorticoids delivered from maternal blood. The inflammatory response evoked at the moment of conception enrols immune cells that participate to the events of trophoblast invasion and early placentation, thereby allowing maternal immune recognition and ability to respond to paternally derived major histocompatibility complex antigens. This active recognition process is required to recruit and regulate uterine NK and T-cell populations supporting the implantation process that persists beyond the first trimester to protect the placenta and the fetus. Thus, exogenous corticosteroids may negatively affect the peri-implantation immune response by damaging the first phase of immune recognition and responsiveness to the embryo; this may in turn impact the quality and strength of the immune tolerance generated and capacity to support placentation with consequences for later pregnancy and fetal growth [6].

Conclusions

The administration of glucocorticoids may have both positive and harmful effects on fertility and pregnancy, possibly related to the immune processes in each and every patient. Nevertheless, up to now, there is no evidence to support the administration of glucocorticoids in infertile patients undergoing IVF. Therefore, well-powered clinical studies are urgently required to identify specific sub-categories of infertile patients who may benefit from glucocorticoids.

References

1. Simón C, Dominguez F, Remohi J, Pellicer A. Embryo effects in human implantation: embryonic regulation of endometrial molecules in human implantation. *Ann NY Acad Sci.* 2001 Sept;943:1–16.

2. Glujovsky D, Farquhar C, Quinteiro Retamar AM, Alvarez Sedo CR, Blake D. Cleavage stage versus blastocyst stage embryo transfer in assisted reproductive technology. *Cochrane Database of Systematic Reviews* 2016, Issue 6. Art. No.: CD002118.

3. Capalbo A, Hoffmann ER, Cimadomo D, Ubaldi FM, Rienzi L. Human female meiosis revised: new insights into the mechanisms of chromosome segregation and aneuploidies from advanced genomics and time-lapse imaging. *Hum Reprod Update.* 2017 Nov 1;23(6):706–22.

4. Romanelli V, Poli M, Capalbo A. Preimplantation genetic testing in assisted reproductive technology. *Panminerva Med.* 2019;61:30–41.

5. Macklon N, Brosens J. The human endometrium as a sensor of embryo quality. *Biol Reprod.* 2014;91(4):98, 1–8.

6. Robertson SA, Jin M, Yu D, et al. Corticosteroid therapy in assisted reproduction-immune suppression is a faulty premise. *Hum Reprod.* 2016;31 (10):2164–73.

7. Boomsma CM, Keay SD, Macklon NS. Peri-implantation glucocorticoid administration for assisted reproductive technology cycles. *Cochrane Database of Systematic Reviews* 2012, Issue 6. Art. No.: CD005996.

14A

DEBATE

IVF Should Be First-Line Treatment for Unexplained Infertility of Two Years Duration

For

Tim Child

Most women conceive within the first 12 months of regular unprotected sexual intercourse. Of the 16% that don't, around half will conceive without treatment during months 12 to 24 [1]. During those first two years of trying the couple should undergo investigations including semen analysis and confirmation of ovulation and tubal patency (by hysterosalpingo contrast sonography [HyCoSy], hysterosalpingogram [HSG] or laparoscopy). If all tests return as normal then, by definition, the couple have 'unexplained' infertility.

Note the 50% pregnancy rate, without treatment, during the 2nd year of trying. Impatience by doctor or patient to 'do something' can lead to the use of unnecessary interventions such as ovarian stimulation (OS) (for ovulating women!) and/or intra-uterine insemination (IUI) (for couples with a normal reproductive tract and sperm function!) as these are often viewed as softer, more natural treatments. Certainly not as natural (or as cheap) as conceiving naturally.

A number of studies comparing outcomes of OS or OS-IUI versus IVF to 'treat' couples with unexplained unfortunately include patients with 12 to 24 months of trying [2]. Unsurprisingly the OS or OS-IUI success rates are high (and therefore falsely close to IVF). I say unsurprising as the woman was likely to conceive anyway even without OS and/or IUI. For couples with less than 2 years of unexplained infertility full investigation, but no treatment is required.

There will still be a chance of natural conception beyond 2 years of trying for couples with unexplained infertility. For a fertility treatment to be offered, it needs to have a chance of success higher than this natural background rate.

It is difficult to understand how OS would increase conception rates in a woman who is already ovulating. I would suggest this is akin to offering spectacles to someone with 20/20 vision. Certainly OS will increase the chance of multiple birth, a significant complication for mother and babies. Similarly, it is difficult to understand how IUI will assist a couple with no psychosexual, anatomical, surgical (e.g. cervical cone biopsy) or semen abnormality who are having regular intercourse. What is the IUI treating? With IUI it is impossible to know whether an egg and sperm actually ever meet, let alone lead to a blastocyst ready to implant in the endometrium. This contrasts with the situation for IVF. During an IVF cycle, oocytes are retrieved following ovarian stimulation, fertilised in vitro, embryos cultured, and (usually nowadays) a single blastocyst transferred into the uterus at the optimal time (elective single embryo transfer [eSET]). Therefore with IVF, regardless of the cause of infertility, nearly all cycles result in an embryo within the endometrial cavity. It is accepted that IVF success rates are very similar regardless of the underlying aetiology of infertility [1].

Fortunately, a recent Cochrane review of 27 randomised trials has analysed interventions for unexplained infertility including expectant management, OS with anti-oestrogens, aromatase inhibitors or gonadotropins, OS-IUI, and IVF/ICSI [2]. Of note, the included studies did not compare one IVF/ICSI cycle versus one IUI or OS-IUI but mostly had a ratio of, for example, one IVF/ICSI to three IUI.

The live birth rate per couple was higher for IVF/ICSI compared to all of the aforementioned interventions (odds ratio compared to expectant management, OS 1.01; IUI 1.21; OS-IUI 1.61; IVF/ICSI 1.88). There was no difference in ovarian hyperstimulation syndrome rates between OS-IUI and IVF/ICSI. In addition, multiple birth is higher for OS and OS-IUI compared to IVF/ICSI (odds ratio for multiple birth compared to expectant management/IUI, OS 3.07; OS-IUI 3.34; IVF/ICSI 2.66 [the only non-significant intervention]). Whilst the multiple pregnancy rate can be very easily controlled in IVF/ICSI using eSET, this is not so for OS. If OS results in a single follicle in an ovulatory woman with unexplained infertility then what is the point of the OS (she would have produced the follicle anyway!). As soon as more than one follicle is produced with OS then there must be an increased multiple pregnancy risk compared to IVF/ICSI with eSET. If three follicles (not at all uncommon with OS) are considered acceptable then triplets become a reality. If three follicles are not considered acceptable then high cancellation rates are an issue.

With recent improvements in IVF including use of short protocol antagonist cycles with an agonist trigger (reducing the ovarian hyperstimulation syndrome [OHSS] rate by 90% compared to long agonist protocol plus hCG trigger), superior embryo culture and supernumerary blastocyst vitrification techniques, and the use of eSET, very high cumulative live birth (and very low multiple birth) rates per egg collection can be achieved. Indeed, a registry database study from Australia and New Zealand [3] shows a higher cumulative live birth rate (CLBR; including all subsequent frozen embryo transfer [FET] cycles) for every extra oocyte retrieved beyond 14 for women <36 years of age, with a CLBR of over 70% when 25 oocytes were collected. Even with lower numbers of oocytes collected the use of blastocyst vitrification and FET still results in a significant extra CLBR [4]. Considering that FET can take place in a natural menstrual cycle with no exogenous hormone supplementation at all [5] this 'one and done' approach is of great interest.

In summary, current IVF techniques allow very high cumulative live birth rates with just one cycle of short protocol antagonist stimulation, eSET, vitrification and subsequent natural FET cycles. The multiple birth rate can be safely kept to low single figures. Even a single IVF-ET cycle has a higher success rate (and lower multiple birth rate) compared to multiple OS-IUI. Why use a treatment such as OS-IUI that hasn't developed since the early days of fertility medicine, and which carries increased risks of the increasingly unacceptable complication of multiple pregnancy, when there is such a quick and effective option as IVF/ICSI?

References

1. National Institute for Health and Care Excellence. Fertility problems: assessment and treatment. Clinical guideline CG156; updated September 2017. www.nice.org.uk/guidance/cg156.

2. Wang R, Danhof NA, Tjon-Kon-Fat RI, et al. *Interventions for unexplained infertility: a systematic review and network meta-analysis. Cochrane Database of Systematic Reviews* 2019, Issue 9. Art. No.: CD012692. DOI: 10.1002/14651858.CD012692.pub2.

3. Law YJ, Zhang N, Venetis CA, Chambers GM, Harris K. The number of oocytes associated with maximum cumulative live birth rates per aspiration depends on female age: a population study of 221 221 treatment cycles. *Hum Reprod.* 2019;34 (9):1778–87.

4. Smith ADAC, Tilling K, Nelson SM, Lawlor DA. Live-birth rate associated with repeat in vitro fertilization treatment cycles. *JAMA.* 2015;314(24):2654–62.

5. Noble M, Child T. The role of frozen-thawed embryo replacement cycles in assisted conception. *Obstet Gynaecol.* 2020;22:57–68.

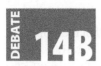

IVF Should Be First-Line Treatment for Unexplained Infertility of Two Years Duration

Against

Gulam Bahadur

That IVF should be first line treatment for unexplained infertility of 2 years duration has widely been accepted as a norm, non-evidence based to suit a profits growth industry increasingly run by hedge fund investors. IVF clinicians naturally have interests and will convince patients to undertake expensive IVF. Despite a plethora of IVF success claims ranging from 15 to 95% via heterogeneous presentation, 70% of women will fail to have a baby [1]. IVF indications have expanded from tubal disorders to many causes of subfertility, including 'unexplained'. It is increasingly convenient to classify unexplained infertility to justify profitable in vitro fertilisation/intracytoplasmic sperm injection (IVF/ICSI) treatments based on erroneously generated evidence by people with interests. Unexplained infertility has grown two-fold from the early 1990s to around 40% in 2020, similar to that experienced for male factor infertility to justify ICSI type treatments. Playing the gallery to untrained stakeholders and fee-paying agencies seems all too common when generating flimsy, smoke and mirrors type evidence to secure lucrative funding in subfertility. Peer reviewing is of course by the same interest groups. UK NICE guidelines have tightened their conflict of interest procedure, but have knowingly continued along the erroneous guidelines pitched in favour of IVF, raising questions of what further interest groups are involved? NICE obtusely asked for evidence to support intrauterine insemination (IUI) despite providing no evidence to dismiss this technique, and as a result good evidence has been published [1]. The politics of healthcare practices has an overbearing presence in assisted reproductive technology (ART) not witnessed in other branches of medicine, thereby eroding patient autonomy, consents and choices.

Securing IVF funding requires influencing how policies and guidance are constructed and this is done in a way not possible for any other medical discipline. It further requires independent third-party bodies such as the World Health Organization (WHO), NICE or the International Committee for Monitoring Assisted Reproductive Technology (ICMART) to support evidence generated by IVF practitioners and peer reviewed by IVF practitioners. This smoke and mirrors approach betrays patients and stakeholders. In the USA, IUI is not considered ART. Classifying infertility as a disease has inherent benefits in attracting state funding [2]. In earlier years infertility was considered a 'non-disease' and even the esteemed Warnock committee could not accept infertility to be classified as a disease. To suit the IVF industry, the years of trying have been conveniently reduced to 1 year from 2 years despite natural pregnancies occurring in this cohort for 35–50% of cases. Second, NICE's erroneous guidelines against IUI have allowed potentially easy cases to gain inflated IVF success rates, much needed to market unnecessary IVF procedures despite a 70% IVF failure rate [1]. Not satisfied, IVF clinics wish to utilise the magnified cumulative IVF success rates for subliminal marketing.

The second major area to understand is what an 'unexplained' condition means? There is no medical discipline like ART which can boldly state the diagnosis as 'unexplained' and proceed in offering costly and often unnecessary IVF without highlighting a high failure rate. Both 'unexplained' and 'infertility' used in combination amount to 'failure in diagnosis'. Critically, the non-evidenced based IVF usage has obfuscated our understanding of the around 70% IVF failure rate, while preventing critical research in unravelling the state of 'subfertility'. Despite prematurely selling unvalidated IVF add-on techniques the success rates have not improved, while the IVF world in is denial of these facts.

Questions on how RCTs and selection biases fare against big data is more relevant for ART where interest exists. Crucially NICE considered IUI with very low dose (25 mg) clomiphene citrate (CC) and without comparative data recommended against IUI, and instead be replaced by three cycles of IVF [1]. The FASST (Fast Track and Standard Treatment) trial serves no purpose with in-built biases omitting IUI/hMG cycles and suggesting the premature use of IVF [3]. That IUI/hMG serves a potential threat to IVF is encapsulated in meta-analyses by focusing on high-risk IUI/hMG papers only, then concluding IUI/hMG should not be practised at all, and this is further supported by a lead commentary [4]. In our opinion almost 100% of cases would have warranted cancellation, but the article appears calculated to dissuade IUI in favour of IVF. None of the limitations were made clear to stakeholders and require more critical analysts. Financial analyses on cost efficiencies have so far been conducted crudely and again overly concerned to show IUI was cost inefficient, thereby playing gallery to the UK Clinical Commissioning Groups (CCGs) and NICE. The data used were unequal and the nature of peer reviewing raises further questions where huge financial interests prevail, making a case of open refereeing. The recent Cochrane review acknowledges IUI in a stimulated cycle may result in a higher cumulative live birth rate compared to IUI in a natural cycle [5].

The latest UK multiple birth rates have reached 10% while the HFEA broad-brushed this to mean unqualified improvement and safety of IVF generally, but this is still five times greater than the background multiple gestation pregnancy (MGP), and higher than IUI. Closer inspection of the data shows an exclusion of 20% of the participant clinics thereby creating a bias and false impression to the public.

The most advanced integrated analyses [1] of live birth levels, risks and costs confirms IUI benefits are dominant over IVF and the data makes a clear case for investing in IUI before IVF. Governments should universally follow this advice, away from IVF clinic countenance and pressures [1]. The success rates for IUI are much closer to IVF than previously acknowledged, with lesser risks of multiple births, severe OHSS, terminations and fetal reduction. The cost-effective analyses confirm IUI was significantly cheaper than IVF to gain one live birth, and that IVF produces a latent and significant cost burden to the NHS for maternal and neonatal care. Based on NICE's own cost-effectiveness guidelines, they should issue urgent instructions to UK CCGs to fund IUI before IVF. Elements of the IVF industry have proactively been generating biased pseudo-evidence to secure IVF practice and funding at the expense of patients and stakeholders. The latest evidence confirms IUI before IVF practice is paramount and beneficial to society.

References

1. Bahadur G, Homburg R, Bosmans JE, et al. Observational retrospective study of UK national success, risks and costs for 319,105 IVF/ICSI and 30,669 IUI treatment cycles. *BMJ Open*. 2020;10:e034566.

2. Zegers-Hochschild F, Adamson GD, de Mouzon J, et al. International Committee for Monitoring Assisted Reproductive Technology (ICMART) and the World Health Organization (WHO) revised glossary of ART terminology, 2009. *Fertil Steril*. 2009 Nov;92(5):1520–24.

3. Reindollar RH, Regan MM, Neumann PJ, et al. A randomized clinical trial to evaluate optimal treatment for unexplained infertility: the fast track and standard treatment (FASTT) trial. *Fertil Steril.* 2010; 94:888–99.

4. Hansen KR. Gonadotropins with intrauterine insemination for unexplained infertility-time to stop? *Fertil Steril.* 2020 February;113(2):333–4.

5. Ayeleke RO, Asseler JD, Cohlen BJ, et al. Intra-uterine insemination for unexplained subfertility. *Cochrane Database Syst Rev.* 2020 March 3;3:CD001838. doi: 10.1002/14651858.CD001838.pub6.

Single Embryo Transfer Should Be Performed in All IVF Cycles

For

Mark Hamilton

Achieving a pregnancy which leads to the birth of a healthy child is the goal of all prospective parents, not least the many who require assistance to become pregnant. In vitro fertilisation (IVF) and embryo transfer (ET) is nowadays increasingly recommended as the treatment of choice in most diagnostic categories of infertility. It is estimated that as many as 2.5 million IVF cycles are carried out in the world each year resulting in over 500,000 births [1].

In many countries the proportion of all births consequent upon IVF, particularly in the developed world, is significant. In the UK in 2016 this figure was 2.5%, while in some countries the proportion exceeds 6%. The practice of IVF should therefore be a matter of significant concern to society.

High rates of multiple pregnancy after fertility treatment are often a result of IVF. Most often these arise after transfer to the uterus more than one embryo. Other treatments, including 'controlled' ovarian stimulation with or without intra-uterine insemination, also carry significant risks of multiple pregnancy.

Twin pregnancies are associated with significant maternal, fetal and neonatal hazard [2]. For the mother these include increased antenatal risks, e.g. pregnancy-induced hypertension, gestational diabetes, pre-term premature rupture of the membranes (PPROM) and infection; intrapartum risks, e.g. haemorrhage at the time of birth, operative delivery; postnatal risks including post-partum depression and psychological stress within the family unit. The relative risk of pre-term birth is increased six-fold with twins and is associated with increased infant mortality and long-term morbidity. Not infrequently, mental and/or physical disability generates considerable costs to society in supporting the care of affected children.

In the last 20 years, initially led from Scandinavia, a drive to reduce the proportion of births derived from twin and higher order multiple pregnancies has gathered pace. Latest data from the UK indicate that in the last 10 years, through regulatory pressure and increased clinical and consumer appreciation of iatrogenic hazard associated with double embryo transfer (DET), the proportion of single embryo transfers (SET) has increased from <10% to more than 25%. As a result the multiple pregnancy rate after IVF in the UK has fallen from around 24% in 2006 to 10% in 2017 [2]. Other countries have embraced SET to a greater degree. In Australia SET rates exceed 70% with a multiple pregnancy rate amongst the lowest in the world.

Resistance to SET in some quarters stems from a concern that pregnancy potential may be threatened by only transferring one embryo where more might be available. However it is important to examine results in terms of the totality of IVF treatment. If one takes account of the utilisation of all embryos, including those cryopreserved, thawed and transferred at a later date, data derived from randomised controlled trials, in good prognosis patients, shows that the chance of a pregnancy leading to live birth is maintained.

An ability to select embryos with the best implantation potential allied to a robust cryopreservation programme are essential prerequisites for the optimal utilisation of SET [4]. Improved understanding of favourable morphological markers of embryo quality have enhanced our ability to select single embryos for transfer. Morphokinetic and pre-implantation genetic analysis of embryos are more recently available tools which arguably have the potential to add further precision though there areas yet insufficient data to routinely recommend their routine use. The use of vitrification has improved freeze–thaw survival rates and implantation potential of vitrified embryos now matches that of freshly transferred embryos. A worry that pregnancy potential might be prejudiced by deferring transfer of good quality embryos is unjustified. Furthermore data suggest that perinatal outcomes may be better where the pregnancy was derived from frozen transfer.

It is conceded that a universal SET policy, inclusive of those with a less favourable prognosis, may provide less certainty in respect of outcome. In older patients and those who have had several failed attempts previously, and indeed some with poor quality embryos, it could be argued that DET may offer a per transfer chance of conception which is higher than SET. Understandable as this concern may be there remains a legitimate concern that a multiple embryo transfer will expose the mother and potential child to avoidable hazard. Multiples can arise after SET but this phenomenon is rare, being seen in <5% of the total number of pregnancies. Recent data in women up to 40 years however suggest that SET-based practice still maintains pregnancy rates.

Some commentators have suggested that twin pregnancy should not be considered an undesirable outcome in comparison with two singleton gestations [5]. The proposition that the cumulative risks of two pregnancies are similar to those of one twin pregnancy however is not supported by published data. Analysis from the Swedish Medical Birth Registry demonstrated that neonatal and maternal outcomes were better for women undergoing two IVF pregnancies consequent on SET, rather than one twin pregnancy following DET. The data included the observations of increased risk of PPROM and pre-eclampsia and a 4× higher caesarean section rate where the DET approach leading to twins was utilised.

Several drivers have a bearing on SET utilisation rates. These include concerns with respect to success rates as above. In some clinical settings, often influenced by limited laboratory resources, IVF success rates may be inferior to those in better equipped facilities. This influences patient choice and arguably clinical practice, particularly where commercial pressures are brought to bear through a fiscal need for clinics to attract self-funding and state-funded patients. Choice of clinic may be influenced by the method of reporting outcomes. It is best practice to report birth rates which take account of all embryos transferred in a treatment cycle including utilised cryopreserved embryos rather than only the fresh transfer. Liberal state funding, permissive of the use of cryopreserved ET and SET, has made an enormous, undeniably favourable, impact on clinical practice in Australia, Belgium and Scandinavia.

A major driver in determining health-care policy in this area relates to the high antenatal, intrapartum and neonatal costs associated with multiple pregnancy. Consideration of cost-effectiveness is essential within the state funded sector and thus there is a moral imperative to ensure that limited resources are used carefully. State commissioning of IVF treatment has been linked to compulsory SET in some countries with maintenance of success rates and low multiple rates. The relationship between an effective multiple births minimisation strategy such as this and adequate state resourcing of multiple treatment cycles is now accepted. Self-funding of treatment however should not be a licence to ignore a recommendation to SET particularly where the state resources neonatal care. While autonomy should be respected to a degree, there is a moral imperative, in considering any request for DET, to avoid the risk of what would be in reality an avoidable pressure on the limited state funds available for wider society in dealing with the consequences of complications. An argument based on a reduction in the financial burden to the individual of treatment costs and shortening time to achieve desired family numbers cannot be supported.

Summary

- Multiple pregnancy, with profound associated hazards, is an avoidable iatrogenic consequence of IVF.
- Adverse outcomes associated with twin pregnancy are costly both to individuals and society.
- With improved cryopreservation capability, similar birth rates, with fewer risks associated, are maintained with SET-based practice.
- Adequate state funding and sound regulatory reporting of outcomes, support SET-based practice.
- Clinical practice must take account of our moral obligations to society as well as to the individual.

References

1. Adamson GD, de Mouzon J, Chambers G, et al. International Committee for Monitoring Assisted Reproductive Technology: world report on assisted reproductive technology, 2011. *Fertil Steril.* 2018;110:1067–80.

2. Human Fertilisation and Embryology Authority. Fertility treatment 2017: trends and figures. (May 2019) www.hfea.gov.uk/media/2894/fertility-treatment-2017-trends-and-figures-may-2019.pdf.

3. El-Toukhy T, Bhattacharya S, and Akande V on behalf of the Royal College of Obstetricians and Gynaecologists. Multiple pregnancies following assisted conception: Scientific Impact Paper No. 22. (2018) www.rcog.org.uk/en/guidelines-research-services/guidelines/sip22.

4. Cutting R Single embryo transfer for all. *Best Pract Res Clin Obstet Gynaecol.* 2018;53:30–37.

5. Adashi EY, Gleicher N. Is a blanket elective single embryo transfer policy defensible? *Rambam Maimonides Med J.* 2017;8(2) (open access) doi: 10.5041/RMMJ.10299.

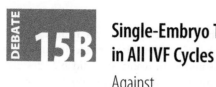

Single-Embryo Transfer Should Be Performed in All IVF Cycles
Against

Lewis Nancarrow

The implementation of single embryo transfer (SET) policies has been ongoing since a Finnish study highlighting the risks and complications that can occur as a result of increased multiple pregnancy rates [1]. This is now common practice in Sweden, Turkey and Belgium, with other countries such as the UK, Australia, Canada and the USA showing increased preference for SET over double embryo transfers [2].

The chance of a multiple pregnancy is significantly increased when comparing a double embryo transfer (DET) (29%) to SET (2%) [3], but is a blanket policy of single embryo transfer suitable for everyone? Meta-analysis showed that in women with a good prognosis, those who had a DET had a significantly higher live birth rate than those who had a SET (42% vs. 27% respectively) [3]. However, when a subsequent SET was performed in the SET group similar live birth rates were found (38% SET vs. 42% DET) [3]. This highlights the similar success rates between the two groups and raises the question, why would we inflict greater risk on this patient group when it is not necessary?

However, this group of patients isn't representative of the entire IVF population. Roughly 20% of patients undergoing IVF in the UK are over the age of 40, this increases to around 30% when including those over 38. This group of patients are known to have reduced implantation rates and live birth rates (26% <35 years old, <15% >40 years old) and they're also on a time sensitive schedule as their chances of conceiving continues to decline as they age. These patients are an example of just one group where DET should be considered.

Adashi et al. summarised discussions previously had by Gleicher and colleagues on why a blanket SET is not appropriate, see Figure 15B.1 [1].

The above points highlight certain aspects favouring the DET. In some cases the option for delay between embryo transfers, due to patient age or those with age-inappropriate ovarian function, is not feasible. These particular patients may wish to accelerate family building and as long as the patients are fully informed of both the maternal and neonatal risks of multiple pregnancies, is it ethical to deny them this option if a blanket SET policy was in place? Particularly in those patients who are >40 years, studies have shown that there is no significant difference between multiple pregnancy rates when comparing SET to DET [5].

For those who have had recurrent implantation failure with good quality SET, why continue offering this option when it is known that DET increases their live birth rate?

There have been conflicting reviews on the cost of multiple pregnancies; one study found that compared with SET, DET ranged from costing an additional £27,356–£15,539 per extra live birth in women aged 32 and 39yearsrespectively [2]. It also stated that in those over 39 there was further reduction in cost due to their reduced chance of multiple pregnancies, highlighting that blanket policies of SET are not the most cost-effective option, particularly for those of advanced maternal age [2]. In contrast to this, another study found that in young women, cost per live-born child with DET was £22,341.70, compared to SET which was £24,647.60 [3]. Further cost-effectiveness studies are required to determine the full impact of DET vs. SET, and should include the lifelong earning potential of additional

1. Paternalistic towards DET-eligible subjects pressed to conceive by prolonged infertility and/or age.
2. Unethical towards DET-eligible subjects in whom successive eSETs could delay or preclude conception.
3. Disadvantageous to DET-eligible subjects whose live birth rates may decline.
4. Inconsiderate of DET-eligible subjects in whom successive eSETs could raise costs and efforts.
5. Incapable of assuring a risk level lower than that displayed by twin pregnancies.

Figure 15B.1 Arguments against a single embryo transfer policy [1].

newborns as a result of DET [1]. Repeated SET also carry the burden of increased cost, both monetary (unless publicly funded) and psychologically to the patient [4].

The majority of data shows more adverse outcomes occur with multiple pregnancies than singleton pregnancies [4]. Adashi highlighted two papers showing no difference between placenta praevia, placental abruption, or gestational diabetes rates between SET and DET groups. Although there was an increase in neonatal complications, there was no difference in perinatal mortality, Apgar scores <7, congenital anomalies, or mortality in the first year of life [1]. The majority of twin complications rates are based on natural conceived pregnancies, however there has been a study showing that IVF twin pregnancies have a reduction of complications by 40% [1] in comparison to those naturally conceived.

But should a multiple pregnancy be seen as an adverse outcome? In some cultures, twins are thought to attract joy, happiness and wealth to a family [4]. This is reflected in numerous surveys with a resounding preference for DET, ranging from 58.7% of Danish couples going up to 94.4% of Nigerian couples wishing DET to achieve a twin pregnancy.

Ultimately, I believe SET should be performed for the majority of patients, but not enforced as a blanket policy. Medical arguments should be attuned to specific characteristics of the patient; such as age, cause of infertility, embryo quality, opportunity for cryopreservation, and the experience of the clinician [4]. Those with advanced maternal age and recurrent implantation failure are examples of those that will be disadvantaged by a compulsory SET policy. This denies patient their autonomy on making a decision which will have a huge impact on their life. Clinicians and patients need to work together to discuss the risks of DET and whether it is appropriate for them, ensuring both sides take responsibility in a shared decision-making approach.

References

1. Adashi EY, Gleicher N. Is a blanket elective single embryo transfer policy defensible? *Rambam Maimonides Med J.* 2017;8(2).

2. Cutting R. Single embryo transfer for all. *Best Pract Res Clin Obstet Gynaecol.* 2018;53:30–7.

3. Wilkinson D, Schaefer GO, Tremellen K, et al. Double trouble: should double embryo transfer be banned? *Theor Med Bioeth.* 2015;36(2):121–39.

4. Ezugwu E, der Burg SV. Debating elective single embryo transfer after in vitro fertilization: a plea for a context-sensitive approach. *Ann Med Health Sci Res.* 2015;5(1):1–7.

5. Tannus S, Son WY, Dahan MH. Elective single blastocyst transfer in advanced maternal age. *J Assist Reprod Genet.* 2017;34(6):741–8.

16A The Freezing of All Embryos Should Be Used for All IVF Cycles

For

Matheus Roque

Among the greatest advances in assisted reproductive technology (ART) in recent years are the improvements made in cryopreservation techniques. The advent and improvement of vitrification protocols have led to high rates of embryo survival after the thawing process, while achieving the same clinical results (or better) when comparing frozen–thawed embryo transfer (FET) to fresh embryo transfer (ET). These advancements in cryopreservation protocols are associated with improvements in the cumulative live birth rate (CLBR) per cycle, and also with the implementation of the so-called freeze-all strategy during in vitro fertilisation (IVF) cycles. In this strategy, fresh ET is not performed and all viable embryos are electively cryopreserved.

Although fresh ET is the norm in ART, there are many concerns about the possible adverse effects of controlled ovarian stimulation (COS) on the endometrium. COS is necessary for the development and maturation of many follicles and oocytes; therefore, it increases the chance of positive outcomes and cumulative pregnancy rates during ART. However, the supra-physiologic hormonal levels that are required for conventional COS are associated with modifications in the peri-implantation endometrium that may be related to decreases in pregnancy rates when comparing fresh ET to FET. Further, endometrial advancement can be observed via histological evaluation during a fresh cycle; when this advancement lasts longer than 3 days, no pregnancies are achieved. There are also changes in the gene expression profiles in the endometrium of patients submitted to COS, suggesting that ovarian hyperstimulation and high progesterone levels on the day of final oocyte maturation might be detrimental to implantation, as it can alter genes that are crucial for the endometrium–embryo interaction. Importantly, all studies presenting differences in endometrial receptivity when comparing a stimulated cycle to a natural cycle are based on endometrial evaluation of hyper-responder patients or of patients with supra-physiologic hormonal levels that occur during COS.

The most widely agreed upon indication for implementing the freeze-all strategy is to avoid the development of ovarian hyperstimulation syndrome (OHSS). OHSS is a potentially lethal complication of COS, and studies have shown that avoiding fresh ET in patients at risk of OHSS was associated with a decrease in OHSS development. Thus, it has been recommended that patients who will be submitted to COS and present risk factors for OHSS (i.e., polycystic ovarian syndrome [PCOS] or previous OHSS) be stimulated under GnRH antagonist protocols with a GnRH agonist trigger, followed by a freeze-all strategy, which aims to decrease OHSS development to almost 0% [1].

When comparing clinical outcomes, the first meta-analysis evaluating the freeze-all strategy was published in 2013 and concluded that this method was associated with improved ongoing pregnancy rates when compared to fresh cycles. However, this conclusion was based on only three randomised controlled trials (RCTs) evaluating a total of 633 IVF cycles. Moreover, after the publication of this meta-analysis, one of the studies was retracted from the literature due to methodological flaws; after the study ended, there were no differences in the ongoing pregnancy rates when comparing the freeze-all to fresh cycles (RR = 1.26; 95% CI 1.00–1.58; $P = 0.05$).In a recent meta-analysis including 5,379 patients randomised to the freeze-all strategy or to a fresh cycle, there was an overall increase of 7% in the live birth rate (LBR) when performing the freeze-all cycle instead of a fresh ET (RR = 1.07; $P = 0.02$). However, when the sub-analysis was conducted, it was shown that the only patient subgroup that presented an advantage when performing the freeze-all strategy was that which included hyper-responders (RR = 1.15; $P = 0.005$) and those who submitted to pre-implantation genetic testing (PGT) in the blastocyst stage (data were only obtained from one study). When evaluating the CLBR, there were no differences when comparing the freeze-all strategy to fresh ET [2].

Concerning progesterone levels on the day of final oocyte maturation, cohort studies and a meta-analysis have respectively shown that elevated progesterone levels are associated with a decrease in implantation rates and pregnancy rates. Some observational studies and a sub-analysis of a recent RCT comparing the freeze-all to fresh ET involving 782 couples showed that the LBR was significantly better with FET compared to fresh ET in patients presenting with elevated progesterone levels on trigger day. There are also other possible indications for the freeze-all, such as patients with slow-developing embryos, leading to an asynchrony between the embryo and endometrium during a fresh cycle; implantation failure; patients presenting with endometrial, tubal and uterine factors; those with endometriosis and adenomyosis; and patients demonstrating oocyte or embryo pooling with a poor ovarian response. However, RCTs specifically examining these factors are lacking [3].

Observational studies and a meta-analysis have highlighted that the obstetric and perinatal outcomes in pregnancies resulting from IVF treatments are different when comparing fresh ET to FET. It has been shown that after fresh ET, patients present with a higher risk of preterm birth, low birth weight, and small for gestational age. However, the FET cycles are associated with pregnancy-associated hypertension, preeclampsia, and macrosomia. Until recently, there was no evidence on whether some of the obstetric and perinatal outcomes favour fresh cycles and other FET [4]. Recent evidence has emerged to show that endometrial priming, and not cryopreservation per se, may underlie some of the adverse obstetric and perinatal outcomes observed in pregnancies after FET. It has been stated that the corpus luteum (CL), which secretes vasoactive hormones, plays a fundamental role in maternal circulation in early pregnancy. Moreover, the absence of CL observed during FET with a programmed cycle, in which hormonal replacement is performed for endometrial preparation, is associated with an increased incidence of preeclampsia. These data are corroborated by the findings of a large, population-based, retrospective registry study that compared the outcomes of singletons after FET to fresh transfer and spontaneous conception singletons. The authors found that FET cycles were associated with increased risk of hypertensive disorders and macrosomia when compared to fresh cycles or natural conception. This increased risk was related to the absence of the CL. Thus, when FET is performed, the to-be-implemented endometrial priming should be evaluated not only for clinical outcomes, but also to assess its degree of safety to the mother and conceptus [5].

In conclusion, although there are many potential advantages associated with performing a freeze-all cycle over fresh ET, it seems that the freeze-all strategy is not designed for all of IVF patients. Based on the findings of available RCTs, it seems reasonable to implement this strategy in patients with a risk of OHSS, hyper-responders/PCOS patients, and when performing PGT in the blastocyst stage. Further, RCTs are needed to evaluate the appropriateness of the freeze-all strategy for all other possible indications. If the freeze-all strategy is performed for unselected and overall populations, there may be increases in the cost of treatment, the time to pregnancy, and the laboratory workflow, without improving clinical, obstetrical, and perinatal outcomes. Thus, implementation of the freeze-all strategy should be individualised and offered to all patients who would most likely benefit from it.

References

1. Devroey P, Polyzos NP, Blockeel C. An OHSS-free clinic by segmentation of IVF treatment. *Hum Reprod.* 2011;26:2593–7.

2. Roque M, Haahr T, Geber S, Esteves SC, Humaidan P. Fresh versus elective frozen embryo transfer in IVF/ICSI cycles: A systematic review and meta-analysis of reproductive outcomes. *Hum Reprod Update.* 2019;25:2–14.

3. Blockeel C, Campbell A, Coticchio G, et al. Should we still perform fresh embryo transfers in ART? *Hum Reprod.* 2019; 34: 2319–29.

4. Maheshwari A, Pandey S, Raja EM, Shetty A, Hamilton M, Bhattacharya S. Is frozen embryo transfer better for mothers and babies? Can cumulative meta-analysis provide a definitive answer? *Hum Reprod Update.* 2018;24:35–8.

5. Roque M, Bedoschi G, Cecchino GN, Esteves SC. Fresh versus frozen blastocyst transfer. *Lancet.* 2019;394:1227–18.

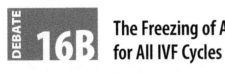

The Freezing of All Embryos Should Be Used for All IVF Cycles

Against

Mark Bowman

Embryo vitrification is a highly successful technique that adds significantly to the cumulative pregnancy rate per initial IVF cycle. Additionally, many women will benefit from the elective freezing of all embryos without fresh transfer. However, the evidence from the published literature, particularly when combined with cost–benefit analyses, indicates that this approach is not indicated in *all* IVF cycles.

Let us examine the literature-based arguments that point to the advantages of embryo freezing to determine if an argument can be made for *never* considering fresh embryo transfer.

Ovarian Stimulation Leads to Abnormally Developed or Out-of-Phase Endometrium That Both Reduces Embryo Implantation and Increases Risk for Fetal Anomalies and Abnormal Perinatal Events -- There is evidence in the literature over many years that particularly high-dose ovarian stimulation will lead to endometrial changes that reduce the rate of embryo implantation, particularly an out-of-phase endometrium following gonadotrophin ovarian stimulation and hCG follicle maturation. This is most likely to occur when there is an excessive response to stimulation and in that circumstance it would always be prudent to consider freezing of all embryos and avoiding fresh transfer – additionally to reduce the risk of ovarian hyperstimulation syndrome (OHSS). However there is little evidence in the literature of adverse endometrial development when mild ovarian stimulation techniques are employed or when IVF is undertaken in poor responder patients. In both of these situations, no evidence has been demonstrated for an improved live birth rate per oocyte collection, whether fresh embryo transfer was immediately instituted when compared to elective freezing and subsequent frozen embryo transfer [1].

Healy and co-workers reported a modest increased relative risk in both rare midline serious congenital anomalies as well as ante-partum bleeding in pregnancies resulting from fresh embryo transfer compared to frozen [2]. However the absolute anomaly rate was exceedingly low and the data was not stratified with respect to degree of stimulation response.

In contrast, there is evidence for an increased risk of other perinatal events in particular pre-eclampsia, in patients with PCOS undergoing frozen embryo transfer compared to fresh [3]. Additionally, IVF per se (either by the nature of the treatment itself or through the application of treatment to already at risk infertile women) increases risk of both perinatal and fetal problems, with no clear direction that leads us to conclude that elective embryo freezing is always advantageous.

Endometrial Preparation for Frozen Embryo Transfer is Always Advantageous in Creating the Best Environment for Implantation – There is sparse literature evidence comparing methods of endometrial preparation for frozen embryo transfer with respect to implantation. Because of small numbers and significant heterogeneity, a recent study [4] struggled to find benefit between the different forms of endometrial preparation but some benefit from largely natural cycle based protocols. However many units use exogenous estrogen and progesterone (often combined with a GnRH agonist), but this remains an artificial environment and leads to a first trimester in the absence of a corpus luteum, which as stated above might in some patient subsets elevate the risk of pre-eclampsia.

For anovulatory women, the only alternative to exogenous estrogen/progesterone is oral or gonadotrophin ovulation induction – usually with hCG trigger – which will presumably risk endometrial changes seen in fresh IVF cycles. For ovulatory women, there is the option of purely natural cycle based frozen embryo transfer but this may add complexity on both the patient's side and on the unit's side with respect to timing of transfer.

Embryo Vitrification Is a Highly Successful Technique with Effectively No Damage to Embryos Either During the Vitrification Step or During Warming -- Unfortunately, there is a known rate of both embryo loss during the vitrification process and failed embryo warming even in the most experienced hands. Whilst these issues are potentially minimised further by automated techniques, there will always be sporadic cases whereby a patient might have conceived through fresh embryo transfer but nonetheless loses that embryo in a program of mandatory vitrification.

Additionally, all IVF units have anecdotal evidence of embryos deemed 'not suitable to freeze' and yet when transferred, lead to successful pregnancies.

Ovarian Stimulation Combined with Elective Embryo Freezing, Allows the Patient to Have Preimplantation Genetic Screening (PGT-A), Which in Turn Improves Both Time-to-Successful-Pregnancy and a Reduction in Miscarriage Rate -- There is no evidence to sustain this argument. The STAR trial [5] found no improvement in either implantation rate or a reduction in miscarriage rate in unselected women undergoing elective PGT-A compared to controls. Furthermore it appears that blastocyst morphology alone is a powerful tool for selecting embryos with a higher likelihood of euploidy, for transfer.

Cost–Benefit Issues and Time Efficiency for Patients

A mandatory program of freezing all embryos implies that every patient's program will last at least two months to pregnancy compared to one month where prudent fresh embryo transfer was undertaken. Additionally there will undoubtedly be added cost for the patient, or if the added expense is borne by the IVF unit, the unit will experience lower margins.

Summary of the Risk–Benefit Trade-Off

For units that operate a system of selected fresh embryo transfers in appropriate cases, for low to medium responders there is little evidence of reduced embryo implantation and a very low risk of OHSS or other morbidity. In ongoing pregnancies with single embryo transfer, perinatal risks may be slightly elevated. In return, for the significant majority of patients prudently selected for fresh embryo transfer, many will achieve success in a shorter time frame and at less cost.

For units that operate a system of mandatory freezing of all embryos, one could expect essentially a zero rate of OHSS and a further reduced rate from an already very low likelihood) of fetal anomalies. Any reduction in some perinatal risks will be offset by an increase in pre-eclampsia rate in a reasonable subset of patients.

In summary, it cannot be argued that placing *all* patients on a mandatory program of freezing all embryos without fresh transfer, given the time delay and cost, in any real way benefits a selected subset of patients, in terms of ultimate outcome.

References

1. Roque M, Valle M, Sampaio M, Geber S. Does freeze-all policy affect IVF outcome in poor ovarian responders? *Ultrasound Obstet Gynecol*. 2018;52(4):530–4.

2. Healy DL, Breheny S, Halliday J, et al. Prevalence and risk factors for obstetric haemorrhage in 6730 singleton births after assisted reproductive technology in Victoria Australia. *Hum Reprod*. 2010;25 (1):265–74.

3. Chen Z-J, Shi Y, Sun Y, et al. Fresh versus frozen embryos for infertility in the polycystic ovary syndrome. *N Engl J Med*. 2016;375(6):523–33.

4. Yarali H, Polat M, Mumusoglu S, Yarali I, Bozdag G. Preparation of endometrium for frozen embryo replacement cycles: a systematic review and meta-analysis. *J Assist Reprod Genet*. 2016;33 (10):1287–304.

5. Munné S, Kaplan B, Frattarelli JL, et al. STAR Study Group: Preimplantation genetic testing for aneuploidy versus morphology as selection criteria for single frozen-thawed embryo transfer in good-prognosis patients: a multicenter randomized clinical trial. *Fertil Steril*. 2019 Dec;112(6):1071–9.

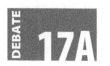

DEBATE 17A

Luteal-Phase Support Should Be Stopped at the Time of a Positive Pregnancy Test

For

Juan A Garcia-Velasco

Introduction

Many interventions in ART are not based on data but are rather empirical. Since ART was carried out in the early times of IVF, we have been trained in these 'classic' protocols, so we 'copy and paste' without critical thinking or analysis of the need of many of them.

What Happens in Nature – Spontaneous Pregnancy

In a spontaneous pregnancy, the corpus luteum produces progesterone after the LH surge. If pregnancy happens, the blastocyst will implant in the endometrium, hCG will be produced and this hCG will support the luteal phase and early days of pregnancy. In a few weeks, the placenta will appear and the steroidogenesis in this placental tissue will begin. In this natural, spontaneous pregnancy there is no need to add or supplement with anything, a perfectly designed and orchestrated steroid production happens in the human body: first the corpus luteum, then, the placenta after week 5/6, a phenomenon called luteo-placental shift [1].

Why Should We Supplement the Luteal Phase Pregnancy?

From the very beginning, it has been pointed out that the luteal phase in IVF after the hCG trigger is defective, and there is a need to supplement it, as much better results were obtained with luteal phase supplementation (LPS). Among the different hypotheses – granulosa cell aspiration after oocyte retrieval, strong pituitary suppression due to the GnRH analogues, luteolysis induced by the GnRH antagonists – the main reason for a defective luteal phase in IVF seems to be the extraordinarily high estradiol and progesterone levels that profoundly inhibit LH levels. At the same time, ovarian stimulation (OS) may alter endometrial maturation and receptivity, compromising the success of a fresh embryo transfer. Today, this is even more complex, as not all cycles are triggered by hCG. In fact, most high responders at risk of OHSS, PGT-A cycles, fertility preservation and donor cycles are triggered by GnRH agonist. And we do know that the luteal phase is absolutely distorted after GnRH agonist trigger, as the LH surge induced is significantly shorter in duration than the effect of hCG.

When Is Endogenous Progesterone Enough to Support the Corpus Luteum?

Physicians usually base their practice on evidence-based protocols, but not always. In fact, the duration of the LPS has been a matter of debate for the last few years. Although the luteo-placental shift happens around week 5/6, when endogenous production of steroids starts in the placental tissue, LPS has 'classically' extended until weeks 10–12. A web-based worldwide survey reported data from 408 IVF units and showed that, even though there is a lack of evidence to continue LPS beyond the luteo-placental shift, there is a tendency to maintain progesterone supplementation up to 8–10 weeks or even 12 weeks of pregnancy [2].

The first RCT on the subject was published in 2002. Nyboe Andersen et al. [3] performed a randomised trial showing that once the pregnancy was established and beta-HCG was detected, no further benefit was obtained by supplementing patients with progesterone. Theoretically, this circulating hCG being produced by the invading tropho-blast in the decidualised endometrium was sufficient to maintain the corpus luteum and the pregnancy till the luteo-placental shift could happen.

A few years later, Aboulghar et al. [4] issued a questionnaire among 21 leading IVF units around the world, trying to understand the current practice around the globe. The study clearly showed the lack of international consensus, as the duration of LPS in the question-naire varied from the day of the positive pregnancy test, up to 12 weeks of pregnancy in different centres [4]. In the same publication, the authors randomised 257 women to either stop LPS at the time of the first ultrasound (around week 6 of pregnancy) versus continuing for three additional weeks. The authors observed comparable miscarriage rates or bleeding episodes between both groups, so they did not support extending the LPS beyond the day of first ultrasound demonstrating fetal heartbeat.

Since then, a few more RCTs have been published. In the USA, Goudge et al. [5] performed a randomised trial using progesterone in oil in good prognosis patients undergo-ing their first IVF cycle with fresh embryo transfer. They randomised 101 women to either the standard protocol of 50 mg of progesterone in oil for at least 6 weeks of LPS vs. only 11 days. The authors found comparable pregnancy rates and live birth rates.

In Europe, Kyrou et al. [6] published a larger study with 200 women who underwent IVF and obtained a positive beta-hCG: they were randomised to standard vaginal progester-one 200 mg t.i.d. for 7 weeks as LPS versus early stopping of progesterone 16 days post embryo transfer. Similar pregnancy rates, miscarriage rates and bleeding episodes were described. The authors concluded that the withdrawal of progesterone supplementation in early pregnancy, with normally increasing β-hCG levels on the 16th day post-ET, had no significant clinical impact in terms of ongoing pregnancy rates beyond 12 weeks.

Almost at the same time, we published a randomised trial with a similar design in which 220 women were randomised to either conventional LPS after a fresh embryo transfer with vaginal progesterone 200 mg b.i.d. for 8 weeks versus stopping the LPS on week 5/6, once the gestational sac was visible [7]. We measured serum progesterone levels on the day of the first pregnancy ultrasound exam (149 ± 108 vs. 167 ± 115 ng/mL). Significantly more bleeding episodes were observed in the first trimester in the group with early cessation of progesterone supplementation (18.0 ± 2.6 vs. 7.2 ± 1.3 episodes). Miscarriage rates among singleton pregnancies were similar in the two groups (5/80 vs. 6/79). So, we could conclude that vaginal progesterone supplementation after IVF/ICSI can be safely withdrawn at 5 weeks' gestation, because cycle outcome was similar to conventional luteal phase support up to 8 weeks of pregnancy [7].

Similarly, in Asia, Liu et al. [8] published a meta-analysis summarising the results of 1201 randomised patients. They concluded that with the currently available evidence, progesterone supplementation beyond the first positive hCG test after IVF/ICSI might generally be unnecessary.

So, all studies were in the same direction, suggesting that we may be over-treating our patients with unnecessary duration of the LPS, with the discomfort that vaginal progester-one may cause, the additional costs and the hypothetical risks.

A more recent questionnaire by Vaisbuch et al. in 2014 [2] analysed data from 408 centres in 82 countries representing a total of 284,600 IVF cycles/year were included. In this particular study, in 72% of cycles, LPS was administered until 8–10 weeks' gestation or beyond. This questionnaire confirmed that, although there is no firm evidence supporting the continuation of LPS after the demonstration of fetal heart beat on ultrasound, this remains the common practice of most assisted reproduction centres worldwide.

So, Why Go Beyond What Is Needed?

First of all, in ART there are a lot of procedures and treatments that are based on empirism, not on data. Doctors and embryologists (and patients) fear to change anything if previous results are good; the uncertainty of a change makes it difficult to take the risk and try new protocols in a very pragmatic practice. Also, the fact that progesterone is an inexpensive drug, with a very low risk (not zero) for the fetus makes it even more difficult not to give it up. And finally, the increased number of frozen embryo transfers, where no corpus luteum exists and there is a need to supplement for the first 10–12 weeks, makes it a bit more complex. However, data is solid, robust, reproducible and we should aim for the most effective treatment for our patients, with the least interventions possible and lowest side effects, including unnecessary drugs.

References

1. Scott R, Navot D, Liu HC, Rosenwaks Z. A human in vivo model for the luteoplacental shift. *Fertil Steril.* 1991;56:481–4.

2. Vaisbuch E, de Zeigler D, Leong M, Weissman A, Shoham Z. Luteal-phase support in ART: real life practices reported worldwide by an updated website-based survey. *Reprod Biomed Online.* 2014;28:330–5.

3. Nyboe Andersen A, Popovic-Todorovic B, Schmidt KT, et al. Progesterone supplementation during early gestations after IVF or ICSI has no effect on the delivery rates: a randomized controlled trial. *Hum Reprod.* 2002;17:357–61.

4. Aboulghar M, Amin Y, Al-Inany H, et al. Prospective randomized study comparing luteal phase support for ICSI patients up to the first ultrasound compared with an additional three weeks. *Hum Reprod.* 2008;23:857–62.

5. Goudge C, Nagel T, Damario M. Duration of progesterone-in-oil support after in vitro fertilization and embryo transfer: a randomized, controlled trial. *Fertil Steril.* 2010;94:946–51.

6. Kyrou D, Fatemi H, Zepiridis L, et al. Does cessation of progesterone supplementation during early pregnancy in patients treated with recFSH/GnRH antagonist affect ongoing pregnancy rates? A randomized controlled trial. *Hum Reprod.* 2011;26:1020–4.

7. Kohls G, Ruiz F, Martínez M, et al. Early progesterone cessation after in vitro fertilization/intracytoplasmic sperm injection: a randomized, controlled trial. *Fertil Steril.* 2012;98:858–62.

8. Liu X, Mu H, Shi Q, et al. The optimal duration of progesterone supplementation in pregnant women after IVF/ICSI: a meta-analysis. *Reprod Biol Endocrinol.* 2012;10:107.

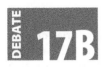

Luteal Phase Support Should Be Stopped at the Time of a Positive Pregnancy Test

Against

Ariel Weissman

The pivotal role of luteal phase support (LPS) in establishing and maintaining IVF pregnancies has been one of the earliest subjects to become evidence-based in clinical ART. Following controlled ovarian stimulation (COS) and ovulation triggering by hCG, pulsatile pituitary LH secretion has been demonstrated to be severely compromised and unable to support normal function of the corpora lutea, resulting in a deficient luteal phase that must be pharmaceutically supported. This was initially demonstrated for GnRH agonist protocols and subsequently confirmed for GnRH antagonist cycles as well. After implantation, embryonic hCG takes over pituitary LH in supporting the corpus luteum (CL) and maintains its function until the establishment of the luteo-placental shift, at around the 8th gestational week. It has been clearly demonstrated that LPS is crucial in filling the gap between the disappearance of exogenously administered hCG for ovulation triggering and the initiation of secretion of endogenous hCG from the implanting conceptus. Early studies have estimated that exogenously administered hCG remains in the circulation for up to 7 days, and that the CL has a remarkable ability to recover after a week of deprivation from gonadotropin stimulation [1]. Thus, LPS in the form of exogenously administered progesterone and/or hCG has become an integral part of fresh IVF cycles. In terms of duration, without clear biological rationale or robust evidence for any clinical benefits, it became common practice to support the corpora lutea of pregnancy until the establishment of the luteo-placental shift, at 8 or even 10 or 12 gestational weeks [2].

Several investigators have questioned the efficacy of LPS beyond the point of pregnancy establishment. Retrospective as well as prospective studies have compared early cessation of LPS either at the time of positive hCG test or early pregnancy ultrasound versus LPS administration until 7–8 gestational weeks. In the majority of studies patients were carefully selected for inclusion based on normal rising hCG patterns, absence of vaginal bleeding episodes, favourable serum progesterone levels, serum estradiol levels, age and even normal early (5 weeks) or 6–7 weeks pregnancy ultrasound. Thus, it appears that carefully selected, good prognosis, rather than treatment naïve patients were studied. Despite the bias and heterogeneity introduced by patient selection criteria, a recent meta-analysis by Watters et al. [3] summarised the results of seven randomised trials including 1627 participants, and found similar live birth, miscarriage and ongoing pregnancy rates with early versus late LPS cessation. The authors concluded that prolonged progesterone supplementation after fresh embryo transfer might be unnecessary.

Most LPS regimens are certainly not patient-friendly and harbour discomfort, side effects and complications as well as added cost to treatment. Therefore, reducing the duration of LPS to a minimum should be considered progress in patient management that may improve patients' convenience and compliance to treatment. While it has been more than a decade that the above RCTs have been published, the scientific community has been reluctant to adopt early cessation of LPS. This can be evidenced from the materials and methods section of the most recent papers and examining the results of a series of web-based surveys (https://ivf-worldwide.com/survey.html) that evaluated the practice of LPS. A close look at four such surveys conducted over the last decade (2009–2019) reveals that the majority (>60%) of clinicians world-wide administer LPS until eight gestational weeks and beyond, without any significant change in trends over the years. These findings represent the 'wisdom of the crowd' and the perception that the quality of data regarding early cessation of LPS is weak and insufficient to allow a change in practice. Clinicians need to obtain a high level of confidence of 'primum non nocere' or 'first do no harm' before routine early withdrawal of LPS.

Griesinger has estimated that for a non-inferiority trial showing a difference of –4% or larger from a live birth rate of 80%, a sample size of 3140 women with a positive pregnancy test would be required [4]. Moreover, an optimal study should be placebo-controlled and all patients with a positive pregnancy test should be randomised and included. Specific patient populations such as high and low responders, young and advanced maternal age, a history of early bleeding episodes or with endometriosis and those with recurrent pregnancy loss should be evaluated separately in detail. The choice of ovulation triggering method, hCG, GnRH agonist or their combination, should also be considered.

Over the years, significant advances have been made in optimising ovarian stimulation protocols, and individualisation has become a major component of COS nowadays. The luteal phase, however, has been neglected in this sense, and practice of 'one size fits all' has become the rule in the majority of ART programs, as most patients receive the same fixed regimen of LPS. There is a crucial need to develop advanced techniques to evaluate and monitor CL function from the mid-luteal phase and the efficiency of CL rescue by the ensuing pregnancy. This could allow individualisation of both the extent and the duration of LPS. With current regimens of LPS, serum progesterone measurements can be used, but are confounded by a lack of distinction between ovarian and exogenously administered progesterone. Serum LH and hCG levels can be monitored as well. Other options include: administration of progestogens such as dydrogesterone that due to its chemical properties does not cross-react with endogenous progesterone measured in the serum, allowing exclusive analysis of progesterone from CL origin [5] or study of other yet undefined non-steroidal substances produced by the CL which may reflect its function or dysfunction.

The quality and quantity of data related to early cessation of LPS in fresh IVF cycles is insufficient to justify a change in the current practice, which includes administration of LPS until the establishment of the luteo-placental shift. Better understanding of CL function following various COS regimens and ovulation triggering agents may allow individualisation of LPS regimens according to specific patients' requirements. Individualisation of LPS should receive high priority of future research in the field of clinical ART.

References

1. Weissman A, Loumaye E, Shoham Z. Recovery of corpus luteum function after prolonged deprivation from gonadotrophin stimulation. *Hum Reprod.* 1996;11:943–9.

2. Vaisbuch E, de Ziegler D, Leong M, Weissman A, Shoham Z. Luteal-phase support in assisted reproduction treatment: real-life practices reported worldwide by an updated website-based survey. *Reprod Biomed.* 2014;28:330–5.

3. Watters M, Noble M, Child T, Nelson S. Short versus extended progesterone supplementation for luteal phase support in fresh IVF cycles: a systematic review and meta-analysis. *Reproduct Biomed.* 2019.

4. Griesinger G. Editorial commentary: is it time to abandon progesterone supplementation of early pregnancy after IVF? *Hum Reprod.* 2011;26:1017–19.

5. Neumann K, Depenbusch M, Schultze-Mosgau A, Griesinger G. Characterization of early pregnancy placental progesterone production by utilization of dydrogesterone in programmed frozen-thawed embryo transfer cycles. *Reprod Biomed.* 2020.

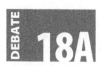

A Natural Cycle Is the Best Protocol for Frozen Embryo Replacement

For

Raoul Orvieto

With the recent trend toward single embryo transfer (ET) or freeze-all strategy adopted in an attempt to reduce the risk of multiple pregnancy and ovarian hyperstimulation syndrome, respectively, the remaining extra embryos are cryopreserved, providing further possibilities for conception after the initial fresh transfer. This trend results in the cryopreservation of the surplus embryos for future replacement.

There are several currently employed replacement protocols for frozen-thawed embryo transfer (FET) [1]. The choice of protocol depends on the individual woman's ovarian function and convenience of the method, as well as on the experience gained with the method by the physicians. According to the meta-analysis of Groenewoud et al. (2017), no compelling advantage for one protocol over another could be demonstrated [2], with a trend toward a higher live-birth rate (LBR) observed in favour of natural cycle FET (NC-FET) over artificial cycle FET (AC-FET) (OR-1.23; 95% CI 0.93–1.62).

Live Birth Rates, NC-FET vs. AC-FET

Since this meta-analysis, several other studies appeared, clearly supporting the use of NC-FET over AC-FET. Orvieto et al. [3] evaluated the outcome of NC-FET with modified luteal support vs AC-FET. Implantation, clinical and ongoing pregnancy rates were found to be significantly higher in patients undergoing the NC-FET cycle with the modified luteal support as compared to AC-FET cycle. In this cohort study, patients undergoing NC-FET were monitored by serial ultrasound for endometrial thickness, follicular development, and LH and progesterone levels, until a rise in LH level (LH level exceeds 180% of the baseline value) and a decrease in E2 level (>25% drop in E2 levels), corresponding to a day prior to OPU/ovulation. All patients were instructed to start a modified luteal support, consisting of daily vaginal progesterone started on the day of ovulation, with two additional injections, one of recombinant hCG (Ovitrelle, Merck Serono, Herzliya, Israel; s.c. 250 mcg) and the other of GnRH-agonist (Triptorelin, Ferring Lapidot, Netanya, Israel; s.c. 0.1 mg), on day of cleaved-stage (Day-3) transfer and 4 days later, respectively.

Even of more interest is the retrospective cohort study by Melnick et al. [4]. They compared pregnancy outcome between NC-FET and AC-FET in patients undergoing *euploid* blastocysts transfer, thus, excluding the embryo quality as a possible confounder. In accordance with the previous study, they also demonstrated significantly higher live birth/ongoing pregnancy rate in NC-FET compared to the AC-FET.

Recently, two large retrospective cohort studies consisting of >100,000 patients have also demonstrated the advantage of NC-FET over the AC-FET. Saito et al. [5] studied pregnancy outcomes of patients who underwent FET and found that patients who conceived by AC-FET (*n* = 75,474) yielded significantly lower pregnancy rate and LBR in comparison to those who conceived following NC-FET (n = 29,760). Another larger study also demonstrated significantly higher clinical pregnancy rate and LBR in the NC-FET group (n = 8425) compared to the AC-FET group (n = 2611).

Obstetrics and Perinatal Outcomes, NC-FET vs. AC-FET

During the last decade, several studies assessed obstetric and perinatal outcomes associated with FET compared to fresh ET and natural conception. FET cycles were consistently shown to be associated with lower risk of prematurity, small for gestational age, and low birth weight and increased risk of large for gestational and/or macrosomia in singletons, when compared with fresh ET. Moreover, higher relative risk of hypertensive disorders in pregnancy, as well as perinatal mortality were also demonstrated to be increased in FET compared with singletons from fresh ET and natural conception.

Recent studies have related the aforementioned pregnancy complications to the endometrial priming and not to the cryopreservation process, with higher risk in programmed FET rather than those following natural and stimulated cycles. A link between the presence or absence of corpus luteum (CL) in ART cycles and pre-eclampsia has been suggested. Higher rates of pre-eclampsia were observed in AC-FET cycles, where no CL is present, compared to natural or stimulated FET cycles where one or more CL occur. They related this observation to circulating relaxin, as the biologically plausible mediator, which is derived solely from the CL. Since relaxin is a known potent vasodilator which increases arterial compliance, the absence of CL during AC-FET, with the consequent undetected circulating relaxin levels, might contribute to the attenuated increase in central arterial compliance and the observed higher preeclampsia risk in pregnant women lacking a CL.

Conclusions

The choice of protocol for FET cycle depends on the individual woman's ovarian function and convenience of the method, as well as on the experience gained with the method by the physicians. It appears, that in ovulatory women, endometrial preparation for FET which includes NC-FET, with or without modified/luteal support, results in the highest LBR with lower obstetric complications. It seems that when considering elective freeze-all policy, in addition to LBR and the risk of OHSS, physicians should also consider the FET cycles' pregnancy complications, including LGA/macrosomia, hypertensive disorders of pregnancy, as well as perinatal mortality. Thus, FET following natural cycle is advised aiming to reduce adverse outcomes.

References

1. Orvieto R, Fisch B, Feldberg D. Endometrial preparation for patients undergoing frozen-thawed embryo transfer cycles. In: *The Art & Science of Assisted Reproductive Techniques*. G. Allahbadia, R. Basuray, R. Merchant, eds. Jaypee Brothers Medical Publishers (P) Ltd. New Delhi, India, 2003, pp. 396–9.

2. Groenewoud ER, Cantineau AE, Kollen BJ, Macklon NS, Cohlen BJ. What is the optimal means of preparing the endometrium in frozen-thawed embryo transfer cycles? A systematic review and meta-analysis. *Hum Reprod Update.* 2017;23(2):255–61.

3. Orvieto R, Feldman N, Lantsberg D, Manela D, Zilberberg E, Haas J. Natural cycle frozen-thawed embryo transfer-can we improve cycle outcome? *J Assist Reprod Genet.* 2016;33(5):611–15.

4. Melnick AP, Setton R, Stone LD, et al. Replacing single frozen-thawed euploid embryos in a natural cycle in ovulatory

women may increase live birth rates compared to medicated cycles in anovulatory women. *J Assist Reprod Genet.* 2017;34(10):1325–31.

5. Saito K, Kuwahara A, Ishikawa T, et al. Endometrial preparation methods for frozen-thawed embryo transfer are associated with altered risks of hypertensive disorders of pregnancy, placenta accreta, and gestational diabetes mellitus. *Hum Reprod.* 2019;34(8):1567–75.

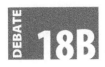

18B

A Natural Cycle Is the Best Protocol for Frozen Embryo Replacement

Against

Ben Cohlen

Introduction

Frozen-thawed embryo transfer (FET) is becoming increasingly important in the armamentarium of assisted reproductive medicine. In the Netherlands, in 2018, 46% of all ongoing pregnancies were the result of a FET cycle. More and more fertility centres offer freeze all cycles to prevent OHSS. Nevertheless, there remains controversy regarding the optimal method of preparing the endometrium of normal ovulatory women before FET. The most applied protocols are the artificial FET cycle, the true natural FET cycle and the modified natural FET cycle. In an artificial FET cycle, the endometrium is prepared by applying oestrogens and progesterone to mimic a natural cycle. Oestrogen is applied until the endometrium reaches a thickness of least 7 mm and then progesterone is added. In a true natural FET cycle the spontaneous LH surge is detected by LH testing in urine or blood to plan thawing and transfer. In a modified natural cycle, hCG is given once the follicle has reached a mean diameter of 16–18 mm with an adequate endometrium thickness. This paper will show that the artificial cycle FET should be offered to all ovulatory women instead of the (modified) natural cycle FET.

Evidence

In this era of evidence-based medicine, we cannot ignore the results of systematic reviews. In 2013, a large systematic review and meta-analysis on this subject was published comparing various methods of endometrium preparation in FET cycles. The authors were clear; no statistically significant differences in clinical pregnancy rate, ongoing pregnancy rate or live birth rate were found [1]. In 2017, a correction on the data was published that did not alter the overall conclusions. However, a subgroup analysis revealed that artificial cycle FET using a GnRH agonist to suppress spontaneous ovulation was superior to natural cycle FET (OR 1.25. 95% CI 1.03–1.52) [2]. In 2016, the first large randomized controlled multicenter non-inferiority trial was published comparing natural versus artificial FET cycles [3]. Again, no statistically significant differences were found with regard to live birth rates, clinical and ongoing pregnancy rates. Furthermore, the costs of both treatment approaches were comparable (just above € 600 per cycle). The authors did find a statistically significant difference in cycle cancellation, with more cycles being cancelled in artificial cycle FET. Introducing a GnRH agonist might prevent these cancellations favouring the outcome of artificial cycle FET further.

Shared Decision-Making

The role of the modern physician is changing from the one who decides what is best for his patients towards a more coaching role, informing the patients about the options, the pros and cons of each option in order to decide together what option to choose. In shared decision-making, the view of the clinical expert is merged with the view of the patient and the evidence from literature.

Evidence shows that artificial FET cycles are at least as cost-effective as true or modified natural FET cycles, making the patient preference and the expertise of a fertility centre more determinative.

From a logistic point of view, the artificial FET cycle has great advantages. One can spread transfers throughout the week, and consider skipping the weekends just by prolonging or shortening oestrogen intake before adding progesterone. One ultrasound check will be sufficient to be able to detect unexpected follicular growth, to measure endometrial thickness and to time the addition of progesterone and thus thawing. Although oestrogen intake in artificial cycles does not suppress follicular development in all cycles, adding a GnRH agonist to prevent this will increase the costs substantially. In a previous study, the cancellation rate of artificial FET cycles was significantly higher compared with modified natural FET cycles due to thin endometrium [3]. However, the influence of endometrial thickness on pregnancy rates in FET cycles is still unclear [4].

The preference of patients might vary tremendously. In a true natural FET cycle, the LH surge has to be detected on time. It is known that LH testing in urine is a source of uncertainty because of the high percentages of false positive or negative testing, due to substantial inter-patient and cycle variation in LH surge amplitude and shape [5]. This can lead to default planning of thawing and transferring. LH testing in urine can be replaced by testing in blood and/or ultrasound monitoring. Besides increasing the costs substantially, patients have to visit the outpatient clinic several times per cycle. The same accounts for the modified natural cycle with ultrasound monitoring and hCG administration once the follicle is 16 to 18 mm. If LH is not determined, spontaneous LH surges might be missed and thawing might be scheduled too late. All these disadvantages of the true and modified natural cycle can be overcome by applying an artificial FET protocol with one ultrasound investigation before the start of progesterone.

Conclusion

Nowadays FET is applied extensively and preparation of the endometrium can be done various ways. There is no evidence of superiority of any of the well-known protocols. Thus, patient and clinic preference is decisive. After listing all advantages and disadvantages of each protocol to make a shared decision, it cannot be otherwise than both patients and fertility specialists choose the artificial FET cycle for optimal preparation of the endometrium.

References

1. Groenewoud ER, Cantineau AE, Kollen BJ, Macklon NS, Cohlen BJ. What is the optimal means of preparing the endometrium in frozen-thawed embryo transfer cycles? A systematic review and meta-analysis. *Hum Reprod Update.* 2013;19(5):458–70.

2. Erratum in: *Hum Reprod Update.* 2017;23(2):255–61.

3. Groenewoud ER, Cohlen BJ, Al-Oraiby A, et al. A randomized controlled, non-inferiority trial of modified natural versus artificial cycle for cryo-thawed embryo transfer. *Hum Reprod.* 2016;31(7):1483–92.

4. Groenewoud ER, Cohlen BJ, Al-Oraiby A, et al. Influence of endometrial thickness on pregnancy rates in modified natural cycle frozen-thawed embryo transfer. *Acta Obstet Gynecol Scand.* 2018;97(7):808–15.

5. Miller PB, Soules MR. The usefulness of a urinary LH kit for ovulation prediction during menstrual cycles of normal women. *Obstet Gynecol.* 1996;87:13–17.

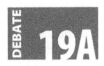

19A All Pregnancies Conceived by IVF Should Be Delivered by Caesarean Section

For

James Hopkisson

Our gold standard aims in the delivery of twenty-first century assisted conception programmes is the delivery of a healthy single baby with a healthy mother. IVF singleton pregnancies are still unfortunately at increased risk of pre-eclampsia, gestational diabetes, placenta praevia, and perinatal mortality. IVF singleton pregnancies also have a higher relative risk of having induction of labour and caesarean section (CS), both emergency and elective. Part of this can be laid at the door of both the obstetrician and patient, with postal surveys of obstetricians confirming this often-held belief. Many studies indicate that rates of caesarean section are significantly higher after assisted than after natural conception. This practice has previously been described as the 'precious baby' effect.

All pregnancies are precious; those that have required the investigation of delayed conception, potential surgical interventions leading up to and then IVF treatment can be considered even more so. With this increased risk I am reminded of the words from one of my old slightly more paternalistic consultant mentors that has stuck with me throughout my career when discussing elective caesarean section: 'My dear boy when deciding on the mode of delivery we must remember that most women will not deliver that often and we must get it right every time as the consequences remain with us all for a lifetime.' Should we opt for the lowest risk strategy for delivery for a group of women who may be pregnant once or twice in their lives with a pregnancy that has been achieved with much 'investment', often physical, emotional and financial?

Much has been written about the right to request elective caesarean section over the last 20 years for those who wish to deliver in a controlled environment, to avoid the anxiety and risks of emergency intervention, perineal trauma or being classed 'too posh to push'. Should we mandate that all pregnancies conceived through IVF and assisted conception should be delivered by caesarean section? This perhaps to some may be a step too far but at least it should be offered to all without the clinician and patient being made to feel that they are deviating from an establishment 'norm' that dictates that unit and national rates of caesarean section are put above autonomy and choice.

What are the risks of elective caesarean section at 39 weeks? These have been minimised over the years, with advances in regional anaesthesia, operative technique, post-operative management and changes in medical staffing. It is indisputable that the risks of an elective procedure are much lower than those of an emergency caesarean section in labour. It is a fact that numerous caesarean sections increase the risks of placenta praevia, morbidly adherent placenta, and miscarriage. Rates of surgical intervention increase with induction of labour, so let us move forward and advocate a policy of caesarean section for all. Many IVF patients will ask for induction of labour and many obstetricians will agree to this intervention, however the process of induction of labour in nulliparous and multiparous women should be seen as carrying a higher risk of obstetric intervention and emergency delivery, something therefore to be avoided.

Concerns have been expressed that multiple deliveries by caesarean section lead to excessive risk. The NICE guideline on caesarean sections for maternal request is clear and we as obstetricians should inform: 'that women who have had up to and including four caesarean sections that the risk of fever, bladder injuries and surgical injuries does not vary with planned mode of birth and that the risk of uterine rupture, although higher for planned vaginal birth, is rare.' Those having IVF rarely get to be lucky enough to go through four singleton pregnancies in a lifetime.

Those women who have an IVF conception and deliver by caesarean section and then go onto conceive spontaneously should be made aware that pregnant women with both previous CS and a previous vaginal delivery have an increased likelihood of achieving a vaginal birth than women who have had a previous CS but no previous vaginal birth. Being informed of risks at the outset is key.

If the question that is asked is: 'Should all women with IVF pregnancies be offered elective caesarean section at 39 weeks?' it would be clear cut and there be no need for debate as the answer would be a resounding 'Yes'. To mandate is to remove choice and that is never a good idea. In the cases of increased maternal age, multiple birth, and egg donation it strikes me that this medical intervention will minimise birth risk and we should be offering an elective delivery by caesarean section.

Unfortunately, at the time of writing there is still little evidence that pre-labour caesarean section as a birth option improves outcomes for mothers and their infants. Obstetricians should continue to support evidenced-based decision-making that includes advocacy for maternal choice on mode of delivery. Overplaying the risks of fever, infection, pneumonia, and thromboembolic events that are increased with emergency caesarean delivery should not be the norm when discussing elective surgical delivery. As for the baby's health, we know when an embryo is replaced in an IVF programme, pre-labour caesarean deliveries should not be performed before 39 weeks of gestation and thus the adverse neonatal outcomes such as mechanical ventilation, newborn sepsis, hypoglycaemia, and admission to the neonatal ICU should be minimised.

As suggested some pregnancies are just 'too precious to push', and we should be open to offering operative delivery in a controlled setting to minimise the well-documented risks of induction and labour.

Further Reading

Braude P. One child at a time. Reducing multiple births after IVF. Report of the Expert Group on Multiple Births after IVF. London: HFEA, 2006. [www.oneatatime.org.uk/images/MBSET_report_Final_Dec_06.pdf]

Hayashi M, Nakai A, Satoh S, Matsuda Y. Adverse obstetric and perinatal outcomes of singleton pregnancies may be related to maternal factors associated with infertility rather than the type of assisted reproductive technology procedure used. *Fertil Steril.* 2012;98:922–8.

NICE. Caesarean section. Clinical guideline [CG132] NICE, 2011.

RCOG. In Vitro Fertilisation: Perinatal Risks and Early Childhood Outcomes. Scientific Impact Paper No. 8, May 2012.

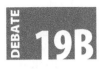

All Pregnancies Conceived by IVF Should Be Delivered by Caesarean Section

Against

Claudia Raperport

'First do no harm.'

Caesarean section has been normalised in a world where birth trauma, bad outcomes and pain are seen as unacceptable despite being a historical reality of child-bearing.

In a society where it is increasingly easy to control most aspects of life, labour and childbirth remain a difficult and unpredictable process. Anxiety surrounding this is high amongst pregnant women but also their care providers who are responsible for the outcomes of both mother and child and who also carry personal risk in this litiginous era. This anxiety seems even more prevalent in pregnancies that were difficult to achieve and long-awaited.

One challenge of caring for the pregnant woman in the NHS as well as many other international health-care systems is the lack of continuity of care. Many obstetricians and midwives will not see women in their next pregnancy or into their following stages of life. They are not responsible for the returning patient with the morbidly adherent placenta or the woman requiring pelvic surgery later in life in whom surgical adhesions make the procedure significantly more dangerous.

What risks are avoided by performing caesarean sections? There has been a general increase in caesarean section rates across the developed world with average rates in the UK and US reaching above 30%.

Anecdotally it is felt that bypassing labour avoids risk of hypoxic injury or traumatic injury, improving the safety of both fetus and mother and that a chosen date of delivery with a calm pre- and intra-delivery period with no imminent emergency is an 'easier way to deliver'.

However, clinicians have a responsibility to practice evidence-based medicine and the evidence does not support this practice.

UK NICE guidance suggests that caesarean section confers no benefit to the baby compared to planned vaginal birth. In fact it increases several maternal risks including length of hospital stay, obstetric haemorrhage, cardiac arrest [1].

In the US, an epidemiological study in 2008 showed an increased neonatal mortality associated with elective caesarean section with an odds ratio of 1.69 compared with planned vaginal birth. Outcomes for both the neonate and mother were worse after caesarean section [2].

The findings of these population studies must of course, be applied with caution to any individual case.

There are certainly factors which make caesarean section the safest mode of delivery, many of which may apply to women after conceiving through assisted reproductive technology (ART). NICE guidance suggests caesarean for pregnancies with placenta praevia or morbidly adherent placenta, breech presentation and maternal blood-borne infection.

Other indications may include multiple pregnancy, fetal compromise associated with intrauterine growth restriction and medical concerns for example pre-eclampsia. Women who conceived with ART may well have a higher incidence of these risk factors compared with spontaneous conceptions especially those with increased maternal age and those receiving donor oocytes. There is no evidence that ART itself represents a risk factor for maternal or fetal morbidity in labour.

Is there evidence that elective caesarean is safest in IVF/ICSI pregnancies? No study has been published specifically comparing mode of delivery within ART-conceived pregnancies. There are several studies investigating perinatal outcomes, all of which are observational. These do support the theory that these pregnancies are higher risk and more likely to involve maternal and neonatal morbidity, however the role that caesarean section plays could be contributing to morbidity rather than reducing it.

The largest meta-analysis to date, comparing IVF/ICSI-conceived pregnancies with spontaneous conceptions, showed small absolute increases in risk of hypertensive disorders, low birth weight and preterm delivery [3]. The risk of perinatal mortality was not significant when results were analysed with random effects to counteract study heterogeneity. The relative risk of neonatal admission was 1.58 (1.42–1.77) but does not report cause for admission.

A study published in 2018 in the *British Medical Journal* showed that maternal morbidities were more common in ART-conceived pregnancies (27.1 versus 5.7%, $P < 0.0001$ for potentially life-threatening conditions; 2.6 versus 0.3%, $P < 0.0001$ for near-miss events) [4]. However, when broken down, two of the three most common reasons for near-miss were peripartum hysterectomy and haemorrhage requiring >5 units of blood transfusion. Caesarean section increases the risk of both of these complications.

Another large study supported the findings of increased risk of pre-term delivery (<32 weeks gestation) and low birthweight in IVF/ICSI conceived pregnancies [5]. It went on to comment that there was a 69% caesarean section rate amongst the study group, with many of the indications for caesarean only being IVF/ICSI conception. There was no difference in rates of stillbirth or neonatal death.

Caesarean sections rates are higher for ART-conceived pregnancies. This is partially iatrogenic and possibly contributing towards the increased risk of preterm birth associated with ART. Caesarean section is an independently recognised risk factor for neonatal unit admission (RR 2.2 (1.4–3.18)) so it is difficult to use this as an argument FOR routine caesarean delivery.

In vitro fertilisation pregnancies can be considered as 'more precious' considering the journey the pregnant woman has taken to arrive at the point of labour. This logic is not, however, extended to single women and same-sex couples who require insemination procedures after spending huge amounts of money on donor sperm, or women who conceive spontaneously or through ovulation induction but might have been trying unsuccessfully for just as many years. If a young woman had one IVF cycle after a year of subfertility, which led to 15 top quality blastocysts and a likelihood of as large a family as she desires, does that warrant the defensive decision for a caesarean section?

The evidence states that caesarean section is not safer for mother or child. I therefore believe that every pregnancy requires assessment according to an evidence-based risk model and that the gynaecological, obstetric, medical and social background of each woman should be considered when forming a birth plan. A blanket policy of caesarean section for all IVF-conceived pregnancies is dangerous, unnecessary and bad medicine.

References

1. National Institute for Clinical Excellence (NICE). Caesarean section Clinical guideline [CG132] Published date: November 2011 Last updated: September 2019.

2. MacDorman MF, Menacker F, Declercq E. Cesarean birth in the United States: epidemiology, trends, and outcomes. *Clin Perinatol.* 2008;35(2):293–307.

3   Pandey S, Shetty A, Hamilton M, Bhattacharya S, Maheshwari A. Obstetric and perinatal outcomes in singleton pregnancies resulting from IVF/ICSI: a systematic review and meta-analysis. *Hum Reprod Update.* 2012;18(5):485–503.

4. Cromi A, Marconi N, Casarin J, et al. Maternal intra- and postpartum near-miss following assisted reproductive technology: a retrospective study. *BMJ.* 2018; 125:12.

5. Szymusik I, Kosinska-Kaczynska K, Krowicka M, et al. Perinatal outcome of in vitro fertilization singletons – 10 years' experience of one center. *Arch Med Sci.* 2019;15(3):666–72.

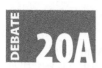

Endometriosis Should Be Suppressed for 6–12 Weeks before Frozen Embryo Transfer

For

Hassan N Sallam

Various management options exist for the treatment of endometriosis-associated infertility. These include medical treatment, surgical treatment and a combination of both. When these options fail to produce a pregnancy, assisted reproduction is resorted to, ranging from intrauterine insemination (IUI) for minimal and mild cases of endometriosis to IVF and ICSI for those who do not achieve a pregnancy with IUI and for more advanced cases [1]. However, the clinical outcomes of IVF in patients with endometriosis-associated infertility seem to be diminished in comparison to patients suffering from tubal or unexplained infertility. In 2016, Senapati et al. published data from 347,185 fresh and frozen ART cycles included in the SART Database, performed between 2008 and 2010. These included data from 39,356 cycles of patients with endometriosis (11% of the study sample), of whom 14,053 cycles were in women who had an isolated diagnosis of endometriosis (4% of the sample). They found that women with a diagnosis of endometriosis had a reduction in oocyte yield (RR 0.91 [0.91–0.92]), implantation rate (RR 0.94 [0.93–0.96]), proportion of blastocyst transfer (RR 0.96 [0.93–0.99]) and a 6% reduction in in live birth rate compared to women without endometriosis (RR 0.94 [0.91–0.97]). Subgroup analyses of data from patients with isolated endometriosis produced similar results although the differences were less dramatic [2].

Numerous explanations were offered for these lower outcomes including a diminished ovarian reserve resulting in a higher cancellation rate, diminished quality of oocytes resulting in a diminished fertilisation rate, a defective endometrium resulting in a lower implantation rate as well as a combination of all these factors. The diminished quality of the oocytes was linked to increased follicular fluid concentrations of progesterone, interleukin-6 (IL-6), lower follicular fluid concentrations of cortisol, insulin-like growth factor binding protein-one (IGFBP-1) and/or an increased expression of tumour necrotising factor-alpha (TNF-alpha) in the cultured granulose cells from women with endometriosis [1]. The rate of apoptosis in the granulose cells obtained from women with endometriosis is also increased and this may be mediated by elevated concentrations of soluble Fas ligand in the serum and peritoneal fluid of these women [1]. In addition, the lower implantation rates were linked to altered HOXA10 gene expression, altered endometrial receptivity and/or progesterone resistance [2].

Consequently, attempts were made to improve the clinical outcomes of IVF in these patients, including surgery as well as medical treatment prior to IVF. Studies have shown that surgery performed by laparotomy or laparoscopy to remove endometriomas or cauterise/ablate endometriosis lesions does not improve the clinical outcome of subsequent IVF and may even be associated with worse results due to their negative effect on the ovarian reserve. Medical pre-treatment was also suggested: for example, in a randomised controlled study (RCT) comparing 54 to 57 endometriosis patients, corticosteroids prior to

IVF was found to improve the clinical pregnancy rate (CPR) in those women, while in another RCT including 41 patients in each arm, treatment with danazol prior to IVF or ICSI was found to increase the CPR significantly in women with repeated IVF failures. Unfortunately these small studies have not so far been replicated probably for fear of the side effects associated with these medications [1]. In another non-randomised study, a 6–8 week course of oral contraceptives preceding IVF in patients with endometriosis was associated with a rise in the CPR from 12.9% to 35.0% per retrieval ($P < 0.01$) [3], but these results have not been confirmed in a RCT.

More importantly, various studies have shown that prolonged treatment with GnRH analogues prior to IVF and ICSI improves the pregnancy and implantation rates. In 2006, we conducted a Cochrane review of the three published RTCs using this approach. They included an Israeli study published in 1992 in which 35 patients with endometriosis who received 6 months of GnRH agonist treatment prior to IVF were compared to 32 patients who received conventional stimulation. The authors found that GnRH therapy prior to IVF was associated with a significantly higher CPR per cycle and per transfer. Similarly, in a German study published in 2002 of 110 patients, half of whom (55 patients) received 6 months of GnRH agonist prior to IVF, the authors found that the CPR per patient was significantly higher among those who received the GnRH therapy. The third study also published in 2002 and conducted in the USA compared 25 patients receiving a 3-month course of GnRH agonist prior to IVF to 26 patients who received the standard long agonist protocol. Again, the authors found that pre-IVF treatment with GnRH agonist resulted in a significantly higher ongoing pregnancy rate (80% vs. 53.85%). Our Cochrane review of these three RCTs concluded that in patients with endometriosis-associated infertility, the administration of GnRH for 3 to 6 months prior to IVF was associated with a significantly higher live birth rate per woman compared to the control group (OR = 9.19; 95% CI = 1.08–78.22). The CPR per woman was also significantly higher (OR = 4.28; 95% CI = 2.00–9.15). In our conclusion, we noted that the studies were heterogeneous and that further trials needed to be conducted taking into consideration the stage of endometriosis, the presence of other infertility factors as well as the type, dose and duration of the GnRH preparation used.

In 2019, we updated our Cochrane review including more studies which have been published since applying stricter inclusion criteria. We concluded that the current evidence was still weak and we repeated our suggestion that further studies are needed to confirm these results [4]. These future studies should standardise the type and dose of the GnRH agonist preparation, the length of the treatment course and the stage of endometriosis. Indeed one such study, a multicentre RCT, is currently being conducted comparing the continuous administration of oral contraceptives to long-term GnRH administration prior to IVF in these patients [5] and the results are eagerly awaited. In addition to the use of GnRH for 6 to 12 weeks prior to IVF, freezing all the embryos and transferring them in a subsequent "more physiologic" cycle was also proposed and this strategy also needs further proper evaluation [4].

Until these studies are conducted and/or completed, current evidence, albeit not totally robust, indicates that patients with endometriosis-associated infertility can benefit from this treatment and it seems unreasonable to deny them this option, particularly if they had one or more IVF failures in the past.

References

1   Sallam HN, Garcia-Velasco JA, Dias S, Arici A. Long-term pituitary down-regulation before in vitro fertilization (IVF) for women with endometriosis. *Cochrane Database Syst Rev.* 2006 Jan 25;(1): CD004635.

2.   Senapati S, Sammel MD, Morse C, Barnhart KT. Impact of endometriosis on in vitro fertilization outcomes: an evaluation of the Society for Assisted Reproductive Technologies Database. *Fertil Steril.* 2016 July;106(1):164–71.

3.   de Ziegler D, Gayet V, Aubriot FX, et al. Use of oral contraceptives in women with endometriosis before assisted reproduction treatment improves outcomes. *Fertil Steril.* 2010 Dec;94(7):2796–9.

4.   Georgiou EX, Melo P, Baker PE, et al. Long-term GnRH agonist therapy before in vitro fertilisation (IVF) for improving fertility outcomes in women with endometriosis. *Cochrane Database Syst Rev.* 2019 Nov 20;2019(11).

5.   Van der Houwen LEE, Lier MCI, Schreurs AMF, et al. Continuous oral contraceptives versus long-term pituitary desensitization prior to IVF/ICSI in moderate to severe endometriosis: study protocol of a non-inferiority randomized controlled trial. *Hum Reprod Open.* 2019 Feb 23;2019(1): hoz001.

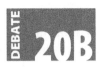

Endometriosis Should Be Suppressed for 6–12 Weeks before Frozen Embryo Transfer

Against

Tom Gunnar Tanbo

Endometriosis associated infertility is a common indication for in vitro fertilisation (IVF). According to the US Society for Assisted Reproductive Technologies (SART) database, endometriosis is the main or secondary diagnosis in 5–15% of all couples and cycles. Results of IVF in endometriosis can therefore be confounded by concomitant diagnoses in the same couple, particularly in the minimal and mild stages with no or little pelvic anatomical distortions. Apart from the advanced cases of endometriosis, it is therefore controversial as to whether endometriosis actually results in lower success rates than other indications like tubal factor infertility. Women with endometriosis have been shown to express a hyper-estrogenic activity in eutopic and ectopic endometrium due to upregulation of the gene encoding for aromatase activity and an inflammation derived resistance to progesterone with subsequent impaired endometrial decidualisation. Both of these might have an adverse effect on the implantation of a high quality embryo. There are also several studies showing different expression of various implantation related factors in the endometrium of women with endometriosis. However, IVF cross-over studies with donated or own oocytes to women with and without endometriosis have shown that endometrial receptivity is not reduced in endometriosis. Inferior results of IVF in patients with endometriosis compared with other indications for IVF must therefore be due to poor oocyte or embryo quality and not a non-receptive endometrium .

Long-term gonadotropin releasing hormone (GnRH) agonist treatment ($>=$ 12 weeks) results in a hypoestrogenic condition and in amenorrhea, both of which have been thought to inactivate endometriotic lesions and therefore be of advantage in IVF for endometriosis. Several observational studies and clinical trials in fresh IVF cycles have been performed, and most of them indicate a beneficial effect of such treatment compared to ordinary luteal phase down regulation. This was the conclusion of a Cochrane review from 2006 stating that although most trials included were of low quality, there seemed to be a beneficial effect of long-term down regulation. Furthermore, ESHRE in their guidelines for treatment of endometriosis-associated infertility advocates such treatment. However, an updated Cochrane review from last year casts doubt on the effect of long-term downregulation with GhRH agonists prior to IVF in endometriosis associated infertility [1].

Additional uncertainty regarding the adverse effect of endometriosis in IVF, came from a large study on almost 350,000 IVF cycles from the SART database for 2016. Admittedly, IVF cycles in couples with isolated endometriosis had lower oocyte yield compared with all other indications. However, implantation rate and live birth rate in fresh as well as frozen embryo transfer cycles were actually as least as good as or higher than in all other indications. On the other hand, couples with endometriosis and one or more additional diagnoses had lower success rates compared with other diagnoses like tubal or male factor infertility [2]. Consequently, endometriosis per se is not an adverse factor in IVF.

Cryopreservation of embryos for later transfer, either surplus embryos after a fresh transfer or in a freeze all strategy is usually based on a selection of the best embryos, those who are most likely to survive the freeze/thaw procedure. Transfer of frozen/thawed embryos (FET) can be performed either in natural cycles, semi-natural cycles with hCG for final follicular maturation, or in substituted cycles with or without a GnRH-agonist. In a meta-analysis it was shown that no endometrial preparation procedure was preferable to another [3].

If progesterone resistance and a hyperestrogenic endometrial environment were supposed to have a negative impact on the results of FET in endometriosis, then GnRH agonist administration in a substituted FET cycle would seem logical for suppression of oestrogen activity. To my knowledge, however, the extent of endometrial decidualisation in natural or substituted FET cycles after weeks of GnRH agonist therapy has not been investigated.

FET has become increasingly more frequent with better embryo culture conditions and thereby embryo survival. Apart from avoiding ovarian hyperstimulation syndrome, some clinics also use the freeze-all strategy with the intention of performing FET in a presumably more receptive endometrium than in a stimulated cycle. In a recent meta-analysis on fresh versus elective FET, there was admittedly a 12% increase in live birth rate with eFET compared with fresh embryo transfer; however, cumulative live birth rate was similar [4].

Endometriosis has been associated with chronic endometritis, and the presence of microbes in a receptive endometrium has been associated with decreased implantation and live birth rates. The occurrence of endometritis has been shown to be higher in GnRH agonist treated women with endometriosis than in untreated endometriosis women; however, to what extent this is a clinical problem is currently unknown [5]. Long-term treatment with a GnRH agonist has significant hypo-estrogenic side-effects, therefore the rationale for such treatment should be strong, and in fresh cycles with extensive endometriosis there may be some evidence for a beneficial effect of such treatment. In FET for endometriosis, however, it is not. On the contrary, there are certain indications that it may actually have an adverse effect.

References

1. Georgiou EX, Melo P, Baker PE, et al. Long-term GnRH agonist therapy before in vitro fertilisation (IVF) for improving fertility outcomes in women with endometriosis. *Cochrane Database Syst Rev.* 2019;11:CD013240.

2. Senapati S, Sammel MD, Morse C, Barnhart KT. Impact of endometriosis on in vitro fertilization outcomes: an evaluation of the Society for Assisted Reproductive Technologies Database. *Fertil Steril.* 2016;106:164–71.e1.

3. Ghobara T, Gelbaya TA, Ayeleke RO. Cycle regimens for frozen-thawed embryo transfer. *Cochrane Database Syst Rev.* 2017;7:CD003414.

4. Roque M, Haahr T, Geber S, Esteves SC, Humaidan P. Fresh versus elective frozen embryo transfer in IVF/ICSI cycles: a systematic review and meta-analysis of reproductive outcomes. *Hum Reprod Update.* 2019;25:2–14.

5. Khan KN, Fujishita A, Hiraki K, et al. Bacterial contamination hypothesis: a new concept in endometriosis. *Reprod Med Biol.* 2018;17:125–33.

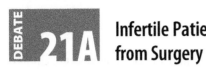

21A Infertile Patients with Endometriosis Benefit from Surgery

For

Stephan Gordts

Increased pregnancy rates, the ease of access to IVF programs in many countries and the low risks for professionals have resulted in very liberal referral to IVF programs. Banning laparoscopy from the exploration, so-called 'unexplained infertility', is hiding an increasing cohort of patients with undiagnosed endometriosis.

Endometriosis is a benign gynaecological disease affecting 25–30% of patients with fertility problems. A diagnostic delay up to 8 years or more in the diagnosis of endometriosis is well-demonstrated. The objectives of treatment of endometriosis are a relief of pain, avoiding recurrences and restoring the patient's fertility when indicated. Nowadays the surgical treatment of endometriosis is balanced against the impact on ovarian reserve and the consequences of a poor ovarian response in case of ovarian stimulation for IVF. The question of surgery increasing the patient's possibilities for a spontaneous pregnancy is outdated. This attitude is reflected in the latest version of the ESHRE guideline stating: *'In women with endometrioma larger than 3 cm, the GDG recommends GPP clinicians only to consider cystectomy prior to ART to improve endometriosis-associated pain or the accessibility of follicles,'* not mentioning the possibility for a spontaneous conception.

As a benign but multifactorial disease, in the absence of any surgery, endometrioma itself has an impaired impact upon ovarian reserve. Micro-vascular injuries and progression through increased interstitial fibrosis have been described in endometriomas smaller than 4 cm [1]. An increased impact with the size of the endometrioma on the ovarian reserve is less clear, but bilateralism has a detrimental effect and is even more pronounced in adolescents. Ovarian reserve is challenged by the disease itself, delaying childbearing and by inappropriate surgery.

Why Surgery?

1. Lack of Diagnosis

As diagnostic laparoscopy is not a routine procedure any more in the exploration of the infertile couple, there are a vast number of undiagnosed cases of endometriosis that are hidden within the population of IVF patients and classified under so-called 'unexplained infertility'. Certainly a majority of these patients with absence of other impairing fertility factors could benefit from a microsurgical reconstructive procedure. Indeed results after surgical correction of endometriosis show a spontaneous pregnancy rate of 50–60% within the first 12 months. It further creates the possibility of a consecutive conception at a later stage without supplementary treatment. A Cochrane review [2] highlighted the improved spontaneous pregnancy rate after surgical treatment of stage I–II endometriosis.

2. Effect of Endometriosis on IVF

Endometriosis as such has a negative impact upon the number of collected oocytes, embryo quality and implantation rates compared to controls. Pre-treatment with GnRha or alternative hormonal suppressive medication seems to ameliorate these negative influences. When laparoscopy was performed to confirm the presence or absence of endometriosis in a group of unexplained infertility, patients with endometriosis were 24% less likely to have a live birth after ART compared to the negative ones and the effect was more pronounced by increased severity [3]. The use of reliable biomarkers like BCL6 recently reported on compromised IVF outcomes in the presence of undiagnosed endometriosis.

3. IVF and Surgery

The absence of a negative effect of surgery on IVF implantation rates, even in the presence of lower oocyte retrieval and less embryos available for transfer is well-documented. A retrospective analysis found that removal of all visible endometriotic lesions at laparoscopy compared with simple diagnostic laparoscopy had a beneficial effect on implantation rates, pregnancy rates and live birth rates after IVF [4]. Higher cumulative pregnancy rates are obtained if surgery is chosen as a first option and if pregnancy is not occurring after surgery, IVF is performed [5]. Several studies report the success of surgery after failed IVF by the occurrence of spontaneous pregnancies.

4. Discussion

Withholding surgery in patients before an IVF treatment carries the risk of difficulty at oocyte pick-up, leakage of the cyst content and infection. No data are available on the further follow-up of these patients after successful or unsuccessful IVF treatments, but they may carry the potential risk of malignancy. Severe complications have been reported in case of pregnancy with acute haemoperitoneum and intestinal perforations in case of DIE (deep infiltrating endometriosis). A lot of studies comparing endometriosis IVF and surgery have been performed, some more than a decade ago; in the meantime new ablative surgical techniques are available with less impact upon ovarian reserve. However lack of training and expertise, certainly in stand-alone centres, will compromise accurate surgical treatments.

Conclusions

There are several reasons for a surgical correction of endometriosis: First there is clear evidence of a spontaneous conception rate of 50–60%; second there is a direct correlation between the severity of the disease and the decreased live birth rates after IVF; third surgery seems to have no negative effect on final pregnancy rates after IVF and when chosen as a first option it results in a higher cumulative pregnancy rate. An individualised approach is mandatory but the question 'Could I conceive without IVF if my endometriosis was properly diagnosed and treated?' should be answered honestly. Lack of expertise and financial benefits should not serve as a prerequisite for referring patients to IVF.

References

1. Kitajima M, Defrere S, Dolmans MM, et al. Endometriomas as a possible cause of reduced ovarian reserve in women with endometriosis. *Fertil Steril.* 2011;96:685–91.

2. Duffy JM, Arambage K, Correa FJ, et al. Laparoscopic surgery for endometriosis. *Cochrane Database Syst Rev.* 2014;4: CD011031.

3. Muteshi CM, Ohuma EO, Child T, Becker CM. The effect of endometriosis on live birth rate and other reproductive outcomes in ART cycles: a cohort study. *Hum Reprod Open.* 2018 Sept 29;2018(4).

4. Opøien HK, Fedorcsak P, Byholm T, Tanbo T. Complete surgical removal of minimal and mild endometriosis improves outcome of subsequent IVF/ICSI treatment. *Reprod Biomed.* 2011;23:389.e95.

5. Barri PN, Coroleu B, Tur R, Barri-Soldevila PN, Rodríguez I.Endometriosis-associated infertility: surgery and IVF, a comprehensive therapeutic approach. *Reprod Biomed.* 2010 Aug;21(2):179–85.

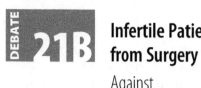

21B Infertile Patients with Endometriosis Benefit from Surgery

Against

Mathew Leonardi

Endometriosis is a chronic, benign inflammatory disease that has been well-established as a cause of pain and infertility, with prevalence rates of endometriosis approaching 50% in women with normal ovulation and normospermic partners [1]. While medications specifically aimed at treating endometriosis may be able to mitigate the pain symptoms, they have not been shown to passively improve fertility outcomes and in many cases, they directly prevent conception. On the other hand, assisted reproductive technology (ART) such as controlled ovarian hyperstimulation and in vitro fertilisation may be effective for patients with infertility but do not address non-fertility concerns.

For some time, operative laparoscopy has been regarded as a viable and evidence-based option for endometriosis-related infertility. This was reinforced in 2014 when a Cochrane review reported that operative laparoscopy was associated with an increased live birth rate (LBR) (grouped with ongoing pregnancy rate) and increased pregnancy rate (PR) [2]. It is important to note that the published RCTs on endometriosis-related infertility compare operative laparoscopy against either diagnostic laparoscopy (i.e. expectant management), operative laparoscopy plus gonadotropin-releasing hormone analogues (GnRHa), or GnRHa alone. There are no RCTs that compare operative laparoscopy to ART. There are a number of observational studies assessing interventions for endometriosis-related fertility outcomes, each with conclusions worthy of critical appraisal. However, the nature of observational studies subjects them to a number of potential problems that may bias their result. When present, clinical guidance should be founded on RCTs, which are an innately higher level of evidence and generally less subject to bias. As such, RCTs are the backbone of the argument made in this chapter.

Based on an updated systematic review and meta-analysis [3] and the studies which comprise the review, operative laparoscopy may *not* be effective at improving fertility-related outcomes in patients with endometriosis-related infertility. Overall, there was insufficient evidence to determine if there was a difference in fertility-related outcomes between operative laparoscopy and diagnostic laparoscopy. Specifically, LBR and PR were assessed in RCTs where patients were recruited for endometriosis-related infertility or endometriosis-related pain with or without infertility. The outcome of 'ongoing pregnancy rate' was grouped with 'PR' rather than 'LBR' in the context of recent evidence demonstrating a greater likelihood of pregnancy complications (pre-eclampsia, antepartum haemorrhage, pre-term premature rupture of membranes, pre-term birth, stillbirth) in patients with endometriosis [4], halting our ability to assume all pregnancies that reach 20 weeks gestational age will result in a live birth.

When we focus on the RCTs that purposely only recruited patients with infertility, there is just one RCT that compares operative to diagnostic laparoscopy assessing the outcome of LBR [5], which is arguably the most reasonably important fertility-related outcome for patients. In this study, women were aged ≤36 years, had laparoscopically confirmed diagnosis of stage I–II endometriosis as per the revised American Society of Reproductive Medicine classification and otherwise unexplained infertility for ≤2 years. The 1-year LBR was comparable at 10/51 women (19.6%) in the operative laparoscopy group and 10/45 women (22.2%) in the diagnostic laparoscopy group (relative risk (RR) 0.88, 95% confidence interval (CI) 0.40–1.92). However, the quality of evidence was rated as very low using the Grading of Recommendation Assessment, Development and Evaluation (GRADE) tool, which equates to a high degree of uncertainty about the findings.

Regarding PR, four RCTs that compared operative to diagnostic laparoscopy were identified with a total of 624. The PR in those who underwent operative laparoscopy was 91/316 (28.8%) compared to 62/308 (20.1%) in those who only had a diagnostic laparoscopy (RR 1.38, 95% CI 0.99–1.92, $P = 0.06$). Despite evidence of moderate quality, the 95% CI suggests that there is insufficient evidence that operative laparoscopy yields a different PR outcome to diagnostic laparoscopy. One reason for the difference in results between reviews is that Duffy et al. [2] did not include the Parazzini et al. [6] study in their meta-analysis for LBR or PR outcomes because a portion of the participants utilized a GnRHa (tryptorelin) within the first year post-operatively at the discretion of the physician (operative laparoscopy: 42.3% versus diagnostic laparoscopy: 53.3%). Interestingly, a portion of the participants in the Marcoux et al. study [7], which contributed the most patients and weighed heaviest on the meta-analysis, underwent ART within the first year post-operatively (operative laparoscopy: 9.3% versus diagnostic laparoscopy: 9.5%) and yet, this study was included.

Amongst the studies that primarily focused on endometriosis-related pain, one did recruit participants with infertility and compared fertility events as a secondary outcome between the following groups: (1) operative laparoscopy; (2) operative laparoscopy plus GnRHa(leuprorelin); and (3) GnRHa. When comparing operative laparoscopy plus GnRHa to GnRHa, there did not seem to be an effect from undergoing operative laparoscopy for LBR ($n = 273$; RR 0.91, 95%CI0.72–1.14) or PR (RR 0.93, 95% CI 0.77–1.12). When comparing operative laparoscopy to GnRHa, there did not seem to be an effect from undergoing operative laparoscopy for LBR ($n = 262$; RR0.82, 95% CI 0.64–1.04) or PR (RR0.84, 95% CI 0.69–1.03).

Though some individual studies may support operative laparoscopy for endometriosis-related infertility, this is not the case for all studies or the most recent synthesis of these studies in a meta-analysis [3]. Moreover, all studies noted have either unclear or high risk of bias in most domains of assessment based on the Cochrane Risk of Bias tool. As such, it is questionable to maintain a sweeping recommendation that patients undergo operative laparoscopy because it is more effective than diagnostic laparoscopy (or 'do nothing', in other words). One must even question the relevance of these studies as 'do nothing' may not be an acceptable 'intervention' for a patient after they have been diagnosed with infertility. It is clear that additional, high-quality studies are necessary to provide clarity on the effectiveness of operative laparoscopy. However, considering that patients with infertility may prefer some form of active intervention, they may be less likely to consent to participate in studies comparing an active intervention (e.g. operative laparoscopy) to expectant management. Rather, RCTs comparing active interventions may be more applicable. Specifically, RCTs that compare operative laparoscopy with ARTs would be very useful. Lastly, distinguishing between the phenotypes of endometriosis (superficial versus ovarian versus deep) in RCTs with these interventions should be considered.

References

1. Meuleman C, Vandenabeele B, Fieuws S, Spiessens C, Timmerman D, D'Hooghe T. High prevalence of endometriosis in infertile women with normal ovulation and normospermic partners. *Fertil Steril.* 2009;92:68–74.

2. Duffy J, Arambage K, Correa F, et al. Laparoscopic surgery for endometriosis. *Cochrane Database Syst Rev.* 2014:79.

3. Leonardi M, Gibbons T, Armour M, et al. When to do surgery and when not to do surgery for endometriosis: a systematic review and meta-analysis. *J Minim Invasive Gynecol.* 2020;27:390–407.e3.

4. Lalani S, Choudhry AJ, Firth B, et al. Endometriosis and adverse maternal, fetal and neonatal outcomes, a systematic review and meta-analysis. *Hum Reprod.* 2018;33:1854–65.

5. Moini A, Bahar L, Ashrafinia M, Eslami B, Hosseini R, Ashrafinia N. Fertility outcome after operative laparoscopy versus no treatment in infertile women with minimal or mild endometriosis. *Int J Fertil Steril.* 2012;5:235–40.

6. Parazzini F, Fedele L, Busacca M, et al. Postsurgical medical treatment of advanced endometriosis: results of a randomized clinical trial. *Am J Obstet Gynecol.* 1994;171 (5):1205–7.

7. Marcoux S, Maheux R, Bérubé S. Laparoscopic surgery in infertile women with minimal or mild endometriosis. Canadian Collaborative Group on Endometriosis. *N Eng J Med.* 1997;337 (4):217–22.

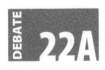

Intramural Fibroids Greater than 4 cm in Diameter Should Be Removed to Aid Fertility

For

Jacques Donnez and Marie-Madeleine Dolmans

Uterine fibroids may cause infertility, depending on their size and their location [1].

The mechanisms linking uterine fibroids and infertility are numerous: uterine cavity distortion according to the FIGO classification; impaired endometrial and myometrial blood supply; increased uterine contractility; hormonal, paracrine and molecular changes; impaired endometrial receptivity and gene expression (decrease in homeobox 10 [HOXA-10] expression); and thicker capsule.

The effect on infertility of fibroids distorting the cavity is easy to understand. We will also review the influence of non-cavity-distorting intramural fibroids.

Uterine Cavity Distortion

Since the publication by Pritts et al. in 2009 [2], this mechanism has been widely documented. There are no doubts that myomas distorting the uterine cavity (type 0, 1, 2, 2–5) impair blastocyst implantation.

Impaired Endometrial and Myometrial Blood Supply

The presence of fibroids close to the uterine cavity (type 3) may interfere with endometrial blood flow. Several studies using contrast MRI have reported reduced blood flow in fibroids and their surrounding myometrium, altering endometrial blood flow.

Increased Uterine Contractility

One of the mechanisms by which non-cavitary intramural myomas may impair fertility is that these fibroids alter uterine peristalsis. Contractile activity plays an important role in the human reproduction process, decreasing in response to progesterone, probably to favour embryo implantation. If the presence of intramural myomas alters uterine peristalsis, it may also interfere with the surrounding myometrium, leading to impaired uterine contractility and subsequently altering blastocyst implantation.

Hormonal, Paracrine and Molecular Changes

We recently stressed in a review the importance of the complex series of interactions that allow successful implantation of the embryo during the window of implantation, which includes apposition, adhesion and invasion [3]. Intramural fibroids can alter expression of genes that are important for implantation, such as glycodelin and bone morphogenetic protein receptor type 2 (BMPR2).

Impaired Endometrial Receptivity and Gene Expression: The Role of Transforming Growth Factor Beta-3 and *HOXA-10*

Endometrial mRNA expression of *HOXA-10* (an important gene regulating endometrial receptivity) is globally decreased in the presence of submucosal myomas [4]. *HOXA* mRNA expression and stromal protein expression were also affected in the intramural group.

As *HOXA-10* expression is regulated by BMP-2, *TGF-β* acts as a diffusible signalling molecule to alter BMP-2, reducing *HOXA-10* expression throughout the endometrium and, subsequently, interfering with implantation. Taylor [4], focused on size and distance, suggesting that larger fibroids produce more *TGF-β3* and those closest to the uterine cavity allow more TGF-β to reach endometrial cells. The amount of *TGF-β3* reaching the uterine cavity would vary by the square of the distance from the cavity ($1/x_2$, where x is the distance between the endometrium and the fibroid). Indirect proof that myomas impair endometrial receptivity is that, after intramural myomectomy, expression of endometrial receptivity genes increases significantly.

Thicker Capsule

A capsule surrounds the fibroid and can be considered a different entity. This pseudocapsule consists of compressed myometrium and contains nerves. It is not clear whether an increase in pseudocapsule thickness also increases the number of neuroendocrine fibres, but their presence may influence muscle contractility and uterine peristalsis.

Effect of Non-Cavity-Distorting Intramural Uterine Fibroids

Taylor [4] wrote an editorial stating that large intramural myomas near the endometrial cavity warrant removal before IVF, as they affect endometrial haemostasis and endometrial receptivity through molecular signalling.

In a meta-analysis totalling 28 studies involving 9189 patients Wang et al [5] conducted an updated systematic review and reported that non-cavity-distorting intramural myomas significantly reduce implantation ($P = 0.04$), clinical pregnancy and live birth rates. Recently, Rikhraj et al. [6] reviewed 15 quantitative studies out of a total of 139 records identified. Among the 15 studies, eight reported live birth rates and five were prospective in nature (with a total of 5029 patients). Their systematic review concluded that patients with non-cavity-distorting intramural fibroids undergoing IVF had 44% lower odds of a live birth and 32% lower odds of a clinical pregnancy than women without fibroids. Focusing solely on patients with intramural fibroids, they removed the potentially confounding effect of subserosal myomas, and also observed lower odds of a live birth and clinical pregnancy in this subgroup, providing a more robust conclusion on the subject.

In conclusion, all published studies and meta-analyses concur that non-cavity-distorting intramural fibroids do have a deleterious effect on IVF outcomes. Two factors seem to be key, namely the size of myomas (if larger, there is greater secretion of TGF-β3), and the close proximity of the uterine cavity [3]. Close to the endometrial lining, a type 3 myoma of 2 cm or more will have a detrimental effect and if a myoma is intramural but not in contact with the underlying endometrium (type 4, 5), a diameter of 3–4 cm is considered the cut-off depending on the study or meta-analysis [6].

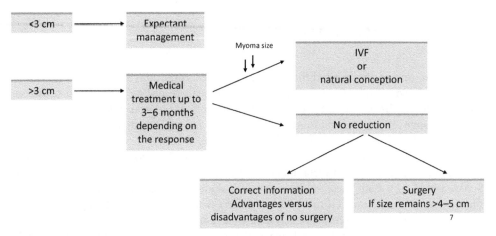

Figure 22A.1 Proposed algorithm for intramural myoma-related infertility. If the myoma measures more than 3 cm, a medical therapy could be proposed as the primary approach in order to (1) decrease myoma size; and (2) induce migration of the myoma as far as possible from the endometrium.
(Adapted from Donnez J, Dolmans MM, 2020 [3])

Several investigators have recommended surgical removal of these intramural fibroids [4]. The crucial question, however, should be that, if the negative effect is related to myoma size and proximity of the uterine cavity, why not try a medical approach to reduce the size of the myoma, and to push it back deeper into the myometrium [1] (**Figure 22A.1**).

References

1. Donnez J, Dolmans MM. Uterine fibroid management: from the present to the future. *Hum Reprod Update*. 2016;22:665–86.

2. Pritts EA, Parker WH, Olive DL. Fibroids and infertility: an updated systematic review of the evidence. *Fertil Steril*. 2009;91:1215–23.

3. Donnez J, Dolmans MM. Hormone therapy for intramural myoma-related infertility from ulipristal acetate to GnRH antagonist: a review. RBMonline. 2020. https://doi.org/10.1016/j. rbmo.2020.05 .017 1472-6483/

4. Taylor HS. Fibroids: when should they be removed to improve in vitro fertilization success? *Fertil Steril*. 2018;109:784–5.

5. Wang X, Chen L, Wang H, Li Q, Liu X, Qi H. The impact of noncavity-distorting intramural fibroids on the efficacy of in vitro fertilization-embryo transfer: an updated meta-analysis. *Biomed Res Int*. 2018;2018:8924703 Online.

6. Rikhraj K, Tan J, Taskin O, Albert AY, Yong P, Bedaiwy MA. The impact of non cavity-distorting intramural fibroids on live birth rate in in vitro fertilization cycles: a systematic review and meta-analysis. *J Women's Health (Larchmt)*. 2020;29:210–19.

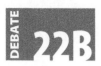

Intramural Fibroids Greater than 4 cm in Diameter Should Be Removed to Aid Fertility

Against

Mostafa Metwally

Fibroids are one of the most commonly encountered conditions in women undergoing fertility treatment. Whilst there is a reasonable consensus regarding the effect of subserous and submucous fibroids on fertility, where most agree that subserous fibroids do not have a direct negative effect and submucous fibroids do have a negative effect, the role of intramural fibroids is significantly more controversial.

Proponents for removal of intramural fibroids, base their conclusion on a series of studies and in particular two meta-analyses. The first by Pritts et al. [1] and the second by Sunkara et al. [2]. Both these studies showed a significant negative effect for intramural fibroids on fertility. However, this evidence suffers from several methodological problems. First and foremost, although meta-analyses are currently viewed as the peak of the evidence pyramid, their results are only as reliable as the quality of the primary studies included. In this case, most included studies, although valiant attempts at answering this clinical dilemma, are mainly of low quality, whether due to their observational nature, small numbers of participants or other methodological problems.

One of the main underlying problems with previous studies is that intramural fibroids are not a single entity. They vary in number, size and proximity to the endometrial cavity. Mostly these variables have not been fully accounted for by existing studies, resulting in significant heterogeneity of analysed data. For example, most clinicians have used a cut off of 4 cm to determine whether or not an intramural fibroid should be removed. This figure is largely arbitrary and is based on the idea that smaller fibroids are probably insignificant with a low chance of encroaching on the endometrial cavity. However, this arbitrary figure does not take into consideration the direction of expansion of a growing fibroid. For example, a fibroid smaller than 4 cm but close to the endometrial/myometrial junction may be more significant than a larger fibroid expanding towards the serosa and clear of endometrium. These two fibroids cannot be compared. Indeed, this absence of clear objective criteria by which to compare intramural fibroids, is one of the main underlying causes for heterogeneity of the evidence.

Furthermore, many of the previous studies use the term 'non-cavity involving fibroids' rather than strictly defined intramural fibroids. This means that inevitably in such studies women with subserous as well as intramural fibroids may have been included. The classification of fibroids into those encroaching on the endometrial cavity and those not encroaching on the cavity when analysing fertility outcomes, presumes that subserous fibroids have absolutely no effect on fertility performance, and that an adverse effect occurs only when there is a space occupying lesion 'i.e. submucous fibroids'. Although the evidence shows that subserous fibroids do not have a significant adverse effect on conception rates, it is impossible to completely exclude an effect when they are numerous, large or combined with intramural fibroids. Furthermore fibroids can affect fertility through mechanisms unrelated to anatomical distortion such as changes in endometrial blood flow, uterine contractility or the release of inflammatory substances [3]. It is therefore impossible to expect that a woman with a single 4 cm intramural fibroid would have comparable reproductive performance to a woman with multiple smaller intramural fibroids combined with a multiple large subserousfibroids. Simply speaking the anatomical variables involved make it impossible to treat all these potential variations in size, number and combination in the same way.

Another major problem, is the certainty by which submucous fibroids have been excluded in previous studies. In many cases cavity involvement was assessed using 2D ultrasound scans rather than more precise methods such as hysterosalpingography or hysteroscopy. This has also contributed to the heterogeneity of the evidence. The misclassification of some women with submucous fibroids as having intramural fibroids may largely explain the skewed evidence towards a negative effect. Indeed, the study by Pritts et al. [1] found that when only studies that performed a hysteroscopy were included, only two studies remained with a consequent loss of power of the analysis.

For the above reasons our group published a meta-analysis in 2011 that after extensively accounting for heterogeneity and confounding variables through sensitivity analyses, we found no convincing evidence that intramural fibroids have a negative effect on fertility outcomes [4]. The main finding of the study however was to emphasise the poor quality of existing evidence and to highlight the importance of pursuing primary rather than secondary research that adequately addressed confounding variables to answer this question. Our conclusion was simply that another meta-analysis was not needed. Since then however, further meta-analyses have continued to be published [5] and we are no closer to answering this important question.

Finally, it is important that we remember that our first role as physicians is to do no harm. Any surgical procedure is potentially harmful and in the absence of good quality evidence for benefits that outweigh the risks, surgery cannot be justified. Even if intramural fibroids did have a negative effect on fertility, this does not mean that myomectomy would necessarily improve outcomes. Myomectomy is a potentially risky procedure with potential adverse effects on fertility such as adhesions and in rare cases even a complete loss of fertility due to hysterectomy. How can we therefore justify such a risk in absence of conclusive evidence for benefit? Only after we have fully addressed the question of whether or not intramural fibroids have a negative effect on fertility can we then consider conducting well designed clinical studies that examine the potential benefit of myomectomy. Until then surgery for all women with intramural fibroids more than 4 cm simply cannot be justified. Rather an individualised approach needs to be adopted on a case by case basis.

References

1. Pritts EA, Parker WH, Olive DL. Fibroids and infertility: an updated systematic review of the evidence. *Fertil Steril.* 2009;91:1215–23.

2. Sunkara SK, Khairy M, El-Toukhy T, Khalaf Y, Coomarasamy A. The effect of intramural fibroids without uterine cavity involvement on the outcome of IVF treatment: a systematic review and meta-analysis. *Hum Reprod.* 2010;25:418–29.

3. Donnez J, Jadoul P. What are the implications of myomas on fertility? A need for a debate? *Hum Reprod.* 2002;17:1424–30.

4. Metwally M, Farquhar CM, Li TC. Is another meta-analysis on the effects of intramural fibroids on reproductive outcomes needed? *Reprod Biomed.* 2011;23:2–14.

5. Wang X, Chen L, Wang H, Li Q, Liu X, Qi H. The impact of noncavity-distorting intramural fibroids on the efficacy of in vitro fertilization-embryo transfer: an updated meta-analysis. *Biomed Res Int.* 2018;2018:8924703.

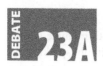

23A All Infertile Women with a Uterine Septum Should Have a Surgical Removal

For

Matt Prior and Nicholas Raine-Fenning

A uterine septum is a congenital abnormality that has been associated with poor reproductive outcome that can be readily corrected by hysteroscopic surgery. For this debate article we argue that all women with a uterine septum should have hysteroscopic septal resection before undergoing any fertility treatment.

A uterine septum is a congenital uterine anomaly arising from the failure of canalisation of the uterus during embryological development. Uterine septa are more prevalent in women with a history of pregnancy loss, but not infertility alone, and are associated with an increased risk of first and second trimester miscarriage and preterm birth [1, 2].

Diagnosis is straightforward with three-dimensional ultrasound. Adequate assessment of uterine morphology requires concurrent imaging of the external and internal controls of the uterus. Three-dimensional ultrasound facilitates such views and is safer and more acceptable to women than surgical assessment with hysteroscopy and laparoscopy which are required to see the internal and external fundal contours.

When considering uterine anatomy, we advise thinking about first principles; how structure is related to function. The pathological mechanisms underlying reproductive outcome in women with a uterine septum are unclear, although several theories have been proposed. Several studies have shown septa consist of fibromuscular tissue, with poor underlying vasculature, which is believed to lead to poor placentation or reduced sensitivity to steroid hormones. Some septa consist of myometrial tissue which may lead to increased contractility, resulting in miscarriage and preterm birth. Research has also shown that a local defect of VEGF receptors in the endometrium covering the septal area may be responsible for the clinical pathology. Reduced uterine capacity, reduced hypertrophy or limited myometrial compliance have all been proposed.

The rationale for septal resection is to attempt to correct the failure of canalisation by removing septal tissue to restore normal uterine anatomy. Restoration of normal anatomy should theoretically improve reproductive outcome. Whatever the mechanism, removal of the septum will restore uterine anatomy. Many observational studies have shown improvement in all reproductive outcomes following septal resection [3].

Traditionally surgical correction of the septate uterus was by transabdominal metroplasty. However, this was a complex procedure associated with significant morbidity. Hysteroscopic septal resection has advantages which we believe outweigh any risk. Resection can be done as a day case procedure and the risk of fluid overload is limited by using a cold scissor technique. Safety can further be improved by operating under ultrasound guidance. Intrauterine adhesions may be prevented by using post-operative oestrogen supplementation and/or the insertion of a coil or an anti-adhesion agent.

A medical intervention should be supported by the highest level of evidence before its widespread adoption by clinicians. Nevertheless, obtaining high quality evidence for surgical interventions is fraught with difficulty and there are no randomised controlled trials of hysteroscopic septal resection. The TRUST trial from the Netherlands and the UK

SEPTUM trial both experienced recruitment problems. Therefore, patient and clinicians must be guided by the observational studies and these do support septal resection.

Uterine septa are no more prevalent in sub fertile women than in the general population but have a stronger association with miscarriage. Some would argue that resection should not be considered until after one, two or even three or more miscarriages. This seems unfair for women who have a fertility problem as they are denied a potentially beneficial treatment unless they endure several pregnancy losses. Furthermore, fertility patients are in a unique position where their reproductive health can be potentially optimised prior to conception. We routinely encourage patients to stop smoking, maintain a healthy body weight and take prenatal folic acid. When a uterine septum is identified, clinicians have a duty to restore anatomy as this will improve potentially the environment for an embryo to implant allow it to develop safely into a successful pregnancy.

References

1. Chan YY, Jayaprakasan K, Zamora J, Thornton JG, Raine-Fenning N, Coomarasamy A. The prevalence of congenital uterine anomalies in unselected and high-risk populations: a systematic review. *Hum Reprod Update.* [Internet] 2011;17(6):761–71. Available from: www.ncbi.nlm.nih.gov/pubmed/21705770.

2. Chan YY, Jayaprakasan K, Tan A, Thornton JG, Coomarasamy A, Raine-Fenning NJ. Reproductive outcomes in women with congenital uterine anomalies: a systematic review. *Ultrasound Obs Gynecol.* [Internet] 2011;38(4):371–82. Available from: www.ncbi.nlm.nih.gov/pubmed/21830244.

3. Valle RF, Ekpo GE. Hysteroscopic metroplasty for the septate uterus: review and meta-analysis. *J Minim Invasive Gynecol.* [Internet] 2013;20(1):22–42. Available from: www.ncbi.nlm.nih.gov/pubmed/23312243.

23B All Infertile Women with a Uterine Septum Should Have a Surgical Removal

Against

Fulco van der Veen

For nearly a century, surgical correction of the septate uterus has been the standard procedure in infertile women with a uterine septum. The simplistic, but intuitively appealing reasoning behind resecting the septum has always been the assumed disturbed implantation within a septate uterus, but actual data on the pathophysiology of the intrauterine septum is extremely limited.

What we do know is that the septum is covered with endometrium corresponding to the lining of the uterine wall and that the majority of septa contains normal myometrial tissue. The glandular cells and stroma have a lower number of glandular cells and cilia, and incomplete ciliogenesis of the ciliated cell and the endometrial septum contains lower levels of VEGF receptors, which are believed to play a role in early embryo implantation and placentation. Also, the gene expression of *HOXA-10* genes, shown to be important in the early implantation of an embryo, seems to be altered in women with a septate uterus [1]. Whether these findings mean that development of the implanted embryo is impaired in the septate uterus remains a moot point. A plausible biological mechanism underpinning the medical intervention has thus not been identified. This in itself should make any practitioner think twice.

What about the existing evidence underpinning surgical removal? Again, also on this topic, data are extremely limited. A Cochrane review to determine whether hysteroscopic septum resection in women of reproductive age with a septate uterus improves live birth rates and to assess the safety of the procedure did not identify a single randomised controlled trial on reproductive outcomes after surgery compared to an expectant management [2]. The review did identify two ongoing trials: the TRUST study (NTR1676) and the pilot randomised controlled trial of hysteroscopic septal resection (ISRCTN2896).

Since publication of this review in 2017, two new and important studies have addressed the value and safety of surgical removal of the septum. The first study is an international multicentre cohort study performed in the Netherlands, the USA and the UK, including women with a septate uterus and a wish to conceive [3]. A total of 257 women were ascertained on the basis of a history of subfertility, pregnancy loss or preterm birth, but they could also have been identified during a gynaecological examination, an ultrasound in pregnancy or during a caesarean section. The women were diagnosed with a uterine septum between 1981 and 2018; the diagnosis was made by the treating physician according to the classification system at that time. A total of 151 women underwent septum resection and 106 women had expectant management. 80 of the 151 women who had surgery (53.0%) had at least one live birth, compared to 76 of the 106 women who had expectant management (71.7%) (HR 0.71 (95% CI 0.49–1.02)). Also, in 88 women with a history of subfertility, there were no differences in reproductive outcomes after adjustment for possible confounders like age, BMI, smoking, ethnicity, country, classification, diagnostic procedure, pregnancy loss, pre-term birth and previous live birth (HR 0.90 (95% CI 0.63–1.28)). On the issue of safety, there were complications in seven women (4.6%); in three women there was a uterine perforation, in one woman the maximal allowed amount of intravasation was reached, and in three women there was more blood loss than was deemed acceptable.

At the time of writing this contribution, data from the TRUST study, in which women were randomly allocated to hysteroscopic septum resection or expectant management, are being analysed. The preliminary data of the intention to treat analysis shows that 12 of 38 women who underwent septum resection (32.4%) had a live birth, compared to 14 of 40 women who had expectant management (37.8%) (RR 0.89 (0.56–1.41). The sample size was based on retrospective studies, anticipating an improvement of the live birth rate from 35% without surgery to 70% with surgery. If the data of the international multicentre cohort study mentioned above were used to recalculate the sample size based, approximately 600 women would need to be recruited. If we then realise that the pilot randomised controlled trial of hysteroscopic septal resection (ISRCTN2896) has stopped after including just six patients, because of poor recruitment, it is not very likely that such a large-scale trial will ever be performed.

So, to conclude: for decades, the recommendation worldwide has been to perform septum resection based on low-grade evidence. The procedure is widely offered, but is associated with financial costs for society, health-care systems or the patients themselves. I feel that I have shown without reasonable doubt that septum resection is not without risks, has no clear benefits and should thus not be performed.

References

1. Rikken JFW, Leeuwis-Fedorovich NE, Letteboer S, et al. The pathophysiology of the septate uterus: a systematic review. *BJOG.* 2019;126:1192–9.

2. Rikken JFW, Kowalik CR, Emanuel MH, et al. Septum resection for women of reproductive age with a septate uterus. *Cochrane Database Syst Rev.* 2017;(1). Art. No.: CD008576. DOI: 10.1002/14651858 .CD008576.pub4.

3. Rikken JFW, Verhorstert KWJ, Emanuel MH, et al. Septum resection in women with a septate uterus: a cohort study. *Human Reprod.* 2020;35(7):1578–88.

24A ICSI Should Be Used for All IVF Cycles

For

John Yovich

As IVF moved from an NHS-supported activity in the UK to private free-standing facilities, fees and careful financial management were required [1]. The underlying fertility profiles became expanded and the age-range of patients was extended. To avoid patient anguish if a live birth was not achieved, IVF clinics moved away from natural cycles to increasingly orchestrated regimens including manipulations. The intracytoplasmic sperm injection (ICSI) procedure was initially introduced in 1992 for male factor due to suboptimal semen profiles, but soon expanded to cases of surgical sperm recovery, thereafter to non-male factors including unexplained infertility, followed by 'precious' scenarios to avoid the risk of failed fertilisation [2].

The Australia and New Zealand Assisted Reproduction Database (ANZARD) shows the annual rate of ICSI across the 10 years 2008 to 2017 has ranged between 59.1% and 62.2% of IVF cycles overall. This is set against a backdrop where embryo vitrification has increased and frozen embryo transfers (FETs), at 56%, are now more common than fresh ETs. The FETs have a significantly higher implantation rate so that 60.2% of the 14,882 live deliveries for 2017 arose from FET cycles. The vast majority of embryo transfers are single, (SETs; 89.4%), and are conducted at the blastocyst stage (82%). Consequently, multiple pregnancies are now at a record low of 3.6% being twins only and the lowest rate recorded around the world. For fresh autologous cycles, ICSI was applied in 67.0% but for donor oocytes, 80.3% were conducted by ICSI representing the desire to ensure fertilisation in this precious scenario. This appears to have been a positive strategy as a higher proportion of the FETs were from ICSI-generated embryos (69.3% of donor oocyte/embryos vs. 60.1% of the autologous). There has been a steady rise in the live birth productivity rate per fresh ET + FETs at 26.8% per initiated cycle (but widely ranging 9.3–33.2% across 91 clinics); unfortunately, ANZARD does not yet assess whether adjuvants or ICSI rates underlie these marked differences.

My own experience with IVF commenced in 1976 in London, assisting Professor Ian Craft establish his pioneer facility [1] and we recognised at an early stage that poor fertilization was often a consequence of some deficient 'sperm factor', despite a normal semen analysis profile. Furthermore, although the advent of sperm DNA fragmentation testing provides some predictive power for ICSI requirement (e.g. DFI $\geq 15\%$), there is no value which assures a normal fertilisation rate for IVF. In recent times this has led to the idea of an IVF-ICSI Split model for all new cases of unexplained infertility [3], i.e. where ICSI is not already mandated (by defined male factor, or for genetic analysis of embryos). The model requires the recovery of ≥ 4 oocytes, enabling at least two with mature oocyte-cumulus complexes (OCCs) to be allocated to IVF. We have shown that ICSI fertilisation rates on randomly allocated oocytes is higher overall, although many cases are equivalent, and occasional cases actually show better fertilisation with IVF. The benefit of this approach is that overall more embryos are generated, the problem of complete failed fertilisation is virtually negated and reduced fertilisation is minimised. This translates to more blastocysts cryopreserved (mostly ICSI-generated), providing a higher oocyte utilisation rate, a parameter which correlates strongly with live birth rate.

The idea of retaining some cases of IVF is fully understandable given the numerous physiological processes bypassed by the ICSI methodology. In particular the recent reports from non-human primate studies do show significant differences in microtubule spindle formation and interaction of the paternal pronucleus at the cortex. There are also orientation differences of the male and female pronucleus between the IVF and ICSI fertilised oocytes [4]. The centrosomes of the developing embryo are purely of paternal origin and contain the microtubule-organising centre, hence these primate findings are potentially concerning. Notwithstanding these observational differences, time has been reassuring in revealing no increase in fetal or developmental abnormalities in children from the ICSI process. The reported difference in congenital anomalies of 4.0% for IVF and 7.1% for ICSI children relates to confounders underlying the male infertility cases, a difference not seen in outcomes from ICSI performed for non-male factors such as donor oocytes, low oocyte numbers and unexplained infertility [5]. However, the notion of ICSI for all is actually not universally required and some allowance should be given for individual preferences of patients, particularly where IVF was favoured in the IVF-ICSI Split insemination model. So too, IVF may be preferred for the potentially fragile single oocyte retrieved from women of advanced age (42–45 years). Alternatively, such precious scenarios may also be managed by 'expert ICSI' applying the PolScope oocyte imaging system to identify the MII spindle and minimise the risk of oocyte destruction. The notion of a near 100% ICSI rate can be accepted in the current day, but our preferred view is to preserve the notion of IVF where 'proven' to be better than or equivalent to ICSI fertilisation; the ICSI rate will then be ~90%. Our emergent data indicates that incorporating the IVF-ICSI Split insemination model into assisted reproduction management accords with happier patients, less distress to the IVF team and no recognisable adverse outcomes.

References

1. Yovich JL, Craft IL. Founding pioneers of IVF: Independent innovative researchers generating livebirths within 4 years of the first birth. *Reprod Biol.* 2018;18:317–23.

2. O'Neill CL, Chow S, Rosenwaks Z, Palermo GD. Development of ICSI. *Reproduction.* 2018;156:F51–8.

3. Yovich JL, Conceicao JL, Marjanovich N, et al. An ICSI rate of 90% minimizes complete failed fertilization and provides satisfactory implantation rates without elevating fetal abnormalities. *Reprod Biol.* 2018;18:301–11.

4. Simerly CR, Takahashi D, Jacoby E, et al. Fertilization and cleavage axis differ in primates conceived by conventional (IVF) versus intracytoplasmic sperm injection (ICSI). *Sci Rep.* 2019;9:15282. doi:10.1038/s41598-019-51815-4.

5. Lamarta C, Ortega C, Villa S, Pommer R, Schwarze JE. Are children born from singleton pregnancies conceived by ICSI at increased risk for congenital malformations when compared to children conceived naturally? A systematic review and meta-analysis. *JBRA Assisted Reprod.* 2017;21 (3):251–9.

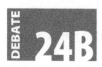

ICSI Should Be Used for All IVF Cycles

Against

Bryan Woodward

Primum non nocere. This Latin phrase means 'first, do no harm.' It is the foundation of non-maleficence, a fundamental principle of medicine and a cornerstone of the Hippocratic Oath. Yet when we perform intracytoplasmic sperm injection (ICSI), the first thing we do is harm the oocyte. We inject a needle through the oolemma, directly into the centre of the oocyte, and aspirate the ooplasm into the needle until we see the cytoplasmic contents rush up indicating oolemma rupture. It is estimated that this process causes irreversible damage to around 10% of oocytes, such that those oocytes are no longer viable [1].

ICSI is justified for male infertility, if there is no chance of fertilisation occurring without it. However, for normospermic men whose sperm are capable of fertilising the oocytes via conventional IVF (cIVF), why should we subject oocytes to this unnecessary risk? Causing lysis in 10% of a patient's oocytes is hardly abstaining from doing harm, particularly when cIVF is a proven viable alternative.

Sadly, unexpected total fertilisation failure (TFF) can result for <5% cycles for normospermic couples having cIVF [1]. Whilst low, this might be considered unacceptable to some, resulting in the doctrine of using 'ICSI for all cycles'. However, let's weigh up the TFF risk against the risks associated with ICSI. For example, it is known that in the cohort of cumulus-oocyte-complexes (COCs), around 10–25% of the oocytes will be immature when they are denuded for ICSI, and are subsequently not microinjected. Oocyte dysmorphisms can also be observed in detail, which can lead to another deselection stage. For instance, many clinics do not microinject oocytes which possess a smooth endoplasmic reticulum aggregate (SERa). Yet, if oocytes are left as COCs, if to be inseminated via cIVF, they remain part of the cohort and are in a better environment for maturation and fertilisation to take place. Healthy babies have been born from SERa oocytes, yet deselection prior to ICSI removes this possibility.

For non-dysmorphic mature oocytes, we need to consider the risks of the actual microinjection process. First, the sperm are arbitrary selected by the embryologist. Whilst we do our best, our visual selection will always be second-rate compared to the natural selection provided by cumulus penetration with cIVF. Second, the ICSI process of cytoplasmic aspiration inevitably disturbs the oocyte ultrastructure which might adversely affect viability. Third, should we really be microinjecting polyvinylpyrrolidone (PVP) into the oocyte? This synthetic polymer is used to make surgical scrub, toothpaste and glue, yet we inject it into oocytes! There are studies that show that reducing the PVP percentage from 7% to 5% might improve embryo viability [3], but should we really be injecting PVP in the first place? Add to this, the risk of lysis mentioned above and we realise there are quite a few risks with ICSI. All of these risks are eliminated by use of cIVF.

Still not convinced? How about we take a mathematical approach to compare the likelihood of success of cIVF vs. ICSI by using internationally accepted performance indicators (see Table 24B.1). Let's take 100 couples, where 10 COCs are collected per couple, and compare the various drop-out stages of cIVF and ICSI, as treatment progresses

Table 24B.1. Reference and key performance indicators for the ART laboratory

		Competence and benchmark values
Failed fertilisation rate (IVF)	no. COCs inseminated / no. of stimulated cycles × 100	<5%
Proportion of MII oocytes at ICSI	no. MII oocytes at ICSI / no. COCs retrieved × 100	75–90%*
ICSI damage rate	no. damaged or degenerated / all oocytes injected × 100	<10%*
ICSI normal fertilisation rate	no. oocytes with 2PN and 2PB / no. MII oocytes injected × 100	≥65**
IVF normal fertilisation rate	no. oocytes with 2PN and 2PB / no. COCs inseminated × 100	≥60**

* Benchmark value.
** Competence value.

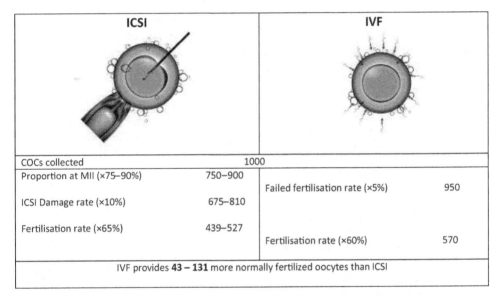

Figure 24B.1 The theoretical difference in success rates between IVF and ICSI for 1000 COCs collected from 100 couples, where each had 10 collected COCs.

(see Figure 24B.1). By doing this, we see that cIVF provides up to 131 more normally fertilized oocytes than ICSI. That figure is staggering, as couples could have 131 more chances of conception with cIVF! This may even be higher, since the simple model has not included ICSI drop-outs from oocyte deselection due to dysmorphism.

Beyond theoretical models, numerous studies have also shown that, when used for non-male factor, ICSI does not increase the cumulative live birth rate or outcomes over cIVF. As a result, some international professional bodies have issued policy statements, such as the ASRM who stated 'There are no data to support the routine use of ICSI for nonmale factor infertility' [4].

Of more concern is a recent study that suggested that conducting ICSI on normospermic couples actually decreased their chance of success compared to cIVF [5]. This Australian group analysed the outcomes in 3363 stimulated cycles (IVF = 1661; ICSI = 1702) between 2009 and 2015. Compared to ICSI, the cIVF group had significantly higher rates of fertilisation (62.3% vs. 67.1%), clinical pregnancy (16.8% vs. 23.1%) and live birth (13.2% vs. 17.2%). The overall pregnancy rate with ICSI was around 30% lower than with cIVF, translating to one less pregnancy in every 15 cycles where ICSI was used without clear indication.

As a final point, we should consider the extra economic burden that comes with ICSI, whether state-funded or paid privately by the patients. ICSI costs more than cIVF in terms of resources, e.g. micromanipulator equipment, microinjection pipettes and PVP, and training. Staggeringly, it has been estimated that over 100,000 ICSI cycles were carried out in Europe for normospermic couples between 1994 and 2014, with over 45 million Euros paid out to clinics [5]. Given that ICSI does not improve success rates over cIVF, we have to ask why did this take place, and was this of economic benefit to patients?

In summary, all of the evidence presented shows that cIVF rather than ICSI offers the best chance of conception for normospermic couples. I will end this debate with another Latin phrase: *Corruptio optimi pessima*, meaning 'corruption of the best is worse'. Performing ICSI for all IVF cycles demonstrates corruption of the optimal treatment for worse. The case is clear. *Quod erat demonstrandum.*

References

1. ESHRE Special Interest Group of Embryology, ALPHA. The Vienna consensus: report of an expert meeting on the development of art laboratory performance indicators. *Hum Reprod Open.* 2017;2.

2. Ding D, Wang Q, Li X, et al. Effects of different polyvinylpyrrolidone concentrations on intracytoplasmic sperm injection. *Zygote.* 2020;14:1–6.

3. Practice Committees of the American Society for Reproductive Medicine and Society for Assisted Reproductive Technology. Intracytoplasmic sperm injection (ICSI) for non-male factor infertility: a committee opinion. *Fertil Steril.* 2012;98(6):1395–9.

4. Sustar K, Rozen G, Agresta F, et al. Use of intracytoplasmic sperm injection (ICSI) in normospermic men may result in lower clinical pregnancy and live birth rates. *Aust NZ J Obstet Gynaecol.* 2019;59:706–11.

5. Focus on Reproduction. Best of ESHRE & ASRM. ICSI: Fertilisation for all or only for male factor indications? Published April 8, 2019. www.focusonreproduction.eu/article/ESHRE-Meetings-BOEA-2019-ICSI.

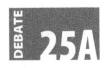

Embryo Morphokinetic Analysis (Time-Lapse Imaging) Is Helpful in Selecting Euploid Blastocysts

For

Zev Rosenwaks

Over the last two decades, embryology laboratories have shifted from using large tissue culture incubators to smaller, streamlined tabletop incubation systems, which appear to allow for more precise control of temperature, pH, and gas homeostasis. A welcome added feature to these incubators has been the ability to continuously photograph embryo development without disturbing culture conditions. This emerging technology has fostered the adoption of time-lapse microscopy (TLM) in many in vitro fertilisation laboratories. Beyond optimising culture conditions, the use of these incubators for continuous observation of embryo development has provided an opportunity to expand our fundamental knowledge of early embryogenesis. Indeed, the adoption of these devices in the ART laboratory is not only invaluable in advancing our scientific understanding of early human development, it also optimises clinical outcomes by enhancing our ability to select morphologically superior (often euploid) embryos for transfer.

It is now well-established that limiting the frequency of embryo evaluations (by reducing embryo exposure to the ambient environment) is associated with an increased yield of high-quality blastocysts and number of embryos frozen. In addition to providing superior culture conditions, time-lapse imaging of embryos allows for the evaluation of developmental events that would otherwise remain unrecognised using a limited, periodic observational approach. Similarly, evaluation of embryo morphokinetics allows the assessment of dynamic parameters that predict implantation; i.e., embryos that cleave at the expected time interval and maintain synchronised developmental speed have the highest potential to reach the blastocyst stage, appear to achieve better morphologic grades, and exhibit higher implantation rates [1, 2]. In our clinic, we evaluate the development of early embryos to day 3 and are able to reliably predict the likelihood that these embryos will develop to the blastocyst stage. The analysis of these data allows for flexible allocation of embryos to either a day-3 or day-5 (blastocyst) transfer, and for selection of the embryo with the highest implantation potential.

Beyond pure morphokinetic analysis, TLM allows for the detection of aberrant developmental events that could not have been appreciated before the inception of this technology. Absent cleavage in the presence of karyokinesis, chaotic cleavage, blastomere fusion, cell lysis, and direct unequal cleavage (DUC) have all been observed and linked to implantation failure. DUC, which occurs when one blastomere divides into three rather than two cells, has been well studied by our centre; embryos that exhibit DUCs have a significantly lower chance of reaching the blastocyst stage and a higher chance of exhibiting chromosomal aneuploidy [3]. DUCs occurring at earlier stages (1–3 cells) are more likely to affect subsequent developmental potential. The earlier the unequal division is observed, the more severe is its impact on development and euploidy. When the first embryo cleavage is unequal (1–3 cells), embryo development beyond day 3 almost always deteriorates, an observation that could not be ascertained by static observation of a seemingly normal day-3 embryo. Moreover, TLM allows for superior detection of multinucleation, which is now known to increase the odds of DUC three-fold [4]. Our centre deselects embryos exhibiting early DUC and uses these data in real-time to discern which embryos are unlikely to reach the blastocyst stage in vitro, thus permitting the selection of patients who are poor candidates for prolonged culture. More investigations are required to identify additional markers of aberrant embryo development.

Our specific use of TLM incubators underscores an important point: their utility largely depends on the approach to patient care taken by the individual clinic or laboratory. For programs that exclusively perform day-5 transfers (which may be to the detriment of certain patients), the use of TLM will assist in the selection of the blastocyst with the highest potential for implantation, but will not be as impactful for programs that interpret data on day 3 to make clinical decisions regarding the timing and the number of embryos for transfer. Less useful still will be the adoption of TLM for programs exclusively performing blastocyst PGT-A. However, TLM may still aid in the selection of the best euploid embryo for transfer; a recent study comparing euploid embryo selection based on morphology alone versus analysis of TLM parameters showed a statistically significant increased clinical pregnancy rate using the latter approach [5].

While detractors of TLM may point to reports indicating that there is no benefit to its use, the bulk of these studies have suffered from methodological flaws. For instance, one retrospective cohort study that concluded a low ability to predict euploidy in 103 consecutive IVF patients did not examine multinucleation or DUCs, the detection of which we have demonstrated to be meaningful predictors of ploidy. Furthermore, a randomised trial by Goodman et al. concluding that analysis of morphokinetic parameters did not improve outcomes suffered several limitations; the average patient age in this study was 33 years old, and more than 75% of patients underwent blastocyst transfer of an average of two blastocysts [6]. The overwhelmingly favourable demographics of the study population limits the generalisability of the findings, but even with these limitations, pregnancy rates were still 5.2% higher overall and 6.3% higher in patients under 40. It should be noted that the study was underpowered to confirm statistical significance. Indeed, a recent meta-analysis suggested an improved clinical pregnancy rate (51.0% vs. 39.9%) and an increased live birth rate (44.2% vs. 31.3%) for TLM as compared to conventional embryo culture and evaluation when five RCTs encompassing outcomes for 1637 patients were analysed [7].

This is not to say that time-lapse microscopy obviates the judicious use of preimplantation genetic testing and next-generation sequencing to assess embryo ploidy. It does, however, allow for further refinement of embryo selection within a cohort of euploid embryos, and also allows for early selection of embryos for fresh transfer that have the highest potential for implantation and successful pregnancy. In spite of some early detractors of this technology, it is my opinion that we have only just begun to harness the clinical benefit of this useful technology for improving ART outcomes.

References

1. Meseguer M, Herrero J, Tejera A, Hilligsoe KM, Ramsing NB, Remohi J. The use of morphokinetics as a predictor of embryo implantation. *Hum Reprod.* 2011;26:2658-71.

2. Dal Canto M, Coticchio G, Mignini Renzini M, et al. Cleavage kinetics analysis of human embryos predicts development to blastocyst and implantation. *Reprod Biomed.* 2012;25:474-80.

3. Chan Y, Zhu B, Jiang H, Zhang J, Luo Y, Tang W. Influence of TP53 codon

72 polymorphism alone or in combination with HDM2 SNP309 on human infertility and IVF outcome. *PLoS ONE.* 2016;11: e0167147.

4. Ergin EG, Caliskan E, Yalcinkaya E, et al. Frequency of embryo multinucleation detected by time-lapse system and its impact on pregnancy outcome. *Fertil Steril.* 2014;102:1029–33, e1021.

5. Rocafort E, Enciso M, Leza A, Sarasa J, Aizpurua J. Euploid embryos selected by an automated time-lapse system have superior SET outcomes than selected solely by conventional morphology assessment. *J Assist Reprod Genet.* 2018;35:1573–83.

6. Goodman LR, Goldberg J, Falcone T, Austin C, Desai N. Does the addition of time-lapse morphokinetics in the selection of embryos for transfer improve pregnancy rates? A randomized controlled trial. *Fertil Steril.* 2016;105:275–85, e210.

7. Pribenszky C, Nilselid AM, Montag M. Time-lapse culture with morphokinetic embryo selection improves pregnancy and live birth chances and reduces early pregnancy loss: a meta-analysis. *Reprod Biomed.* 2017;35:511–20.

25B Embryo Morphokinetic Analysis (Time-Lapse Imaging) Is Helpful in Selecting Euploid Blastocysts

Against

Christine Leary

Introduction

One of the most challenging aspects of IVF is selecting the embryo(s) most likely to implant and result in live birth. Traditional methods of embryo selection are limited to daily assessments of development and morphology. Time-lapse (TL) technology permits frequent imaging and analysis of embryos, without disturbance to culture conditions and many of the latest models are capable of complex algorithms to aid embryo selection.

Asides from trying to demonstrate that TL incubators offer superior culture conditions many studies have sought to identify morphokinetic markers that correlate with clinical pregnancy rates (CPRs), live birth rates (LBRs) and euploid status of embryos; seeking to compare TL with more traditional invasive methods of preimplantation genetic testing for aneuploidy (PGT-A).

Depending on female age, over half of all embryos maybe aneuploidy, which is a possible cause of implantation failure, miscarriage and birth defects. Aneuploidy has a weak association with conventional morphology grading, but TL could provide a breakthrough in identifying discreet markers, predictive of ploidy and implantation potential. This review seeks to demonstrate that the current technology is not yet suitable for this application.

Main Argument

Premise 1 TL Selection Doesn't Improve CPRs

The evidence that morphokinetic analysis has resulted in the identification of viable and therefore presumably euploid embryos is low quality; insufficient studies support the use of TL to increase CPRs. Many studies have been retrospective and confounding factors, such as different culture conditions and patient populations were not controlled for.

The results are also open to other interpretations; one of the few prospective randomised controlled trials (RCT), reported 10% increased CPR when TL selection criteria were applied, but embryo quality was higher under TL compared to conventional incubation; findings may be unrelated to the mophokinetic analysis. A Cochrane review from 2019 (2955 patients from 9 RCT), attempted to address this factor, but even accounting for the better culture conditions combined with the use of TL technology there were no significant differences in CPRs [1].

There have been numerous meta-analyses, but all inherently flawed; as studies have used different start/end points, kinetic markers and morphology criteria, resulting in multiple algorithms. As such, it has not been possible to collate, replicate and externally validate the findings.

It could be argued that whilst it may not be possible to improve outcome per treatment cycle started, TL could be used to prioritise embryos for cryopreservation and transfer, therefore reducing the time to pregnancy and loss rate. The counter argument to this is that the analysis of development to the blastocyst stage, relies on a misconception that TL conditions are superior for supporting development of viable embryos, but these conditions may actually be supporting the development of less viable embryos, resulting in more aneuploid embryos in the selection cohort and few of the studies conducted so far have looked at miscarriage or LBR.

Premise 2   Aneuploidy Screening Doesn't Improve Clinical Outcomes

Expert groups are in agreement there is no quality evidence that aneuploidy screening results in improved clinical outcomes. On this basis, any study seeking to correlate embryo mophokinetics with embryo ploidy status as identified by PGT-A, will also lack any evidence basis for improving clinical outcomes. Identifying that an embryo has the correct number of chromosomes is no guarantee of implantation.

It has been suggested that aneuploid embryos follow a less strict division pattern than healthy embryos, but it is highly improbable that this will be irrespective of patient characteristics, based on the findings of studies reviewed in the previous section.

The accuracy of prediction and quality of evidence is low and there are limited RCT. Several retrospective studies have identified differences in the morphokinetics of cleavage stage embryos based on ploidy status. Others have observed differences in timings of blastocyst formation between euploid and aneuploidy embryos and related these differences to CPRs. These studies have been based on low numbers (25–530 cycles), at single centres and many cofounding factors such as patient age were not considered. Reignier et al. [2]) attempted to combined the data from 13 such smaller studies, many of which had suggested differences, however the overall findings were not statistically significant.

To date there are only two prospective studies; the first by Chavez et al. [3] reported that euploid cleavage stage embryos show less variability in duration of divisions than aneuploid. However, the study included only 45 research allocated embryos. The second study by Yang et al. [4], included 285 biopsied blastocysts allocated to TL or conventional incubation. TL used in conjunction with PGT-A resulted in significantly higher CPRs. A further retrospective analysis [5], has similarly reported that PGT-A combined with TL can be used to effectively select embryos. From these studies, it has been suggested that whilst TL cannot substitute PGT-A, once euploid embryos have been identified TL could be used to identify morphokinetics specific to gene expression patterns related to embryo viability.

Ultimately, other confounding factors, not just ploidy status affects kinetics and much of the variability in morphokinetics could be patient related, something which the above studies have failed to account for. Using the embryo as the 'experimental unit' for statistical analysis rather than the patient, means that the findings were not appropriately adjusted for patient cohort effects and these studies thus lack both sensitivity and specificity.

It could be argued that TL has permitted the characterisation of dysmorphisms, associated with lower euploidy rates, which may have previously gone undetected. However, clear interpretation of the findings is not possible and conclusive evidence of which deviations from the norm negatively impact embryo competence and which are benign variations is still lacking.

Premise 3 Using TL, Either Singularly or in Combination with PGT-A for Embryo Selection is Not Cost-Effective

There is insufficient evidence that either technology can be used individually to identify viable embryos capable of successful implantation and stringent testing of the combined use of these technologies is yet to be performed. Introduction into a clinical setting, would be inappropriate, as both technologies require significant financial investment (equipment, consumables, staff time) and costs should not fall to the patient or the funding authority until efficacy has been demonstrated.

Frequent operator discrepancies during TL image annotation, which will likely limit the accuracy of any prediction models. It is also yet to be established if different timings may be peculiar to different subgroups of patients requiring different predictive models, with some patients more likely to benefit from TL than others. The technologies may not be appropriate for all patients, as in some instances the patient may have no embryos from which to choose, resulting in cycle cancelation. In other cases, the patient may have a higher number of embryos, than can be accommodated on one TL slide and comparisons across the full cohort may not be possible. As a general point, the complexity of the information relayed to patient may cause unnecessary anxiety.

As a final point, it could be argued that TL has operational advantages and whilst the benefits of TL for audit and training are not contested, this should not be provided at a financial burden to the patient. Furthermore, TL should not be introduced into clinical practice until it is clear that it is free of any potential harm. During imaging embryos, may be frequently exposed to light, heat, electromagnetic and shearing forces. Whilst these risks have largely been allayed, TL is a new technology, the first reported pregnancy in 2010 and follow-up studies from live births are currently lacking.

Conclusion

At present judgement on the efficacy of TL to select viable euploid embryos should be suspended. Evidence is not available to support the use of morphokinetics as a surrogate/replacement for PGT-A to determine ploidy. Whilst it may be possible to combine selection techniques to identify putative biomarkers of embryo viability, robust kinetic predictors of embryo viability in euploid embryos is currently lacking, as illustrated by the lack of consensus amongst studies. To appropriately validate TL, RCTs within multiple clinical settings, with standardised patient groups, culture conditions and biopsy protocols are required. There is a need to identify proper clinical aims, such as time to pregnancy, miscarriage, LBR and long-term safety.

The on-going iteration of improvements to TL will likely result in advanced software automation and the development of deep learning/artificial intelligence to select embryos that are not only likely to be euploid, but which display characteristics associated with increased probability of implantation and live birth. This could lead to different conclusions, but at present the evidence is not available to support the routine widespread application of TL to select euploid embryos. It is also clear that chromosome status is only one factor associated with embryo implantation potential and TL remains only a promising selection tool, however further development of software will likely increase its future application value.

References

1. Armstrong S, Bhide P, Jordan V, Pacey A, Marjoribanks J, Farquhar C. Time-lapse systems for embryo incubation and assessment in assisted reproduction. *Cochrne Database Syst Rev.* 2019;(5). Art. No.: CD011320.

2. Reignier A, Lammers J, Barriere P, Freour T. Can time-lapse parameters predict embryo ploidy? A systematic review. *Reprod Biomed.* Online. 2018;36(4):380–7. DOI: 10.1016/j.rbmo.2018.01.001.

3. Chavez SL, Loewke KE, Han J, et al. Dynamic blastomere behaviour reflects human embryo ploidy by the four-cell stage. *Nat Commun.* 2012;3:1251.

4. Yang Z, Zhang J, Salem SA, et al. Selection of competent blastocysts for transfer by combining time-lapse monitoring and array CGH testing for patients undergoing preimplantation genetic screening: a prospective study with sibling oocytes. *BMC Med Genom.* 2014;7:38.

5. Rocafort E, Enciso M, Leza A, Sarasa J, Aizpurua J. Euploid embryos selected by an automated time-lapse system have superior SET outcomes than selected solely by conventional morphology assessment. *J Assist Reprod Genet.* 2018;35:1573–83.

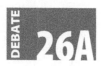

Time-Lapse Imaging Should Be a Routine Procedure in Clinical Embryology

For

William Ledger

Assisted reproductive technology has moved from the cottage industry of the 1980s to a global business that treats millions of patients using advanced treatments and cutting-edge science. The landscape shifts constantly and it is incumbent upon those who work in this area of medicine to stay up to date and provide their patients with the best possible chance of a healthy child. In my opinion it is incontrovertible that the best currently available laboratory technology for culture of optimal quality and number of blastocysts involves time lapse imaging systems with use of artificial intelligence (AI) in image analysis. As with many rapidly moving areas of medical technology, it has taken time to develop efficient systems for time lapse imaging of embryos in culture but there are now several mature and stable options available for purchase. Time lapse systems obviously allow the embryologist to assess development to blastocyst without disturbing the embryo incubation, and offer significant shortening in time to pregnancy over conventional incubation methods [1]. This is important to patients as a shorter time to pregnancy reduces the emotional burden of treatment that leads to implantation failure and reduces the financial and psychological costs involved in repeated embryo transfers. Patients are also reassured by the intensity of information that can be gleaned about their embryo development from the time lapse images and can be provided with a copy of the video loops as part of the feedback from the clinic at the end of their cycle.

Until recently, time lapse systems were held to be no more beneficial than conventional embryo culture with assessment of blastocyst quality at a single point on day five, possibly with incorporation of information from assessment at one or two points earlier in embryo development. There has been much research and debate over which are the most significant developmental check points to select from the information from the time lapse system in order to identify the blastocyst with the best potential for successful implantation [2]. This debate has now been resolved with a move away from reliance on assessment at set points by human embryologists towards use of AI [3].The AI system simply compares the entirety of the images captured for each embryo against its known paradigm, giving each blastocyst a percentage chance of livebirth. Selecting the embryo with the highest score, with or without the added reassurance of pre-implantation genetic testing for aneuploidy, offers the highest chance of a successful outcome. Incorporation of AI into the time lapse system circumvents the need for an embryologist to scan through the video recordings to identify progress at pre-determined check points, saving embryologist time, avoiding possibility of human error and giving a superior assessment of the progress of each embryo as it develops.

Time lapse imaging provides other benefits. Most of the embryos that we transfer will not implant. Most women will go on to have a negative pregnancy test. They then return to their doctor to explore what went wrong and to discuss next steps. Data from the time lapse images provide powerful support when suggesting that patients do not have further IVF cycles, giving visual justification for the clinician's advice to stop. Conversely the images can be used to encourage women to have another go if they confirm good development to blastocyst.

High quality data from randomised trials that support this model as 'best practice' are lacking [4]. There have been false dawns before [5] but in the real world of reproductive medicine, patients are very reluctant to take the risk of being randomised into the 'wrong' arm of a randomised study that compares a conventional with a 'new' treatment option, and any study that uses livebirth as primary outcome requires large numbers of participants, long-term follow-up and becomes prohibitively costly for all but pharma company supported research. Hence as in so many other areas of practice, including use of ICSI in male infertility, we must rely on less high-quality evidence, using evidence from case series and cohort studies to allow us to move forward. Use of time lapse imaging in embryology is currently at this point of its development. The body of evidence that supports its use is growing and it is not in the best interest of our patients to continue to rely on outmoded methods for embryo culture and classification. Those who feel otherwise must identify drawbacks to use of a time lapse system, which I find difficult to define.

Time lapse technology has come of age. Costs have fallen and will fall further with increased uptake of these systems and entry of new companies into this market. Whilst adequately powered randomised trials are lacking, there seems little reason for high quality assisted reproduction laboratories not to move to non-invasive time lapse as their preferred approach to embryo culture.

References

1. Pribenszky C, Nilselid AM, Montag M. Time-lapse culture with morphokinetic embryo selection improves pregnancy and live birth chances and reduces early pregnancy loss: a meta-analysis. *Reprod Biomed Online*. 2017 Nov;35(5):511–20.

2. Storr A, Venetis C, Cooke S, Kilani S, Ledger W. Time-lapse algorithms and morphological selection of day-5 embryos for transfer: a preclinical validation study. *Fertil Steril*. 2018 Feb;109(2):276–83.e3.

3. Tran D, Cooke S, Illingworth PJ, Gardner DK. Deep learning as a predictive tool for fetal heart pregnancy following time-lapse incubation and blastocyst transfer. *Hum Reprod*. 2019 June 4;34(6):1011–18.

4. Armstrong S, Bhide P, Jordan V, Pacey A, Marjoribanks J, Farquhar C. Time-lapse systems for embryo incubation and assessment in assisted reproduction. *Cochrane Database Syst Rev*. 2019 May 29;5:CD011320.

5. Mastenbroek S, Twisk M, van Echten-Arends J, et al. In vitro fertilization with preimplantation genetic screening. *New Engl J Med*. 2007;357:9–17.

Time-Lapse Imaging Should Be a Routine Procedure in Clinical Embryology

Against

Virginia N Bolton

Assisted reproduction technology (ART) is no different from any clinical therapy, in that for the inclusion of a particular treatment in the portfolio of those offered to patients, there must be sufficient evidence that whilst doing no harm, it actually enhances the chance of a successful outcome. Once that evidence is available, it should be offered universally, with all patients having equal access to the best possible treatment wherever it is undertaken. To offer any element of ART treatment selectively, when it has been shown to lead to a better outcome, is morally indefensible.

In order to incorporate time-lapse imaging (TLI) into routine ART treatment it must first be supported by evidence that it harms neither the developing embryo nor the patient, and that its use increases the chance of achieving the birth of a healthy child. If that evidence is available, TLI should be incorporated routinely into all ART treatments and the cost absorbed accordingly. Currently, TLI technology meets neither of these criteria, and its use, whether selective or routine, cannot justify the expense that may be incurred.

Regarding *direct harm* to the embryo, there is no published evidence to suggest that exposure to TLI technology, taking digital images at intervals (up to every 5–15 minutes), impairs development. In terms of *direct benefit*, using TLI incubators is theoretically beneficial, through enabling assessment of embryo morphology without disrupting stable culture conditions. Using conventional incubators, embryos are exposed to the risk of physical accident and environmental disturbance during repeated removal of culture dishes, for embryo assessment using conventional light microscopy.

This theoretical benefit is not upheld by any published evidence. Different TLI systems vary technically, in terms of gas mixtures and temperatures used, and whether they use dark- or light-field microscopy. Moreover, different laboratories use different culture media and culture practices with different TLI systems. Any one of these factors may influence embryo viability and, ultimately, treatment outcomes. There are no published data that distinguish specifically between the impact of different incubator types and the numerous other variables in embryo culture techniques on treatment outcome.

The most recent Cochrane Review (2019) [1] of TLI examines this theoretical incubation advantage of TLI technology, looking at the evidence of RCTs where patients (not oocytes or embryos) were randomised, and where clinical (post-implantation) outcomes were reported. Only four RCTs (875 participants) were identified where the study design examined whether there is any overall benefit from culturing embryos in TLI incubators compared with conventional incubation. Yet these studies included participants with varying diagnoses, and with embryo transfer carried out on days 2, 3 or 5–6 of development, thus exposing embryos to different lengths of time in the respective incubators. The review concludes that the available evidence is low-quality, and fails to establish whether there is any advantage in using TLI over conventional incubation, in terms of rates of live birth/ongoing pregnancy, miscarriage/stillbirth, or even clinical pregnancy. Clearly, there is no compelling evidence to suggest this theoretical culture advantage has any effect, and therefore the routine use of incubators incorporating TLI technology during ART treatment with a view to improving embryo culture conditions is not justified.

A second potential *direct benefit* of TLI technology resides in its theoretical ability to improve accuracy in selecting those embryo(s) from a given cohort that are most likely to implant and lead to a successful pregnancy, through use of algorithms developed by analysis of time-lapse images of embryo development (morphokinetic analysis). The same Cochrane review (2019) [1] examines the evidence for improved embryo selection through use of such algorithms, rather than with conventional embryo selection using 'snapshot' observations at intervals during development. Only five eligible RCTs (1841 participants) were identified from the published literature, and even amongst these there were major methodological differences, including the transfer of varying numbers of embryos on day 3 or day 5 of development, and not all the studies reported live birth data. The review concludes that the available evidence is very low-quality, and fails to establish whether there is any difference between treatment outcomes with either method of embryo selection, irrespective of the type of incubator used, in terms of ongoing pregnancy, miscarriage, or clinical pregnancy, or even livebirth where these data were reported.

Of the four systematic reviews published to date examining the question of improved embryo selection, all are flawed (as detailed in the same Cochrane review, 2019) [1]. Only one concludes that use of TLI-generated algorithms for embryo selection confers any benefit in terms of treatment outcome [2]. The major weaknesses in the methodology, data inclusion and analysis of this review, compounded by the authors' possible conflict of interest in its findings, render its conclusion unreliable. Therefore, the routine use of incubators incorporating TLI technology during ART treatment with a view to improving embryo selection is not justified.

Finally, we must consider the *indirect harm* caused to patients by offering to use TLI technology during their treatment, presenting them with a significant additional financial burden (up to £750 or more in the UK), combined with the emotional burden of misplaced expectation. Vulnerable and highly suggestible patients embarking on ART need to know that there is no good evidence that using TLI technology, with or without associated embryo selection algorithms, will give them a better chance of achieving the birth of a healthy child than conventional methods of embryo incubation and assessment.

Therefore, due to the lack of robust studies and any definitive evidence, the only conclusion that can be drawn is that TLI technology should not be incorporated routinely into ART, and that its promotion may in fact cause indirect harm to patients.

References

1. Armstrong S, Bhide P, Jordan V, Pacey A, Marjoribanks J, Farquhar C. Time-lapse systems for embryo incubation and assessment in assisted reproduction. *Cochrane Database Syst Rev.* 2019; Issue 5. Art. No.: CD011320. DOI: 10.1002/14651858.CD011320.pub4.

2. Pribenszky C, Nilselid A-M, Montag M Time-lapse culture with morphokinetic embryo selection improves pregnancy and live birth chances and reduces early pregnancy loss: a meta-analysis. *Reprod BioMed.* Online 2017;35:511–20.

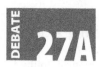

27A Artificial Intelligence Is Useful for Embryo Selection in IVF

For

Rachel Smith

Embryo selection is critical for optimising IVF outcome by identifying the embryo with the greatest chance to achieve a live birth (LB). There are several methods utilised, assessment of chromosomal copy number, application of time-lapse models based on temporal changes in development, or microscopical analysis of the embryo's morphological features. Identifying the single 'best' embryo does not improve the cumulative pregnancy or birth outcome, but reduces time to pregnancy, in turn reducing emotional and financial burdens by minimising the number of interventions needed. Here we debate whether artificial intelligence (AI) can improve our ability to select an embryo with the optimum potential to implant?

The use of artificial intelligence in medicine has risen with a recent explosion in reproductive technology with the promise to reduce errors, save time, remove bias and improve consistency, as AI follows a defined set of rules. Improvements in computer processing and the availability of big data sets to train and validate AI systems have driven this expansion. Deep learning (DL) is a subset of machine learning, requiring large amounts of quality data; it is suited to analysing digital images using multiple layered neural networks to detect complex structures or patterns. As machine learning is based on known outcomes, consideration of the quality of the input is imperative to ensure a robust outcome. Wang and colleagues recently identified seven areas of focus for AI in reproductive medicine: robotic surgery, sperm classification, oocyte selection, individualised outcome prediction, cost-effectiveness, clinical decision-making and embryo selection [1].

Emerging AI technologies aimed at embryo selection hold the promise of more detailed analysis of the morphological features from an image that would otherwise be impossible for a human to compute, and in a timeframe that allows the information to be used in cycle. Many laboratories already have access to a light microscope image or access to thousands of images generated using time-lapse; AI is an attractive selection tool which may be accessible without the need for additional equipment. To date, the focus has been on developing AI systems that can accurately predict the embryo grade, its viability (chance of achieving a pregnancy), and its ploidy status (aneuploid or euploid).

Conventional morphological embryo grading is generally performed by embryologists based on a microscopical static observation, at a specific time point. Morphological grading, of the blastocyst, is largely based on the inner cell mass, the trophectoderm and the degree of expansion exhibited by the embryo. To date there is no universally adopted classification system or consensus on the best time for this assessment to be performed. Morphological assessment is time-consuming and an insufficiently reliable indicator of implantation, due to its subjectivity and bias, as embryologists may be influenced subconsciously by various factors.

AI has the potential to increase the determining factors for classification by using image segmentation, deep neural networks (DNNs) and in particular, convolutional neural networks (CNNs) which contain neurons in three dimensions, enhancing the ability of DL algorithms to analyse images. An image can be static or a sequence of temporal images and the aim is to predict the quality or viability of the embryo better than an embryologist. Once the algorithm is trained and validated it is consistently applied and not open to inter- or intra-observer variation; it therefore has the potential to more accurately select embryos, thus improving pregnancy outcomes.

Recently, Khosravi and co-workers, graded time-lapse images as good or poor quality to train an application named STORK, with a reported 97.53% prediction accuracy [2]. Manually scored embryos, where at least three embryologists agreed on the grade, were compared to STORK with a precision prediction of 95.7%. Blastocysts graded by multiple embryologists to provide a majority agreed score, is the gold standard training data set, but large data sets of this type do not exist, and are time-consuming to create. AI prediction of embryo grade is therefore potentially at least as good as an embryologist classification, with the benefit of being consistent, rapid and not open to bias. The limitation is that predictive grading may be mimicking an existing classification system which is not strongly predictive of outcome. This could be improved by training an AI model to predict pregnancy or birth, rather than morphological grade.

Time-lapse derived morphokinetic algorithms are designed to improve the selection of embryos using known outcomes of ploidy, fetal heart (FH) or LB. Largely built on in-house clinical data, models are not necessarily transferable, and the potential improvement in outcome over morphological classification and standard incubation remains hotly debated, with a call for further randomised controlled trials. With many morphokinetic markers being linked to implantation outcome there is scope for AI to interpret where human interpretation is not possible.

A number of recently published AI models were trained on images from transferred embryos with a known FH (positive or negative). Using a defined outcome such as FH, instead of subjective embryo grading, improves clinical applicability of an AI model. Predicting FH is determined largely by embryo quality (80%) but patient factors and clinical indicators also play a role (20%); a theoretical prediction is assumed to be ~80%.

Static 2D images from light microscopy from 11 clinics were used to train an AI application called Life Whisperer, using ground truth outcomes from transferred embryos [3]. Life Whisperer reported an increase of 24.7% over predictions of viability made by the embryologist, with an 64.3% overall accuracy of prediction. Using images from light microscopy might have the widest application, but sequential images from time-lapse, spanning the development of the embryo, will provide substantially more data and may improve the prediction accuracy.

An alternative AI model named ERICA was trained on static, day 5 embryo images from three clinics with known ploidy or FH outcome, with the aim to rank embryos, predict ploidy and pregnancy outcome [4]. This study obtained a euploid, positive predictive value of 0.79 and a negative predictive value of 0.66; outperforming random classification and prediction by two embryologists and therefore demonstrating the potential for AI to rank embryos according to ploidy prediction.

Artificial intelligence has the potential to link factors beyond human interpretation within an image or sequence of images, and incorporating meta data, to pregnancy or ploidy outcome with prediction accuracy that outperforms an experienced embryologist. The same is not true for prediction of embryo grading, that only replicates an existing subjective classification system and is not currently reliably predictive of outcome. AI is reproducible, without bias, potentially low cost and time-saving. If trained on high quality, large compiled data from collaborators from multiple clinics has the potential to be transferable, unlike some time-lapse algorithms. Commercial AI models for embryo selection are emerging. Designed for use with blastocyst culture, they hold the promise to further enhance outcomes for IVF patients, with a more reliable, easily accessible, non-invasive, sequential embryo assessment of viability.

References

1. Wang R, Pan W, Jin L, et al. Artificial intelligence in reproductive medicine. *Reproduction*. 2019;158(4):R139–54.

2. Khosravi P, Kazemi E, Zhan Q, et al. Deep learning enables robust assessment and selection of human blastocysts after in vitro fertilization. *NPJ Dig Med*. 2019;2(21).

3. VerMilyea M, Hall JMM, Diakiw SM, et al. Development of an artificial intelligence-based assessment model for prediction of embryo viability using static images captured by optical light microscopy during IVF. *Hum Reprod*. 2020;35 (4):770–84.

4. Chavez-Badiola A, Flores-Saiffe-Farías A, Mendizabal-Ruiz G, Drakeley AJ, Cohen J. Embryo Ranking Intelligent Classification Algorithm (ERICA), an artificial intelligence clinical assistant with embryo ploidy and implantation predicting capabilities. *Reprod BioMed*. Online 2020;41(4):585–93.

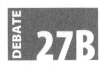

Artificial Intelligence Is Useful for Embryo Selection in IVF

Against

Lucy Wood and Helen Clarke

The use of artificial intelligence (AI) aims to revolutionise the way we work within the clinical IVF laboratory by offering invaluable assistance to the scientists selecting embryos for transfer. AI does this by removing the human operator from the process, allowing digital systems to feed on the data through a process called datamining. The AI system establishes artificial neural networks and essentially learns which embryo parameters are associated with desirable or undesirable outcomes [1]. The aim is to accurately detect the viability of embryos and rank them according to their implantation potential, thus increasing confidence in single embryo transfer and time to pregnancy. By performing entirely objectively, with precise scrutiny and with a wealth of data not accessible to the scientist, this computerised approach is designed to outperform the embryologist.

However, despite efforts to establish a firm place for AI during routine IVF, to date there is little evidence it will serve as a useful clinical tool. Although the non-invasive nature of AI appeals to professionals and patients as being seemingly harmless, the technology has multiple flaws that currently prevent its promotion to anything other than yet another useless and risky IVF 'add-on'.

Preceding AI embryo selection, time-lapse imaging within the IVF laboratory has provided over a decade's-worth of detailed morphological and morphokinetic data on undisturbed human embryo development in vitro. Since its implementation researchers have been attempting to associate aspects of this data with reproductive outcomes in efforts to make more accurate predictions on the viability of individual embryos. Sadly, statistical algorithms involving manual embryo annotation have so far failed to improve reproductive outcomes for IVF patients, with authors of a recent Cochrane review concluding there is no evidence to support their use over conventional morphological assessment of a static image by the embryologist [2]. The glaring lack of high-quality studies or evidence produced following a decade of time-lapse use leads us to the conclusion that morphokinetic annotation data is not useful in predicting live birth.

Tran et al. recently published a paper introducing an AI model based on such morphokinetic data collected during the development of over 8000 embryos [1]. Deep learning methods were employed to predict the likelihood of an embryo giving rise to a clinical pregnancy, measured by the presence of a foetal heart, with 93% accuracy. There is no denying this is an impressive leap for those in favour of automated embryology. However, the evidence falls short of holding clinical significance. Not only is the model based on retrospective data, but the all-important live birth data is lacking. A prospective randomised controlled trial is required to determine whether or not this AI application will be of any use in future.

A clinically relevant application of AI has been attempted by analysing static images of blastocysts, which resulted in a predictive value of 0.65 for ploidy status [3]. Although the researchers seemed satisfied with this value, it actually highlights the major flaw of the potential for AI to make the wrong call. Low accuracy outputs are not useful and cannot benefit the decision-making process. More of a hindrance than a help, at worst AI could lead to the deselection and disposal of perfectly viable embryos, or transfer of an aneuploid embryo with improper counselling or consent of the patient. This raises the issue of who takes responsibility for the calls made by the computer? It is currently impossible to understand how the AI makes its predictions based on the parameters it is given, therefore the embryologist would be expected to blindly trust the output. Given the far from perfect accuracy of the AI model, this would not be a wise choice. Acknowledging that other reproductive factors, such as uterine health, play a major role in the outcome of the cycle may explain the lack of precision and suggests that even attempting to perfect embryo selection using AI may ultimately be futile.

Convincing patients, medical clinicians or healthcare managers that the embryologists' fundamental role can be replaced by AI risks devaluing the scientists' highly specific skills. These capabilities are crucial for the success of the cycle and for providing information and specialist advice to patients. Patients deserve a detailed explanation of their embryo quality; with AI the embryologist is removed from the process and is unable to offer extra information other than 'computer says poor'. It is disheartening for the field. The personal touch, so important in an IVF cycle, is lost.

Crucially, the process of grading embryos provides insight for the scientific team about the health of their culture system. Embryologists become attuned to the behaviour of embryos under their watch to notice aberrations that feed directly into quality control systems. By skipping this robust monitoring step and relying solely on AI, the laboratory quality management system is compromised.

Replacing scientific skill with relatively cheap AI technology may seem attractive in a climate increasingly obsessed with financial gain. Similarly, charging patients high fees for unproven assisted reproductive technology has somehow become acceptable in the UK, damaging the reputation of the field. The HFEA traffic light system does not advocate the use of unproven technologies but many clinics nevertheless choose to sell such technology as an 'add on' [4]. Following this trend, vulnerable patients could easily be persuaded to pay for AI embryo selection in the misguided hope of improving their chances of having a baby.

The embryologist brings more to embryo selection than AI will ever achieve. By focusing on tiny scientific observations AI fails to comprehend the bigger picture. There is often more than one viable embryo produced per cycle, so why does it matter which is selected first? If the AI predicts a low chance of success, which patient would decide not to take the chance? The bottom line is that no matter how many embryo-selection tools we invent, we cannot use them to improve embryo viability. Considering the lack of robust evidence available and the ethical issues surrounding AI in the IVF laboratory, the conclusion is clear: artificial intelligence is not useful for embryo selection.

References

1. Tran D, Cooke S, Illingworth P, Gardner D. Deep learning as a predictive tool for fetal heart pregnancy following time-lapse incubation and blastocyst transfer. *Hum Reprod.* 2019;34(6):1011–18.

2. Armstrong S, Bhide P, Jordan V, Pacey A, Marjoribanks J, Farquhar C. Time-lapse systems for embryo incubation and assessment in assisted reproduction.

Cochrane Database Syst Rev. 2019(5). 10.1002/14651858.CD011320.pub4.

3. Miyagi Y, Habara T, Hirata R, Hayashi N. Feasibility of artificial intelligence for predicting live birth without aneuploidy from a blastocyst image. *Reprod Med Biol.* 2019;18(2):204–11.

4. HFEA. Treatment add-ons 2019. Available from: www.hfea.gov.uk/treatments/explore-all-treatments/treatment-add-ons/

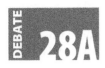

28A There Is No Need to Take Embryos Out of the Incubator until the Day of Embryo Transfer

For

Karen Thompson

The aim of any assisted reproductive technology (ART) cycle is ideally the delivery of a single healthy baby. This has led to clinics developing a robust single embryo transfer (eSET) policy in order to minimise the risk of multiple pregnancy without reducing the chance of having a live birth in any individual cycle. Of course this does rely on the ability to grow good embryos and the selection of the best embryo with the most potential for implantation for transfer. It is now common practice for women to have a single blastocyst transfer in order to maximise their chance of a successful implantation per embryo transfer [1].

The culture environment is critical for embryo development and studies using single step media without interruption combined with time lapse imaging (TLI) incubators have demonstrated similar rates of blastocyst development compared with a sequential system [2]. Historically a concern of culturing embryos for a prolonged period of time without a refresh of the media was the accumulation of ammonium ions which can have a negative impact on embryo development. This has been negated by advances in culture media design, particularly the use of the dipeptide form of glutamine which results in fewer ammonium ions being produced. A recent study also showed a trend to increased live birth rates and cumulative pregnancy rates with single step culture using TLI compared to standard culture [3]. This may in part be due to the use of morphokinetic data to enhance selection of the embryo for transfer. However an increase in cumulative pregnancy rates with this group suggests that the undisturbed culture may contribute to this uplift. The choice of culture media used is clearly important but successful embryo development also relies on a stable laboratory environment.

These laboratory controlled variables can impact on media efficacy and embryo development resulting in significantly different outcomes [4]. It is well-known that a change in temperature can influence the development of the early embryo by altering the meiotic spindle and possibly embryo metabolism, thus maintenance of a stable optimal temperature is absolutely crucial. Changes in intracellular pH can also impact embryo metabolism and therefore culture media contain buffers which help to regulate the pH. The majority of buffers in commercially available media contain bicarbonate buffer and this relies on the CO_2 in the incubator environment to maintain this pH. Finally it has been demonstrated that embryo development improves when embryos are cultured in low O_2 (5%) when compared to atmospheric O_2. Prolonged exposure to light and atmospheric volatile organic compounds (VOCs) may also contribute to impaired development, although most laboratories try to negate this effect by using sophisticated air filtration systems and filtered lighting.

Modern incubators have been designed to control all of these variables to optimise embryo development and therefore it makes no sense to remove embryos from the incubator, as this can lead to changes in the embryo environment which may have a deleterious effect on development and outcome. The use of TLI is clearly a handy tool as embryo development can be assessed without the need to remove the embryos from the incubator; however some laboratories do not have access to these incubators which are expensive. Therefore in these clinics, the embryos would need to be removed from the incubator in order to assess embryo development at an early stage, but is this really necessary?

A recent study demonstrated that assessment on day 2 and day 3 of embryos cultured in standard incubators without TLI may give an indication of predicted blastocyst formation [5]. This however does not necessarily aid selection of the best embryo as multiple embryos may have the potential to develop to the blastocyst stage, and therefore it is selection at the blastocyst stage which is really useful for successful outcome. Assessment at an earlier stage of development may however help to avoid cancellation of cycles where no blastocysts developed. In some scenarios, such as when patients only have one or two embryos available, then it may be appropriate to transfer at an earlier stage as blastocyst transfer does not convey any additional selection benefit. However, it could be argued that the transfer of a day 5 embryo may offer better uterine synchronicity. Cancellation rates remain low for patients where embryos are cultured to day 5, and if patients are counselled appropriately it would make sense not to remove them from the incubator in order to minimise disturbance to the embryo environment.

In summary, the advantages of maintaining a stable embryo environment by their remaining in the incubator outweigh the benefit of assessments of development made at an earlier stage by removing the embryos from culture. In addition, fewer assessments and manipulation of the embryos reduces the risk of any adverse incidents.

References

1. Glujovsky D, Farquhar C, Quinteiro Retamar AM, Alvarez Sedo CR, Blake D. Cleavage stage versus blastocyst stage embryo transfer in assisted reproductive technology. *Cochrane Database Syst Rev.* 2016; Issue 6. Art.No.: CD002118. DOI: 10.1002/14651858.CD002118.pub5.

2. Ciray HN, Aksoy T, Goktas C, Ozturk B, Bahecci M. Time lapse evaluation of human embryo development in single versus sequential culture media – a sibling oocyte study. *J Assist Reprod Genet.* 2012;29:891–900.

3. Mascarenhas M, Fox SJ, Thompson K, Balen AH. Cumulative live birth rates and perinatal outcomes with the use of time lapse imaging incubators for embryo culture: a retrospective cohort study of 1882 ART cycles. *BJOG.* 2018; https://doi.org/10.1111/1471-0528.15161.

4. Swain JE, Carrell D, Cobo A, Messeuger M, Rubio C, Smith GD. Optimising the culture environment and embryo manipulation to help maintain embryo developmental potential. *Fertil Steril.* 2016;105:571–87.

5. Van HK, Segal T, Epstein D, Liu J, Rossi B, Goldfarb J. Predicting blastulation rate with day 2 and 3 morphology: evaluation of cost limited embryo assessment. *Fertil Steril.* 2018;109(3) sup e54–5.

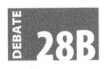
There Is No Need to Take Embryos Out of the Incubator until the Day of Embryo Transfer

Against

Catherine Pretty

The clear goal of any embryologist is to minimise the stress placed on the embryos in their care, thereby maximising the chance of healthy pregnancies by replacing high quality, euploid embryos. The means to attain this goal however, aren't always so clear.

The evolution of single-step culture media, and the increasing use of time-lapse technology to monitor embryo development has intensified interest in a 'hands-off' approach to culture. Leaving the embryos undisturbed is certainly appealing to the lab manager organising the workload, but does it always benefit the embryos?

There are several reasons why an embryo may need to be removed from the incubator during the period of culture – namely observation, manipulation or to optimise their environment. Each of these can be examined independently.

Observation of embryos is vital, both for selection of the embryo to transfer, and for information during the culture period. Where more than one embryo is available for transfer, the embryologist aims to replace whichever embryo has the highest chance of creating a healthy pregnancy. Conversely, when embryo development during the cleavage stage is suboptimal, and the chance of even a single embryo continuing to develop for transfer are reduced, most patients would prefer to be advised and counselled appropriately. Five days between fertilisation and transfer could be an unbearable wait for the patient, especially if the outcome was a cancelled transfer due to embryo fragmentation or arrest days earlier. The possibility that an embryo would have formed a viable pregnancy if transferred earlier in the culture period is a thought that might haunt patients and embryologists alike.

Of course, the advent of time-lapse technology allows assessment of both morphology and developmental timing without the need to remove the culture dish from the incubator. However this equipment is costly to install and run, and many patients and clinics do not have access to this technology. Indeed, further work is needed to determine whether use of time-lapse imaging is effective in terms of cost per live birth [1]. The introduction of time-lapse technology requires excellent training and quality control to maintain standards [2]. In cases without time-lapse observation, the removal of the embryos from the incubator to assess development during culture would generally be considered necessary.

Second, any embryo manipulation during the period of culture would necessitate removing the embryo from culture. Prior to biopsy for pre-implantation genetic testing for aneuploidy (PGT-A), embryos may undergo laser assisted hatching on day three. This allows cells to herniate through the zona pellucida through internal pressure caused by blastocyst expansion, and facilitates biopsy at the blastocyst stage [3]. Such a process would clearly necessitate removal from the incubator, for hatching to occur.

Finally, and perhaps most controversially, undisturbed embryos would by definition require single-step culture conditions. The media that fertilised eggs are placed into on day one of culture would be unchanged through the cleavage stages of development, compaction and eventually blastulation. The use of single-step culture media has the potential to reduce stress to the embryo, and it can certainly simplify laboratory processes and reduce associated costs. On the other hand, five-to-seven days of uninterrupted culture has the potential to exacerbate the effect of any sub-optimal culture conditions [4]. Laboratory-based stressors such as changes in osmolality due to evaporation, build-up of toxins or changes in pH may negate any potential benefits seen from well-implemented single-step culture. If a laboratory refreshes culture media on day three, the chance for accumulation of volatile organic compounds or for degradation of culture media is reduced. The stress caused by build-up of ammonia, or other negative effects from degradation of culture media or oil could significantly impact the implantation potential of embryos. Sequential culture systems of course also provide the benefit of providing each substrate at a developmentally appropriate stage, mimicking the in vivo environment more closely.

Overall, there are benefits and drawbacks to single-step culture. More research is required to clarify whether single-step culture is preferable to sequential, and ultimately both systems may have their place [5]. In the future, microfluidic systems may allow the growth of embryos in a dynamic culture environment. Until that time, one thing is clear, that use of a sequential culture system and moving embryos from one culture dish to another will require their removal from the incubator.

To conclude, new developments in assisted reproductive technology such as time-lapse imaging can reduce the need for embryos to be disturbed during the culture period. Conversely the implementation of other new technologies such as PGT-A may require embryos to be removed from the incubator for manipulation. Future developments such as microfluidics may negate the need for moving embryos into fresh dishes, while maintaining the benefits of refreshed culture media, but for now there are significant benefits of sequential culture systems. In short, embryos clearly do still need to be removed from the incubator – and there is still work for an embryologist!

References

1. Mascarenhas M, Fox SJ, Thompson K, Balen AH. Cumulative live birth rates and perinatal outcomes with the use of time-lapse imaging incubators for embryo culture: a retrospective cohort study of 1882 ART cycles. *BJOG* 2019;**126** (2):280–86.

2. ESHRE Working Group on Time-Lapse Technology: Apter S, Ebner T, Freour T, et al. Good practice recommendations for the use of time-lapse technology. *Hum Reprod Open.* 2020;**2020**: Issue 2.

3. Singh S, Hobeika E, Knochenhauer ES, Traub ML. Pregnancy rates after pre-implantation genetic screening for aneuploidy are only superior when trophectoderm biopsy is performed on hatching embryos. *JARG.* 2019;**36** (4):621–8.

4. Swain J. Controversies in ART: considerations and risks for uninterrupted embryo culture. *RMBO.* 2019:**39**(1):19–26.

5. Sfontouris IA, Martins WP, Nastri CO, et al. Blastocyst culture using single versus sequential media in clinical IVF: a systematic review and meta-analysis of randomized controlled trials. *JARG.* 2016;**33**(10):1261–72.

29A Blastocyst Culture Should Be a Routine in All IVF Cycles

For

Louise Kellam

In IVF treatment an embryo can be transferred to the uterus at the blastocyst-stage or earlier at the cleavage-stage. Here we debate the merits of blastocyst transfer over cleavage-stage, and the case for routine blastocyst culture in all IVF cycles.

We know that the single embryo transfer of a blastocyst is more likely to result in a live birth compared to a cleavage-stage embryo [1]. This is not surprising as a blastocyst is the consequence of self-selection and by definition has conquered many morphogenetic hurdles of early embryonic development, including the activation of its own embryonic genome. Its unique morphology provides a visual marker of its biological journey over an arrested or degenerate embryo; only the most viable embryos develop to blastocyst. It is postulated that similarly, in vivo, up to half of embryos fail to develop and this may explain the low fecundity rates of humans relative to many other species. Moreover, the improved uterine and embryonic synchronicity with a blastocyst transfer, prevents premature exposure to the uterine environment. Human embryos in vivo reach the uterine cavity on day 4–5 of development, so for cleavage-stage embryos, particularly following ovarian stimulation and elevated oestrogen, the endometrium may not provide the appropriate physiological environment. Whereas blastocyst culture offers time for the oestrogen levels to subside and enhances embryo–endometrium synchronisation, with reduced uterine contractility.

Extended culture to blastocyst is a common first-line approach to embryo selection in many IVF laboratories. UK HFEA clinic data shows that the proportion of blastocyst embryo transfers rose steadily from 10% in 2006 to 61% in 2014 [2]. This is likely to be part of an active decision to only transfer one embryo even if more are available. Consequently, the incidence of multiple births, the single biggest health risk from IVF, declined from 24% in 2008 to an unprecedented low of 10% in 2019.

The improved survival of blastocysts in vitro is attributed to advances in the understanding of the nutritional requirements and physiology of embryos. Today the use of superior culture media, reduced oxygen concentration and strict temperature control minimises the stress imposed on embryos. The use of uninterrupted culture, integrated time-lapse microscopy, and single-step media has grown in popularity, reducing the handling and disturbance involved in blastocyst culture and permitting assessment of morphokinetic markers of embryo development to blastocyst stage, a concept not feasible with cleavage-stage checks. In addition, information gained from time-lapse imagery of abnormal cleavage, fragmentation, multinucleation, degeneration and mitotic arrest, provide further indicators for embryo selection.

For patients with a good prognosis, the transfer of a blastocyst over a cleavage-stage embryo is more successful, as concluded by a Cochrane meta-analysis of 27 randomised controlled trials in 2016 [1]. This analysis reported a higher implantation and live birth rate per transfer in the blastocyst transfer group compared to cleavage-stage transfer, with no evidence for a difference in the rates of miscarriage and multiple pregnancy. In poorer prognosis patients, high-quality studies are lacking in number and hence no strong conclusions can be made. However, the meta-analysis suggested only 2–4% of patients will have no embryos transferred, compared to 1% of women that planned cleavage-stage transfer. To advocate extending culture to improve success, it may be suggested that patient expectations can be managed by counselling pertaining to this outcome. Besides, whilst it cannot be proven, it may be considered that embryos may not have developed any differently in vivo. Appreciating that the surrounding microenvironment of the embryo in vivo is dynamic; muscle movement, epithelial cilia movement and maternal respiration, and that this is not easily reconstructed in a lab, the development in vivo *could* be superior to that in vitro. This is hard to determine and natural pre-implantation embryo loss from cleavage-stage to blastocyst remains quantitatively undefined [3]. Embryos that fail to continue to develop in extended culture have been shown to have multiple aneuploidies although the development to the blastocyst stage is not a guarantee of chromosomal normality [4]. A further advantage of having a laboratory blastocyst culture strategy is that for pre-implantation genetic testing (PGT), an important embryo selection tool used to determine the karyotype or genetic disease status of the embryo, blastocysts withstand the stress of a biopsy procedure better than cleavage-stage embryos, have less mosaicism to confound results, and are more likely to survive a freeze–thaw process.

Comparative information on embryo utilisation and cumulative pregnancy and birth rates, by developmental stage of the embryo, are lacking but may well prove to highlight other benefits of blastocyst culture and transfer. Vitrification of blastocysts is commonly employed due to the high survival and implantation success compared to early stage embryos. Robust data is required, but an earlier time to pregnancy requiring fewer cycles, would be preferable to patients, physically, emotionally and financially, and would further promote a blastocyst culture strategy.

Finally, and importantly, it is accepted that an embryo may be vulnerable to alterations of environmental factors, but evidence of epigenetic changes in blastocyst culture is weak, nevertheless the health of live births has been investigated. A study in 2019 showed that babies born following blastocyst transfer have a similar chance of being healthy as those born after cleavage-stage embryo transfer, concluding that perinatal outcomes in singleton live births following the transfer of fresh blastocysts are no different from those of singleton live births after cleavage-stage embryo transfer [5]. However further evidence is needed before drawing a definitive conclusion about perinatal safety of extended embryo culture.

As extended culture is gaining popularity across the world, there is little doubt that it is the best strategy for selecting embryos for their implantation potential, particularly in elective single-embryo transfers to reduce the risk of multiple pregnancies, with no evident detrimental impact on live birth outcomes or health of babies born.

References

1. Glujovsky D, Farquhar C, Quinteiro Retamar AM, Alvarez Sedo CR, Blake D. Cleavage-stage versus blastocyst stage embryo transfer in assisted reproductive technology. *Cochrane Database Syst Rev.* 2016; Issue 6.

2. HFEA. Fertility treatment in 2014–2016, trends and figures. Human Fertility Embryology Authority: UK, 2018.

3. Jarvis GE. Early embryo mortality in natural human reproduction: What the data say. *F1000Res.* 2017;5:2765.

4. Delhanty JDA. Mechanisms of aneuploidy induction in human oogenesis and early embryogenesis. *Cytogenet Genome Res.* 2005;111(3–4):237–44.

5. Marconi N, Raja EA, Bhattacharya S, Maheshwari A. Perinatal outcomes in singleton live births after fresh blastocyst-stage embryo transfer: A retrospective analysis of 67 147 IVF/ICSI cycles. *Hum Reprod.* 2019;34(9):1716–25.

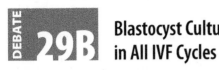

29B Blastocyst Culture Should Be a Routine in All IVF Cycles

Against

Jason Kasraie

Introduction

Improvements in embryo culture techniques combined with the need to maximise pregnancy rate per embryo transferred whilst minimising the multiple pregnancy rate have, in the last decade or so, led to a huge increase in the number of blastocyst transfer cycles undertaken in IVF [1]. However, whilst reductions in time to pregnancy have been made and single blastocyst transfer is useful in reducing multiple pregnancy rates, the drive towards blastocyst culture and transfer has not been clearly demonstrated to be beneficial for all patients. There is an assumption in clinics that culture all patients' embryos to the blastocyst stage that any embryo that does not reach the blastocyst stage in vitro would not do so in vivo, but there remains a lack of robust evidence to support this.

Discussion

There are many putative advantages of blastocyst transfer, these include:

- Not exposing the embryo to the environment of the uterus earlier than normal.
- Transferring the embryo to the uterus when the endometrium is more receptive and potentially more synchronous to the embryo.
- Increased time for embryo selection leading to increased implantation and pregnancy rates.
- Reduction in multiple pregnancy rates if a single blastocyst is transferred.
- Trophectoderm biopsy is possible when performing pre-implantation genetic diagnosis or screening [2].

The possible disadvantages of blastocyst transfer include:

- Higher cycle cancellation rate (8.9% for blastocyst culture vs. 2.8% for cleavage stage culture [3]).
- Reduction in the rate of cryopreservation.
- Poorer obstetric and perinatal outcomes including:
  o Increase in preterm birth.
  o Monozygotic twinning.
  o Increase in congenital anomalies.
  o Increased imprinting disorders and large for gestational age babies.
  o Increased miscarriage rate.

- Altered sex ratio [4].

There is a remarkable lack of certainty on a number of the issues listed above. Blastocyst transfer probably results in increased pregnancy rates when equal numbers of embryos are transferred and is key to the selection of a single embryo to transfer for the reduction of multiple pregnancy rates. It is undoubtedly key to modern pre-implantation genetic diagnosis (PGD) and pre-implantation genetic screening (PGS).

There is not enough evidence to determine the effects of blastocyst transfer on monozygotic twinning rates, rates of congenital abnormality, imprinting errors or cumulative pregnancy rates [3]. There are some disadvantages associated with blastocyst transfer including increased cycle cancellation rates, an altered sex ratio (favouring males), a reduction in embryo cryopreservation rates and an increase in preterm birth rates [2].

Cumulative pregnancy rate is key for many and it is clear that less embryos are frozen following blastocyst culture. There is no convincing evidence that blastocyst culture is not inferior to cleavage stage culture in terms of cumulative pregnancy [3], so blastocyst transfer may be detrimental to some patients.

The advantages of blastocyst transfer are seductive and lead to instant gratification for the IVF clinic, which, if it implements a policy of blastocyst culture for all patients, experiences an increase in pregnancy rates per cycle completed and can advertise it. The importance of this cannot be underestimated in the ultra-competitive IVF sector, where centres may be perversely incentivised to report higher pregnancy rates and thus may favour, albeit subconsciously, a system that deselects patients with a lower prognosis (i.e. those whose embryos fail to blastulate). It is easy to forget the 9% of cycles that are abandoned.

A 'one size fits all' approach such as blastocyst transfer for everyone, potentially limits our flexibility as scientists and clinicians and undermines our ability to offer individualised patient care. It also assumes that in vitro embryo culture is now as good as, if not superior to in vivo culture, as it infers that embryos that fail to reach the blastocyst stage in vitro would do so in vivo. Are we at the stage, after just over 40 years of clinical IVF that we can claim our laboratories and our clinical protocols are superior to millions of years of evolution?

Is it fair to advise a couple that they will never achieve a pregnancy through IVF because they fail to develop blastocysts in the laboratory or is it better to advise patients, based on their specific circumstances, what the most appropriate treatment plan might be? Is it fair to rob couples of an embryo transfer and the chance of a pregnancy, no matter how remote that might be, because they fail to develop a blastocyst?

Surely, rather than having the decision taken out of their hands when there is no convincing evidence of the superiority of blastocyst transfer across the patient population as a whole, patients should be informed of the relative advantages and disadvantages of cleavage stage versus blastocyst culture and involved in the decision making process? If time to pregnancy is paramount and there is a good chance of blastocyst formation then blastocyst culture is perfectly appropriate. If there is a need to maximise embryo utilisation and cumulative pregnancy rates whilst minimising the number of invasive egg collections and/or the risk of ovarian hyperstimulation syndrome (OHSS), then cleavage stage transfer with the chance of more frozen embryo transfers may be appropriate.

Conclusions

Ultimately, can we categorically advise patients that do not develop blastocysts in vitro that they would not have achieved a pregnancy if we transferred embryos at the cleavage stage? Quite simply the answer is currently *no*, which is why a treatment algorithm that includes both blastocyst transfer and cleavage stage transfer is optimal at this time.

References

1. Human Fertilisation and Embryology Authority. Fertility treatment in 2014: Trends and figures. HFEA, 2016; available from: www.hfea.gov.uk/10243.html.

2. Kasraie J. (2019) Cleavage stage or blastocyst transfer: which is better? In: G Kovacs, L Salamonsen (eds.) *How to Prepare the Endometrium to Maximize Implantation Rates and IVF Success.* Cambridge: Cambridge University Press, pp. 91–103.

3. Glujovsky D, Farquhar C, Quinteiro Retamar AM, Alvarez Sedo CR, Blake D. Cleavage stage versus blastocyst stage embryo transfer in assisted reproductive technology. *Cochrane Database Syst Rev.* 2016, Issue 6.

4. Maheshwari A, Hamilton M, Bhattacharya S. Should we be promoting embryo transfer at blastocyst stage? *Reprod BioMed.* Online, 2016;32(2):142–6.

30A Sex Selection Should Be Permitted for Family Balancing

For

Jigal Haas

When a couple decides to conceive, many emotions, hopes and expectations are involved. For most of the future parents, the gender of the child is the least significant concern. All the parents hope is for a healthy child.

In the minority of the cases, for various reasons, there is a preferred particular sex. The parents may want to reduce sex-linked and sex-limited disease risk for their future children or to balance the sex ratio among their children.

Pre-conception sex selection for non-medical reasons raises serious moral, legal and social issues. The main concern relies on the assumption that a freely available service for sex selection will distort the natural sex ratio and lead to a severe gender imbalance.

There are different methods proposed for pre-conception sex selection. The most natural method is trying to change the pH of the vagina. It has been suggested that the pH of the vagina at the time of fertilisation may have a differential effect on X- or Y-bearing sperm and thereby affect the sex of the offspring. Various studies demonstrated an impact of pH on sperm viability, motility and capacitation, but whether changing the pH of the vagina may affect the sex ratio is still debatable. In mammals, different studies have shown non-significant and contradictory results for impact of altering the pH on the migration of X- and Y-bearing sperm. Different diets were shown to change the vaginal pH, but still studies didn't show an increase in the desired gender by changing the diet.

Whether the timing of intercourse may influence the sex of the baby is another enigma. One of the theories is that couples who wish to have a male should time their intercourse to coincide with ovulation, with up to 85% success claimed for the selection of males and 80% for the selection of girls. In contrast, another theory is that if there is any tendency, it is for more females than males to be conceived when coitus occurs close to ovulation. A study published by Wilcox et al. in the NEJM, aimed to assess the association between timing of intercourse and the sex of the infant. They didn't find any differences between the patterns of intercourse that produced boys nor those that produced girls [1].

Human sperm sorted by flow cytometry may increase the likelihood that a child so conceived will be of a particular sex. The intensity of the fluorescence emitted by the DNA of chromosomally normal sperm varies depending on the presence of the X- or the Y-chromosome. The X-chromosome contains more DNA than the Y chromosome. In sperm stained with a DNA specific fluorochrome, this difference in DNA content is made evident by the intensity of the fluorescent signal emitted by the stained sperm, thereby allowing the differentiation of X- from Y-bearing sperm such that enriched populations of X- or Y-bearing sperm may be generated using flow cytometric sorting. Karabinus et al. [2] found that sorted specimens averaged $87.7 \pm 5.0\%$ X-bearing sperm after sorting for X and $74.3 \pm 7.0\%$ Y-bearing sperm after sorting for Y. They concluded that flow cytometric sorting of human sperm shifted the X:Y sperm ratio. IUI, IVF/ICSI and FET outcomes were consistent with unimpaired sperm function. Results provide evidence supporting the effectiveness of flow cytometric sorting of human sperm for use as a pre-conception method of influencing a baby's sex.

All the previously described methods are non-invasive and performed prior to the formation of the embryo, and are therefore more acceptable for ethical reasons, but the only 100% accurate method for sex selection is IVF (in vitro fertilisation) and PGT-A (pre-implantation genetic testing for aneuploidy). After performing IVF, the embryo can be biopsied, genetically tested, and the patients will be able to know the gender of the embryo. There are countries in the world where sex selection is permitted for different non-medical indications. In Israel for example, sex selection for non-medical reasons is basically prohibited. Exceptions are granted by a committee appointed by the director general of the Ministry of Health, where married couples with four children of same sex can apply if they feel there would be significant psychological distress to one of the family members following the delivery of another child with the same sex. Kirshenbaum et al. described the pre-implantation embryos' sex ratios in couples with four or more children of same sex, undergoing sex selection for non-medical reasons, and surprisingly found that only 35% were of the desired sex [3].

Sex selection can be performed pre-conception – by sperm selection, post-fertilisation using pre-implantation genetic diagnosis (PGD), or prenatally, using sex selective abortion, methods that should avoid the worst cases of neglecting undesired-sex babies. Moreover, since the latter is less acceptable due to the need for late first trimester abortion with its consequent complications, the combination of PGD with flow cytometric sorting of human sperm might be the preferred choice.

Although it's medically possible to perform sex selection, it does raise serious moral, legal and social issues, but even so, shouldn't the parents decide whether to perform the sex selection or not? In a world where early abortions are performed daily for non-medical reasons, is it so non-ethical to perform sex selection? In some cultures, the gender of the child can be extremely important for the family, and there may be a significant psychological distress to the parents following the delivery of another child with the same sex.

I believe that every country should have their own ethical committees deciding what is appropriate for their citizens, and what the criteria should be for sex selection in their region, and by that, the sex balance between the genders will stay stable.

References

1. Wilcox AJ, CR Weinberg, DD Baird. Timing of sexual intercourse in relation to ovulation. Effects on the probability of conception, survival of the pregnancy, and sex of the baby. *N Engl J Med.* 1995;333 (23):1517–21.

2. Karabinus DS, Marazo DP, Stern HJ, et al. The effectiveness of flow cytometric sorting of human sperm (MicroSort(R)) for influencing a child's sex. *Reprod Biol Endocrinol.* 2014;12:106.

3. Kirshenbaum M, Feldman B, Aizer A, et al. Preimplantation embryos sex ratios in couples with four or more children of same sex, what should be expected from a preimplantation genetic diagnosis cycle? *Gynecol Endocrinol.* 2019;35(6):515–17.

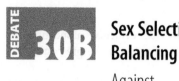

Sex Selection Should Be Permitted for Family Balancing

Against

Shirley Eve Levitan

There are four arguments against sex selection: (1) It encourages 'parenting by stereotype', where the desire to have a child of a certain gender may be based on a stereotypical ideal of what that gender is *supposed* to be like. (2) It is typically done in favour of males, leading to a significant shortage of females, which causes a myriad of serious problems. (3) It gives pre-implantation genetic diagnosis (PGD) a bad name. PGD is utilised to screen out a panoply of genetic disorders such as Lou Gehrig's disease, breast cancer, and cystic fibrosis. Using it to screen out an unwanted *gender* is a poor way to deploy scarce medical resources and know-how. (4) It could be a gateway to eugenics, the widely condemned theory of improving humanity by preventing inferior people from reproducing while encouraging reproduction of those judged to be superior.

Introduction

Sex selection is illegal in Canada, but in the United States 73% of fertility clinics offer it. Of those, nearly 84% offer it to couples who do not have fertility problems, but are doing in vitro fertilisation solely as a means of controlling the pregnancy's outcome. Sex selection is not new – the ancient Greeks and Romans attempted it with various methods, involving things like heat and cold, left and right testicles, left and right sides of the body, and sperm crossing or not crossing from one side of the womb to the other. In ancient China, a Gender Chart was utilised to predict and select a baby's sex, based on Yin-Yang, Five Elements, Eight Diagrams, and time. Today, sex selection is accomplished by creating embryos, sorting out the male and female ones, then implanting only the desired gender. Many arguments have been made on both sides of this controversial issue. Below are my views against sex selection.

1. **Parenting by Stereotype** –– The desire to have a child of a certain gender may be based on a *stereotypical* ideal of what that gender is supposed to be like. This could lead to difficulty if, say, the longed-for boy asks for ballet lessons, or the longed-for girl becomes a 6' 4", 250-pound basketball champion who wears nothing but jeans and boots. Not that there's anything wrong with that, but someone who pre-selects their child's sex might think there is. In other words, having a preference for one sex over the other may suggest a kind of parental sexism.

The child, of course, cannot be sent back for a refund, and the 'failure' of the child to conform to gender-prejudice norms might become a source of higher-than-normal parental scorn. It's bad enough to be told by your parents that, 'We were hoping for a girl, but we love you just the same,' but family dysfunction rises to a new level if you're told, 'We made sure you were a girl, but nevertheless we are very disappointed in you.' The emotional and psychological impact of this type of parental rejection cannot be quantified.

2. **'Missing' Females** –– In certain parts of the world, notably China and India, sex selection in favour of boys has led to a significant shortage of females. (Boys are said to be

preferred because they are seen as the earners who will support their parents throughout their life, inherit property, and carry on the family name. Plus, boys do not have to provide dowry payments – rather, they are on the receiving end of this practice.) A recent Indian government report found that about 63 million women were statistically 'missing' from the country's population.

This leads to obvious problems. When there are more men than women in a society, there will be a lot of men who will *never* be able to marry or otherwise have a female life partner. Violent crimes like rape may become more frequent, and a society of single men with a steadily diminishing mating pool can lead to human trafficking and prostitution. There are reports of women in poor areas being drugged, kidnapped, and transported elsewhere to satisfy the shortage of young females.

3. **Giving PGD a Bad Name** –– In the past, the only way to sex-select was to become pregnant, do an ultrasound to discover the gender, then abort if it's not the one you want. Nowadays sex selection has piggybacked onto a legitimate disease-prevention technique known as pre-implantation genetic diagnosis (PGD), where embryos are created and scrutinised for a panoply of genetic disorders such as Lou Gehrig's disease, breast cancer, and cystic fibrosis. While they're at it, the technicians can see what gender the embryos are. The undesired sex can be put aside, and later discarded or frozen for future use.

This represents a corruption of a lifesaving clinical procedure, and it might turn public sentiment against PGD generally. It may be viewed as unseemly that sex selection is carried out during the PGD disease-purging process, and it may invite the conflation of the critical with the superficial: 'We got rid of the embryos suffering from Huntington's disease, and while we were at it, we chucked the ones suffering from femaleness.'

After all, it's easy to respect a dermatologist who does nothing but heal the sick, but it might be less easy to respect a mere 'cosmetic' dermatologist. It's the same with 'cosmetic' PGD – is this *really* how we want to deploy scarce medical resources and know-how?

4. **Eugenics** –– Eugenics, which is the attempt to improve humanity by preventing inferior people from reproducing while encouraging reproduction of those judged to be superior, is widely considered to be a bad idea. For one thing, who's to say what's inferior? The recent film *Peanut Butter Falcon* stars an actor with Down's syndrome who many perceive to be an interesting man with a fulfilling life.

While sex-selection is not eugenics, it might be a *gateway* to it: if you're going to make a boy, while you're at it why don't you make a boy with blonde hair, blue eyes, and – more importantly – a genius IQ?

This flies in the face of the idea of equality, and invites discrimination and stigmatisation of those who do not want, or cannot afford, the technology. It could lead to genetic 'castes'. More disturbingly, some believe it could create human sub-species, with no ability to cross-breed, and with as much interest in each other as a current human would have for a chimpanzee.

It has also been argued that it is morally wrong to tamper with universal human constraints, such as aging, and limitations on physical and cognitive ability. These constraints provide a necessary context for the experience of meaningful human choice, and human lives would no longer seem meaningful in a world where such limitations could be overcome with technology. Also, eugenics involves the elimination of traits, and therefore reduces genetic diversity. A loss of genetic diversity could lead to increased vulnerability to disease, a reduced ability to adapt to environmental change, and other problems that cannot be anticipated.

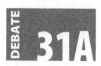

Reproductive Medicine Should Be Publicly Funded

For

Jeff Nisker

I have argued ever since the April Fool's Day declaration in 1994 that took away public funding of in vitro fertilisation (IVF) in Canada, that all women in Canada should have equal access to reproductive medicine [1, 2]. I have argued ever since the April Fool's Day declaration in 1994, no woman in Canada should have to undergo suboptimal and risky medical strategies in order to have IVF or related technologies to achieve having a child [1, 2]. These suboptimal and risky strategies include having to sell half their oocytes in exchange (or barter) for access to an IVF cycle [1, 2]. What I mean when I refer to having access to appropriate reproductive medicine, including IVF and related technologies, is that all women in Canada with appropriate indications should be able to have multiple publicly funded IVF cycles if they so wish, rather than women in Canada being confined to having only one cycle in some provinces, and only if the woman has blocked (rather than otherwise incapacitated) fallopian tubes as demonstrated by imaging techniques [1]. There are scientifically proven medical indications for IVF and related technologies other than damaged fallopian tubes [2].

I will argue here by taking the affirmative to re-instating public funding of scientifically proven reproductive medicine in Canada, including IVF and related technologies, that in a social justice-based democracy such as Canada's all women ought to receive equal access to health promotion and care, which includes reproductive medicine. I will argue here by taking the affirmative to re-instating public funding of scientifically-proven reproductive medicine in Canada, that this view is consistent with the Canada Health Act [3] that insists all Canadians out to receive equal access to health promotion and care. I will argue here that for women in Canada to whom it is important to have a child for their social and psychological health, access to appropriate reproductive medicine ought to be publicly funded. I will argue here that access to the best reproductive-medicine strategies, including for many women access to IVF and related technologies, must be equal for all women in Canada.

The Canada Health Act makes no distinction regarding access between Canada's socially-economically advantaged and socially-economically disadvantaged women [3]. For example, the Canada Health Act states:

> that continued access to quality health care without financial or other barriers will be critical to maintaining and improving the health and well-being of Canadians [3].

Further, the Canada Health Act states:

> that the primary objective of Canadian health care policy is to protect, promote and restore the physical and mental well-being of residents of Canada and to facilitate reasonable access to health services without financial or other barriers [3].

In addition, Section 12 (1) of the Canada Health Act specifically addresses accessibility when it states that:

> to satisfy the criterion respecting accessibility, the health care insurance plan of a province (a) must provide for insured health services on uniform terms and conditions and on a basis that does not impede or preclude, either directly or indirectly whether by charges made to insured persons or

otherwise, reasonable access to those services by insured persons; (b) must provide for payment for insured health services in accordance with a tariff or system of payment authorized by the law of the province; (c) must provide for reasonable compensation for all insured health services rendered by medical practitioners or dentists ... [3]

Although health promotion and care in Canada is funded by provincial rather than federal governments, the spirit of the Canada Health Act must still apply. Provinces have enough wealth, and should have enough medical resources, to afford women access to IVF and related technologies. This statement is valid particularly considering public funding of IVF will actually decrease health spending because women will not be forced to have controlled ovarian hyperstimulation with intrauterine insemination and risk multiple pregnancies, or tubal pregnancies and subsequent medical treatment [1, 2]. This view is supported by the many other jurisdictions in the world that fund IVF [1, 2], and emphasised by the World Health Organization. Indeed the World Health Organization emphasises that, 'Many studies have established that in vitro fertilisation (IVF) may be cost-effective and feasible in developing nations' [4], and argues further that the highest pregnancy rate and safest way to pursue having a child is through IVF [5]. This research, and these statements, continue to be true, although current health resources in jurisdictions all over the world have been stretched by the COVID-19 pandemic.

Those who would declare that the choice to have the ability to pursue becoming pregnant has nothing to do with the health of a woman, argue that infertility does not kill or in any way physically harm a woman. However, there is more to health than prevention of death or physical ill health. In fact psychological and social health are important parameters as described in the World Health Organization's social determinants of health [5]. Further, the World Health Organization draws attention to the fact that

> Equitable access to affordable, quality MAR [medically assisted reproduction] care should contribute to public health and become government policy in all countries with summary data, as a minimal standard, to be regularly published.

In summary, who has the right in a social justice-based democracy, and in light of the Canada Health Act and the World Health Organization's declarations, to deny women who believe their good health includes their fulfillment of having a child the right to have a child in our public health system? Who has the right to suggest that socially-economically disadvantaged women should be denied access to social and psychological health, while socially-economically advantaged women can buy their way into such health fulfillment? Who has the right to suggest that social and psychological health is not covered in the Canada Health Act, or in the World Health Organization's social determinants of health? [5] Who has the right to suggest that in Canada, national and provincial jurisdictions are so ungenerous as to deny socially-economically disadvantaged women the right to have a child?

Canadians are generous people, and I believe none of us ought to desire to deny the opportunity to pursue having a child any woman in Canada who desires having a child.

References

1. Nisker JA. Rachel's ladders or how societal situation determines reproductive therapy. *Hum Reprod.* 1996 June;11(6):1162–7.

2. Nisker JA. Anniversary of injustice: April Fool's Day, 1994. Will the Enactment of Bill C-6 be the birthday of equitable reproductive health care in Canada?

J Obstet Gynaecol Can. 2004 April 1;26 (4):321–4.

3. Minister of Justice. Canada Health Act, RSC, 1985, c. C-6. Available from: https://laws-lois.justice.gc.ca/PDF/C-6.pdf.

4. WHO. 2002. Current Practices and Controversies in Assisted Reproduction Report of a meeting on 'Medical, Ethical and Social Aspects of Assisted Reproduction,' held at WHO Headquarters in Geneva, Switzerland. Available from: https://apps.who.int/iris/bitstream/handle/10665/42576/9241590300.pdf;jsessionid=6F5FA04D8407B19F4A6527EC188A48F7?sequence=1.

5. WHO. Social Determinants of Health. 2020. Available from: www.who.int/social_determinants/en.

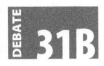

Reproductive Medicine Should Be Publicly Funded

Against

William D Schlaff

If only the world were ideal, I would be passionately in favour of public funding for reproductive care. Given that the majority of people throughout the world define themselves and their lives in the context of family, a responsive body politic would emphatically insist that medical care that enables family building should be one of the highest priorities for health care coverage. Perhaps I would find myself as avidly supportive of this viewpoint were I living somewhere other than the United States. Alas, the world is not ideal, and I am privileged to live in the U.S. where the burden of public funding for reproductive medicine would outweigh the advantages for both providers and patients.

Let me first address the more obviously disadvantaged party in this analysis – the providers. The United States has had a national system of paying for (some) medical care for well over five decades. Over these many years there is a glaring record of increasingly bureaucratic and administratively burdensome requirements that providers must satisfy in order to receive ever-skimpier payments for the services rendered. There is absolutely no doubt that a system of publicly funded reproductive care would produce mountains of demands for medical records, pre-authorisations, case reviews, and other documentation, the likes of which we can only imagine at present. The predictable increase in necessary clinical and office staff would likely be paralleled by increases in frustration, delays, and dissatisfaction for all involved. Equally expected would be a dramatic decrease in compensation to providers despite this exploding administrative cost. Indeed, I doubt that anyone would be surprised if the cost of providing reproductive care in such a system proved to be higher than the reimbursement received. Few providers could survive in such a setting.

Perhaps the various ways that patients would also be disadvantaged by public funding of reproductive care are less obvious, though I would suggest more numerous. It is fair to speculate that public funding of reproductive medicine would make fertility care and family building feasible for many who cannot presently afford treatment. I will leave the financial modelling to actuaries with far more robust computers than my own, but the concerns expressed above are critical to this analysis – if providers cannot afford to be in business there is no care for anyone.

What, then, are the predictable dilemmas and decisions that lead me to my position against public funding? First, the practical reality is that even if public funds are to be used to pay for reproductive care, there is no doubt that the amount of money available will be insufficient to meet the demands of all those who are experiencing infertility. Government will of necessity need to make policy decisions regarding what will or will not be covered and how much will be paid for. It does not seem like a stretch to suggest that the least expensive treatments will be prioritised. Ovulation induction cycles may abound, but what impact do we suppose this will have on more expensive treatments such as assisted reproductive technologies? Furthermore, one could anticipate that the rationing of reproductive care that will be necessary could make treatment impossible for many patients such as older women or those with a poor prognosis for successful treatment.

Second, the scope and practice of reproductive care would most certainly become a political target for elected representatives or their appointees rather than remain in the domain of medical providers and their patients. Sweeping legislative efforts directed at constraining or eliminating reproductive options and fraught with unintended consequences are virtually daily occurrences in the United States. If public officials are given the opportunity to design and enact legislation that defines the parameters of the care that will be covered, they will also be able to invoke their own personal beliefs and values in defining the care that will be declared unlawful. Said more directly, if reproductive care were publicly funded, patients in some states could enjoy significant benefit, but those in many other states would have access only to the care condoned by those opposed to reproductive freedom. We have often contemplated the potential impact of laws that define a fertilised egg as a human being or bring into question the legality of embryo biopsy, cryopreservation, disposal of embryos and many other procedures in reproductive medicine. Were public funding to open the door to political edict this speculative discussion would become a reality for patients in many, and perhaps in the majority of states in the U.S.

Third, certain classes of individuals who presently have insurance coverage for the care that they need could find that their coverage has evaporated. It is easy to guess that single patients, same sex couples, or those whose relationships are inconsistent with traditional 'family values' might be excluded from coverage. Indeed, it is easy to see how many of these patients could be completely barred from obtaining any reproductive care at all for reasons similar to those just described.

Finally, public funding of reproductive care could have a grave effect on discovery and innovation in fertility treatment. The impact of political intrusion into reproductive research has been felt since the inception of in vitro fertilisation in the United States, perhaps most compellingly with passage of the Dickey-Wicker amendment in 1996. This law prohibited the use of federal funds for research in which human embryos are destroyed, discarded or knowingly subjected to risks of injury or death. Because governmental decision-makers outlawed federal funding of human embryo research, the financial burden of critical research in the U.S. has largely been borne by programs or foundations that rely on revenue from clinical practice and philanthropy. Some of the resulting research has been extraordinary and some shoddy, but all will be existentially threatened if public funding is invoked to both constrain the funds available to support research and to define the limits of acceptable exploration.

There is no doubt that public funding of reproductive care in the United States could make access to care feasible for many who would otherwise be disenfranchised. However, on balance, far more patients and providers would be hurt rather than helped, and the age of scientific exploration and discovery could well end with a whimper, not a bang.

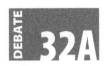

Gamete Donation Should Be Anonymous

For

Guido Pennings

Whether or not gamete donation should be anonymous depends on the existence of a right to know one's genetic origin. This right has been created in a number of countries in the last two decades on the request of a small group of donor conceived persons who stated that they were harmed by not knowing one of their genetic parents. However, this claim is neither a natural right, nor a human right. Rights are social constructions meant to protect important interests. The defenders of this so-called right must show that there is an interest worth defending. This group of donor-conceived has very successfully campaigned for their wish to be recognised as a right by making a connection between genetic origin and personal identity. They claim that knowing their genetic origin is necessary to know who they really are and what their true identity is. Although knowledge of one's genetic parents may be part of some people's identity, one's identity is generally composed of numerous other elements (such as gender or race, nationality or ideology). One's genealogy is a possible but not an essential part. We will not analyse this complex concept but focus on the main point: the claim that knowing one's genetic origin is necessary to be a psychologic-ally healthy person. The literature on family building through gamete donation has shown that donor offspring (both those who do and those who do not know that they are donor conceived) do not differ in term of socio-psychological characteristics from other children [1]. There is no empirical evidence that lack of this information harms a person or results in lower psychological well-being and inadequate family functioning [2].

Then how to explain that some people suffer from not being able to find their donor's identity? The explanation is that they wrongfully attribute the cause of their suffering to the lack of knowledge while the cause lies in the belief that the name of the donor is crucial for their identity. To use an analogy: some people believe that some part of their body prevents them from being their real self. The solution according to them is cosmetic surgery to correct the flawed body part. In general, as a society we do not believe that cosmetic surgery for this reason (with some exceptions) is appropriate. This belief underlies the refusal to provide public funding for such interventions. The right solution would be to offer these people counselling to explain that, even if there is a flaw in the body part, it is not important or crucial for their identity. Following this line of reasoning, the solution for the donor offspring's suffering is not to provide the name of the donor but to explain to the person that the lack of information on his or her genetic origin is not essential or necessary for his or her identity. Not knowing one's genetic origin does not cause harm unless people have been told and/or believe that this is important. This is corroborated by the fact that the suffering is entirely knowledge-dependent: people who do not know that they are donor conceived, do not suffer.

A new argument advanced by the opponents is that with the use of large genetic databases, anonymity no longer exists. Although this is an overstatement, it is clear that donor anonymity can no longer be guaranteed by the clinics or gamete banks. However, this fact has no implications for the right to know and neither does it lead to the conclusion that anonymity should be abolished. To use another analogy: a country has a speed limit of 100 kpm even though very few cars are able to drive at that speed. Now suppose car manufacturers introduce new cars on the market that can easily drive faster. Would we then argue that we should abolish the speed limit or that there is a right to drive as fast as one likes? I don't think so. Anonymity maintains the same function that it had before: it signals a wish for privacy and distance, both by the parents and by the donors [3]. Now more than ever, this function should be strengthened rather than weakened. The arrangement agreed upon between donor and recipient(s) should be respected by both parties.

An important reason to oppose the creation of a right to know one's genetic origin is that such right reinforces the geneticisation of our social and psychological world. Identity is genetic identity, parents are genetic parents and relationships are genetic relationships. This evolution will eventually lead to the abolition of the practice of gamete donation. The emphasis on the essential contribution of the donor to the child's well-being contradicts the basic idea underlying gamete donation. As such, the battle over donor anonymity has very little to do with the welfare of the child. It is a strategy in an ideological battle about the role of genetics in family building and relationships in general.

A final specification should be made: the fact that there is no right to know one's genetic origin does not imply that donors should obligatory be anonymous. Parents can opt for a known or identifiable donor if they believe that their child should later have the possibility to find out the donor's identity. It is part of the parental freedom and responsibility to make such choices for their child. But that does not imply or support a right to know of the donor offspring.

References

1. Golombok S, Blake L, Casey P, Roman G, Jadva V. Children born through reproductive donation: a longitudinal study of psychological adjustment. *J Child Psychol Psyc.* 2013;54:653–60.

2. Pennings G. Disclosure of donor conception, age of disclosure and the well-being of donor offspring. *Hum Reprod.* 2017;32:969–73.

3. Pennings G. Genetic databases and the future of donor anonymity. *Hum Reprod.* 2019;34:786–90.

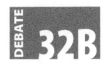

Gamete Donation Should Be Anonymous

Against

Carl Laskin

Third party reproduction is a significant proportion of the undertakings of most reproductive medicine clinics and practitioners. Whether the clientele wishes to use donor sperm or donor oocytes, many considerations remain the same. Perhaps one of the most prominent concerns is the issue of anonymity of the gamete donor. This issue potentially impacts the intended parent(s), the donor and perhaps most importantly, the offspring as a result of the treatment.

The Intended Parent(s) (IP)

The IP will may desire certain information about the donor. Although the IP may want to know why the donor donated their gametes, this may be difficult to obtain and likely less relevant to more important issues. The appearance of the donor and a listing of physical traits may be important when considering the appearance of the future child. The IP will want to know the health and genetic history of the donor and the donor's family. If there is a history of genetic disease, then the IP needs to know the details and may insist on screening of the donor(s) for recessive genes. The IP needs to know if there are others to whom this donor has donated and if so, how many others. Coupled with this information would be the geographic location of the donor. What is the possibility that the child or children from the IP could meet other children conceived from this donor? What is the possibility that the IP's child as an adult could meet and become romantically involved with other children conceived with this donor's gametes? Does the gamete donor desire contact with the donor-conceived child? How will the IP answer these major questions when posed by the donor-conceived child? The answers to these questions and scenarios are incompatible with anonymous gamete donation.

The Gamete Donor (GD)

The GD and/or the family of the GD may want contact with the offspring from a gamete donation. Although this is an unlikely scenario at present, health issues may arise in the donor or donor's own children where it is essential that all donor-conceived offspring must be notified of a recently discovered medical issue. Should the GD's own children become aware that the GD did donate, they may wish to find their half-siblings. These situations are also incompatible with anonymous gamete donation.

Donor-Conceived Children

Currently, disclosure to donor-conceived children of their biological origins is expected and every IP must be prepared for this discussion. The offspring from gamete donation are unlikely to simply accept the fact that their genetic origins are not entirely from the parent(s) to whom they have related. They will likely be very motivated to discover details of the donor and if there are others who are half-siblings. The questions that arise are: (i) what is the harm in not informing the child and avoiding what may be a difficult conversation;

(ii) if the child is to be told, when is the best age to introduce the discussion; and (iii) how might the child pursue the search for the gamete donor?

Some investigators will argue that there is little if any evidence supporting the disclosure of donor conception to the offspring. That is, the offspring's emotional and psychological adjustment depends upon their family and the environment in which they grew up. In contrast, other studies have shown that the children and adults who are informed regarding their gamete donor origins are emotionally and psychologically as well-adjusted when compared to individuals conceived naturally. In addition, better psychological development was seen the earlier the child is informed of their genetic origin. Those children informed as pre-schoolers showed better adjustment in later childhood with better child–parent relationships compared to those informed in adolescence and later. Those informed later in life may display evidence of psychological harm. Similar findings have been shown in adopted children where they are informed at an early age compared to those informed when older.

Considering the above arguments favouring disclosure, my opponent may argue that not disclosing would avoid any future issues of psychological harm. At the very least, disclosure may result in neutral psychological consequences whereas failure to disclose the genetic origins has greater potential for psychological harm and identity issues. Therefore, it is simply better for the IP to be open and disclose as this is in the best interests of the child.

Some suggest that the above arguments regarding psychological harm are not based on evidence but on the morals of the investigators. Let us assume that this argument is correct, and that the IP decides not to disclose to the child thinking that the child will never become aware of their genetic origin. These are erroneous assumptions as they ignore genealogy testing and the growth of direct-to-consumer genetic testing. The child/adolescent/adult now decides to explore their origins with a cheek swab. This individual's genetic makeup may suggest that they are the offspring of an anonymous gamete donor with possible half siblings and relatives that have been previously unknown. Not only is the privacy and anonymity now gone, but what will be the emotional and psychological consequences to the individual? What happens to the relationship with the parent(s) that have raised them? Therefore, it is not simply a parental choice whether to tell their child regarding genetic origins; it is an obligation.

In summary, disclosure of a gamete donor carries less risk of harm to the donor-conceived child than non-disclosure. Furthermore, whether the child is informed or not by the parent, in time, that older child/adult will discover there is an inconsistency in their genetic origins. How will you as the parent then answer those very awkward questions?

Further Reading

Golombok S. Disclosure and donor-conceived children. *Hum Reprod.* 2017;32:1532–3.

Harper JC, Kennett D, Reisel D. The end of donor anonymity: how genetic testing is likely to drive anonymous gamete donation out of business. *Hum Reprod.* 2016;31:1135–40.

Illioi E, Blake L, Jadva V, Roman G, Golombok S. The role of age of disclosure of biological origins in the psychological wellbeing of adolescents conceived by reproductive donation: a longitudinal study from age 1 to age 14. *J Child Psychol Psychiatr.* 2017;58:315–34.

Pennings G. Disclosure of donor conception, age of disclosure and the well-being of donor offspring. *Hum Reprod.* 2017;32:969–73.

Skoog Svanberg, A, Sydsjo G, Lampic C. Psychosocial aspects of identity-release gamete donation – perspectives of donors, recipients, and offspring. *Upsala J Med Sci.* 2019, Online https://doi.org/10.1080/03009734.2019.1696431.

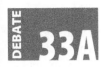

33A

Uterus Transplantation Is a Step Too Far

For

Francoise Shenfield

According to the American Society for Reproductive Medicine (ASRM) Practice Committee [1], uterus transplantation (UT) is 'an experimental procedure that may allow women with absolute uterus factor infertility to achieve a pregnancy,' and which 'should be performed within a research protocol.' We know that the uterus may be obtained from living or deceased donors and there is no certainty as yet as to which approach is optimum.

What Are the Facts and Why Is It Still 'A Step Too Far'?

The first live birth after uterus transplantation was achieved in Sweden in 2014 and since then more than 30 uterus transplantations have been performed worldwide with 11 reported deliveries, all through IVF [2]. The technique of this vascularised composite allograft (VCA) transplant necessitates access to a large medical and surgical multidisciplinary team including psychological support for both recipient and donor. Furthermore, the offspring of the transplant recipient is often born prematurely, which necessitates special care at delivery and in the neonatal period, if not longer.

Thus, several aspects of the endeavour warrant the ASRM caution statement and there are several obstacles to a successful outcome for women with uterine agenesis or severe malformation who wish to be a gestating mother. Furthermore, there is already a well-practised technique which may help such women, surrogacy, although not legal in all countries practising reproductive medicine. Surrogacy is not without problems, but a major advantage of it is that it is not research. In order to validate the statement that uterus transplantation is a 'step too far', our objections will be analysed according to the different parties involved taking into account that there are only two options currently available, i.e. adoption or childlessness.

We will thus consider in turn the pros and cons of both alternatives for the future/intended mother (and partner), the collaborator, the future offspring as well as societal consequences.

For the gestating recipient of this VCA, one should consider the psychological benefits of carrying the pregnancy, an extremely satisfying experience for most women with infertility seeking a much wanted pregnancy where bonding benefits both the foetus and herself. This should be contrasted with the dangers of major surgery for transplantation, taking anti-rejection medication, undergoing caesarian section for delivery and then further surgery to remove the graft. In addition, there is the possible psychological burden of the feeling of shared responsibility if complications occur to the live donor.

If the gestating woman is a surrogate carrier, with potential concerns of higher risk of hypertension as well as post-partum bleeding, the intended mother (and her partner) may have the same concerns about her health during pregnancy and its effect on the foetus. They may also worry about the possible legal problems documented worldwide especially in cross-border reproductive care when they return to their country of residence with the much wanted child [3]. There is, however, a trend for giving a national legal status to the child born abroad when the parents return home, even if this may be a difficult process.

In this complex balance, the comparative provisions and complications with regards to the third party, either the uterus donor or the surrogate should also be taken into account. In the case of a dead donor for UT there is obviously no risk, and the risk for the live donor may be small. Counselling is required for both alternatives and it may be demanding to determine whether the balance favours uterus transplantation or surrogacy.

With regards to the offspring, we lack strong data to compare outcomes for babies born from UT versus surrogacy on health grounds, but many babies delivered after UT are premature, generally less than those born from surrogacy. Research, albeit limited, has shown good psychological outcome for all parties involved in surrogacy, but a benefit may ensue from a simpler birth story after UT, whether from a dead or live donor.

Finally, with regards to society in general, there is no doubt that where surrogacy is forbidden because it is viewed as an assault on 'women's dignity' and a planned abandonment of the offspring such as in France, UT is a welcome possible solution for women who otherwise would need to seek, and be able to afford, surrogacy abroad.

But further concerns here include the need for considerable investment in resources for the multidisciplinary teams involved in UT, pregnancy care if successful, as well as follow-up care of mother and child, including the long-term unknown risks of immunotherapy. Whilst there is a struggle worldwide to achieve universal health care, it is doubtful that starting a program of uterus transplant may be seen as a priority, certainly whilst it is still deemed research. Uniquely, major concerns about the possible draining of medical resources in low and moderate income countries applies to both UT with its heavy multidisciplinary demands, and surrogacy arrangements for cross-border patients from higher income countries [4], although the latter is likely to demand less resources.

Thus, on balance, and taking into account all parties involved in UT and its only alternative to date, surrogacy, this VCA appears to be 'a step too far', at least whilst it is still experimental. Whether this will change in the near future depends on further data gathered during worldwide research on the health of the prospective mothers and their children and the donors. The main obstacles remain the cost of setting up the multidisciplinary team, and the effect of prematurity on the child to be.

References

1. ASRM. Position statement on UT: a practice committee opinion. *Fert Ster.* 2018;110:605–10.

2. Kvarnstrom N, Enskog A, Dahm-Kähler P. Live versus deceased donor in uterus transplantation. *Fert Ster.* 2019;112:24–27.

3. Whittaker A, Inhorn MC, Shenfield F. Globalised quests for assisted conception: reproductive travel for infertility and involuntary childlessness. *Global Public Health.* 2019;14(12):1669–88.

4. FIGO Committee for the Ethical Aspects of Human Reproduction and Women's Health. Cross border reproductive care. *Int J Gynaecol Obstet.* 2010;11:190–1.

Uterus Transplantation Is a Step Too Far

Against

Mats Brännström

Uterus transplantation (UTx) is the first available treatment for absolute uterine factor infertility (AUFI), which is caused by absence of a uterus or presence of a non-functional uterus. Women with AUFI may in a limited number of countries achieve genetic mother-hood by gestational surrogate carrier arrangements, and after adoption from the birth-giving mother, also obtain legal motherhood. However, gestational surrogacy is non-approved in a vast majority of countries/societies of the world because of ethical, legal and/or religious reasons. Thus, gestational surrogacy is not an available option for most women with AUFI.

The first live birth after UTx occurred in 2014 and this was after a live donor (LD) UTx procedure 1.5 years prior to the birth [1]. This LD UTx birth has been replicated several times within the initial Swedish trial and also at other centres in the world. Moreover, deceased donor (DD) UTx proved its feasibility by the first birth from that procedure in 2017 in Brazil [2]. Today, around 75 UTx procedures have been performed worldwide and there are more than 25 live births reported in the literature, in media or by personal communication. Notably, the UTx procedure should only be counted as successful, when a healthy baby is born. Thus, there is a waiting period of at least 1.5 years from UTx to the first possible indication of success.

Within the initial Swedish LD UTx trial, with laparotomy technique in both donor and recipient, nine women underwent UTx and seven out of these women had functional (menstruating) grafts during the one-year follow-up period before pregnancy attempts by embryo transfer [3]. During the 6-year period after UTx, six of these seven women gave birth to nine totally healthy babies. One woman did not give birth but had several miscarriages, some as late as gestational week 16. The clinical pregnancy rate of the intention-to-treat population ($n = 9$) was 7/9 (78%) and of the treated population 7/7 (100%). The respective take-home-baby rates were 6/9 (67%) and 6/7 (86%). Importantly, long-term follow-up of donors and recipients, both concerning psychology and medical issues, have not showed any long-term complications or negative issues [4, 5]. Although clinical trials with similar LD-UTx techniques are under way in several countries, including USA, Czech Republic, France and Germany, these trials started some years after the Swedish trial and full results are not yet available. However, it is important to point out that it is highly likely that the take-home-baby rates in the ongoing clinical UTx trials will be comparable to the Swedish trial and that the future developments in the field of UTx will lead to even increased efficiency and safety concerning the procedure. These advances include minimal invasive surgery of LDs by robotic-assisted laparoscopy, improved pre-operative imaging of the LDs to exclude donor uteri with insufficient vascularisation, and developments of harvesting techniques in DD UTx.

One essential factor behind the encouraging results during introduction of UTx, which is still at an experimental stage, is that first clinical trials came after more of a decade of systematic animal-based research, first in rodents, later in domestic species and lastly in non-human primates. The experimental UTx research in animals is also pointed out to be important by the first ethical guidelines in the UTx field, published by FIGO, but as late as 2009 [6], when our group had worked along those lines for more than a decade. Moreover, the commencement of UTx complies with the IDEAL guidelines for introduction of major surgical innovations [7]. The IDEAL concept points out the necessity of pre-clinical research to optimise and safeguard any new major surgical procedure and this should be followed by clinical introduction in restricted observational studies. This developmental stage, with observational studies, is the stage where UTx is today. The IDEAL concept also emphasises the importance of long-term follow-up of study populations, a pre-requisite existing in the UTx field already today, with published donor follow-up for three years after UTx [4].

Uterus transplantation has unlike many procedures in assisted reproduction been introduced as a translational project with a solid base of preclinical research to stand on. This life-creating transplantation/infertility treatment, with proved initial high success rate, is the only chance for hundreds of thousands of women with AUFI around the globe, to acquire genetic motherhood. There also exist a sound motivation of leading groups within the field to perform further developments and adjustments of UTx, according to highest scientific standards. The results of ongoing trials, with both negative and positive results scientifically published, and registry data of the International Society of Uterus Transplantation (ISUTx), will guarantee a transparent and safe transition from the present experimental stage to a clinical stage, when UTx will be a routinely offered procedure. In Sweden it is quite likely that UTx will be included as an alternative within the area of infertility treatments, which then will be covered fully within national health system for women under the age of 40.

When initially offering UTx, the availability of this procedure should be restricted to women with AUFI that cannot for financial, legal, religious, or availability reasons pursue another less risky option to acquire motherhood. Whilst UTx will be further developed, with reduction of initial development-associated risks, this restriction should be eliminated.

In conclusion, UTx is a great step forward in infertility treatment and not at all a step too far.

References

1. Brännström M, Johannesson L, Bokström H, et al. Livebirth after uterus transplantation. *Lancet*. 2015;14:607–16.

2. Ejzenberg D, Andraus W, Baratelli Carelli Mendes LR, et al. Livebirth after uterus transplantation from a deceased donor in a recipient with uterine infertility. *Lancet*. 2019;392:2697–704.

3. Johannesson L, Kvarnström N, Mölne J, et al. Uterus transplantation trial, 1-year outcome. *Fertil Steril*. 2015;103:199–204.

4. Järvholm S, Kvarnström N, Dahm-Kähler P, Brännström M. Donor´s health-related quality-of-life and psychosocial outcomes 3 years after uterus donation for transplantation. *Hum Reprod*. 2019;34:1270–7.

5. Järvholm S, Johannesson L, Clarke A, Brännström M. Uterus transplantation trial: psychological evaluation of recipients and partners during the post-transplantation year. *Fertil Steril*. 2015;104:1010–15.

6. Milliez J. Uterine transplantation FIGO committee for the ethical aspects of human reproduction and women's health. *Int J Gynaecol Obstet*. 2009;106:270.

7. McCulloch P, Altman DG, Campbell WB, et al. No surgical innovation without evaluation: the IDEAL recommendations. *Lancet*. 2009;374:1105–12.

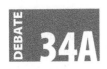

Meta-analysis Should Not Be Considered Class A Evidence

For

A Albert Yuzpe

Meta-analyses aim to combine the results of a number of smaller studies, looking at similar outcomes, in order to draw support for or against the use of a therapeutic intervention. Some consider meta-analyses as the highest form of evidence yet, their clinical value is limited to summarising aggregated data that cannot distinguish between patients with different clinical profiles.

I will begin my position that meta-analysis should not necessarily be considered as Type A evidence with the analogy of a dying fire on a cold winter night and the desire to reignite the flames to warm oneself. If one were to place a large dry log on the glowing embers, it will eventually ignite and the flames will certainly erupt. On the other hand, if one chooses a wet log it almost certainly will not ignite and the fire will die. Fanning the fire will not help and adding paper to the mix will only result in a temporary flare-up of the flame until the paper burns away. This analogy, although perhaps not the best, still serves to support my point of view. There are good or appropriate logs and inappropriate or poor logs from which one can choose. The same is true of meta-analyses. Meta-analyses are meant to provide a summary effect and to gather statistical support to prove or to disprove a specific hypothesis by combining the results of a number of studies or trials. My analogy therefore, is comparing the meta-analysis to the fire (the desired end-point) and the studies included in the meta-analysis to the logs (the fuel). In simple terms, not every meta-analysis can be considered to provide Type A evidence that will fuel the fire of true knowledge gained. As such, not every meta-analysis can be considered as Type A evidence.

There are many well-designed and well-performed meta-analyses, but there are equally as many that are constructed from 'poor logs' as in my analogy. Therefore, the purpose of my position in this debate is not to dissuade individuals from conducting or reading meta-analyses, but simply to awaken them to the fact that not every meta-analysis is of the quality that can be considered as Type A evidence. My goal, in other words, is to reinforce the importance of critical assessment of a meta-analysis including its design, its statistical methodology and its conclusion(s). A conclusion of a meta-analysis is not necessarily gospel.

What I am really saying is that there some meta-analyses that can be considered to be of high quality, by meeting the rigorous criteria for selecting the studies included in the analysis, while there are others that lack some of the essential requirements considered important in a powerful meta-analysis. In other words, some meta-analyses do qualify as Type A evidence, the pinnacle of the evidence pyramid, whereas others should not and therefore, cannot be regarded in the same light. Publication of a meta-analysis, in itself, does not qualify it as an irrefutable source of Type A evidence. How can this happen? Simply put, the conclusions of different trials often disagree. By including a number of these studies on a particular subject, the author(s) of the meta-analysis set out to produce a summary effect by combining the results of the studies included. However, therein lies the problem.

A number of factors influence the quality of a meta-analysis and must be considered when undertaking, formulating or assessing the conclusions proposed by a meta-analysis. A well-designed meta-analysis that includes poorly designed studies in order to draw its conclusions results in a poor meta-analysis with questionable conclusions. Studies are never identical in all respects and thus, selection criteria for the primary studies included in the analysis must be rigorous. Carelessness in abstracting and summarising appropriate studies, failure to consider important co-variates, bias on the part of the meta-analyst and overstatement of the strength and precision of the results can all contribute to an invalid meta-analysis [1].

Other drawbacks associated with meta-analysis exist making another analogy applicable at this juncture. 'You need both a good chef and good ingredients to make a high-quality meal.' The fact that the overall treatment effect could be overstated due to the combination of excluded patients and short duration of follow-up may not be the same across patient sub-groups, e.g. an intervention may be more or less effective in different age groups. In response to these shortcomings related to meta-analyses, Broeze has proposed the addition of 'Individual patient data meta-analysis – IPD' to supplement the findings of a meta-analysis of randomised clinical trials [2].

It is also essential that the meta-analysis consider the differences or heterogeneity that exist among studies and study populations. There is also an issue referred to as 'publication bias'. There are many studies can never be included in a meta-analysis because they were never published simply because they did not show the benefit or a statistically significant benefit of a treatment or procedure. Finally, studies reported in languages other than English are often not considered.

Dhont analysed meta-analyses and systemic reviews involving failed implantation (10 different suggested interventions) and ovarian response to stimulation (four different interventions) [3]. He points out that, 'Not withstanding the fact that many clinical trials have been performed, very few procedures can as yet stand the critical test of evidence based medicine.' The lack of sufficiently powered trials in these analyses, he points out, leads to the lack of solid evidence for a number of interventions employed in IVF programs.

In conclusion, I have presented evidence to support the fact that some, but definitely not all, meta-analyses can be considered as Type A evidence. It is up to authors, reviewers and readers to critically consider the shortcomings as well as the strengths associated with a meta-analysis before drawing any worthwhile conclusions. By doing so, we can only strengthen our resolve in delivering the highest quality of medical care to our patients based upon high quality evidence-based medicine derived from strong meta-analyses and systematic reviews and perhaps the addition of individual patient data meta-analysis. Not until all meta-analyses include large, sufficiently powered trials will we be able to state that meta-analyses can be considered as Type A evidence.

References

1. Esterhuizen TM, Thabane L. Con: Meta-analysis; some key limitations and potential solutions. *Nephrol Dial Transplant.* 2016;31:882–5.

2. Broeze K, Opmeer BC, van der Veen F, et al. Individual patient data meta-analysis: a promising approach for evidence synthesis in reproductive medicine. *Hum Reprod Update.* 2010;16(6):561–7.

3. Dhont M. Evidence-based reproductive medicine: a clinical appraisal. *Facts Views Vis Obgyn.* 2013;5(3):233–40.

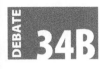

Meta-analysis Should Not Be Considered Class A Evidence

Against

William Buckett

Introduction

Judgments about evidence and the resulting recommendations in healthcare are complex, especially in rapidly evolving fields such as reproductive medicine. Case reports have transformed the treatment of infertility from the first reported case of successful IVF, through ICSI and PGD to uterine transplantation, and in many of these cases there is no need to conduct a prospective trial. Indeed, in many cases it would be impossible or unethical [1].

However, there are many interventions where the benefit, if any, is less clear. Recent examples in the treatment of infertility are the use of endometrial scratching or the use of PGT-A in IVF where initial enthusiasm has ultimately been replaced with disappointment. The reason for this change is the inherent bias (both known and unknown) in lower evidence level studies – such as cohort studies or 'big data' studies where the different interventions compared are often applied to groups with different prognostic profiles.

Classification of Evidence

Levels of evidence were originally described in a report by the Canadian Task Force on the Periodic Health Examination in 1979 [2]. The authors developed a system of rating evidence when determining the effectiveness of a particular intervention. The evidence was taken into account when grading recommendations. For example, a Grade A recommendation was given if there was good evidence to support a recommendation. Randomised controlled trials (RCTs) were considered the highest level and case series or expert opinions at the lowest level. The hierarchies rank studies according to the probability of bias. RCTs are given the highest level because they are designed to be unbiased and have less risk of systematic errors. For example, by randomly allocating subjects to two or more treatment groups, these types of studies also randomise confounding factors that may bias results. A case series or expert opinion is often biased by the author's experience or opinions and there is no control of confounding factors.

However, if the RCT sample size is too small (which it often is in infertility – as usually over 2000 couples will need to be randomised to show any meaningful effect), RCTs will suffer from a lack of precision. This can be overcome by combining data from several RCTs and collectively analysing this (*meta-analysis*) allowing a more precise measurement of effect. An example of this would be the use of ultrasound guidance for embryo transfer where initial RCTs were underpowered to demonstrate an effect but the systemic review and meta-analysis of over 3000 randomised patients demonstrated a clear effect [3].

Therefore systemic review and meta-analysis can be regarded as the highest evidence (Class A) and sit at the top of the hierarchy pyramid (see Figure 34B.1).

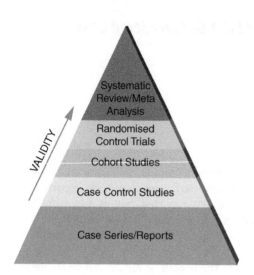

Figure 34B.1 The hierarchy of evidence pyramid.

Systemic Review/Meta-analysis and Study Quality

Obviously, the quality of any meta-analysis depends on the quality of the original RCTs – and when this is low, combining the data will also result in a low-quality meta-analysis – the commonly quoted 'garbage in; garbage out'.

As it became increasingly apparent that the study design alone does not necessarily confer high certainty or quality of evidence, about ten years ago the Grading of Recommendations Assessment, Development and Evaluations (GRADE) approach was developed [4]. GRADE offers a transparent and structured process for assessing the evidence, and developing and presenting evidence summaries.

This structured assessment of evidence should be an essential of any systemic review and is already an established part of all Cochrane reviews where the assessment of the quality of evidence for each individual study is clearly displayed with the resulting meta-analysis (see Figure 34B.2) [4].

Newer Techniques – Network Meta-analysis and IPD Meta-analysis

In the same way that understanding quality of evidence changes with time – an example would be the first group to classify evidence (the Canadian Task Force on the Periodic Health Examination) now use GRADE – so too do the techniques and practice of meta-analysis evolve over time. How RCTs are assessed and analysed is very different today compared to 20 years ago.

Network meta-analysis [5] is possible where indirect comparisons can be made to allow simultaneous comparison of multiple interventions, including comparing outcomes that were not directly compared in the original RCTs. Also, individual participant data (IPD) meta-analysis is feasible, where row-by-row, participant-level data is requested for each eligible trial and used to control for participant-level covariates, thus improving the consistency and precision of network meta-analysis.

Provided key assumptions are satisfied, these techniques could be considered in the future as an essential part of evidence synthesis and further facilitate clinical decision-making in reproductive medicine.

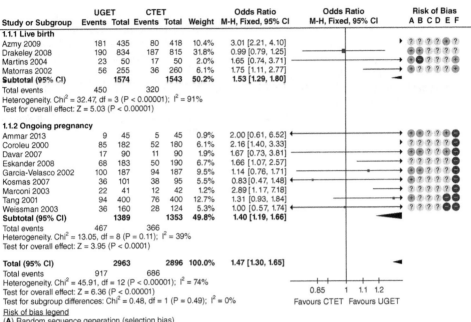

Study or Subgroup	UGET Events	Total	CTET Events	Total	Weight	Odds Ratio M-H, Fixed, 95% CI	Odds Ratio M-H, Fixed, 95% CI	Risk of Bias A B C D E F
1.1.1 Live birth								
Azmy 2009	181	435	80	418	10.4%	3.01 [2.21, 4.10]		
Drakeley 2008	190	834	187	815	31.8%	0.99 [0.79, 1.25]		
Martins 2004	23	50	17	50	2.0%	1.65 [0.74, 3.71]		
Matorras 2002	56	255	36	260	6.1%	1.75 [1.11, 2.77]		
Subtotal (95% CI)		1574		1543	50.2%	1.53 [1.29, 1.80]		
Total events	450		320					

Heterogeneity. Chi² = 32.47, df = 3 (P < 0.00001); I² = 91%
Test for overall effect: Z = 5.03 (P < 0.00001)

Study or Subgroup	UGET Events	Total	CTET Events	Total	Weight	Odds Ratio M-H, Fixed, 95% CI	Odds Ratio M-H, Fixed, 95% CI	Risk of Bias A B C D E F
1.1.2 Ongoing pregnancy								
Ammar 2013	9	45	5	45	0.9%	2.00 [0.61, 6.52]		
Coroleu 2000	85	182	52	180	6.1%	2.16 [1.40, 3.33]		
Davar 2007	17	90	11	90	1.9%	1.67 [0.73, 3.81]		
Eskander 2008	68	183	50	190	6.7%	1.66 [1.07, 2.57]		
Garcia-Velasco 2002	100	187	94	187	9.5%	1.14 [0.76, 1.71]		
Kosmas 2007	36	101	38	95	5.5%	0.83 [0.47, 1.48]		
Marconi 2003	22	41	12	42	1.2%	2.89 [1.17, 7.18]		
Tang 2001	94	400	76	400	12.7%	1.31 [0.93, 1.84]		
Weissman 2003	36	160	28	124	5.3%	1.00 [0.57, 1.74]		
Subtotal (95% CI)		1389		1353	49.8%	1.40 [1.19, 1.66]		
Total events	467		366					

Heterogeneity. Chi² = 13.05, df = 8 (P = 0.11); I² = 39%
Test for overall effect: Z = 3.95 (P < 0.0001)

Total (95% CI)		2963		2896	100.0%	1.47 [1.30, 1.65]	
Total events	917		686				

Heterogeneity. Chi² = 45.91, df = 12 (P < 0.00001); I² = 74%
Test for overall effect: Z = 6.36 (P < 0.00001)
Test for subgroup differences: Chi² = 0.48, df = 1 (P = 0.49); I² = 0%

0.85   1   1.1 1.2
Favours CTET Favours UGET

Risk of bias legend
(A) Random sequence generation (selection bias)
(B) Allocation concealment (selection bias)
(C) Blinding of participants and personnel (performance bias)
(D) Blinding of outcome assessment (detection bias)
(E) Incomplete outcome data (attrition bias)
(F) Selective reporting (reporting bias)

Figure 34B.2 GRADE Structured assessment of evidence.

Conclusions

Assessing the certainty of any published evidence is essential in synthesising the best evidence from which to make decisions about the care of individual patients and also to determine the strength of any recommendations for care.

Injudicious use of meta-analysis by just putting numbers from published studies into a statistical programme to generate a forest plot without the appropriate rigour needed to assess the quality of the studies has led to justified concerns about the validity of meta-analysis as Class A evidence. Combined with the improving statistical techniques used to reduce bias in some 'big data' studies, many have questioned the pre-eminence of meta-analysis.

However, where RCTs are appropriately assessed for bias and when improving techniques are used, a good systematic review and meta-analysis still remains the best available evidence and is still used widely by many authorities, such as the WHO and the United Kingdom's National Institute for Health and Care Excellence (NICE), in order to determine best evidence and formulate guideline recommendations.

References

1. Smith GC, Pell JP. Parachute use to prevent death and major trauma related to gravitational challenge: systematic review of randomised controlled trials. *BMJ.* 2003;327(7429):1459–61.

2. Canadian Task Force on the Periodic Health Examination. The periodic health

examination. *Can Med Assoc J.* 1979;121:1193–54.

3. Brown JA, Buckingham K, Abou-Setta A, Buckett W. Ultrasound versus 'clinical touch' for catheter guidance during embryo transfer in women. *Cochrane Database Syst Rev.* 2007 Jan 24;(1):CD006107. doi: 10.1002/14651858.CD006107.pub2.

4. Guyatt G, Oxman AD, Akl EA, et al. GRADE guidelines: 1. Introduction-GRADE evidence profiles and summary of findings tables. *J Clin Epidemiol.* 2011;64 (4):383–94.

5. Wang R, Seidler AL, Askie L, et al. Network meta-analyses in reproductive medicine: challenges and opportunities. *Hum Reprod.* 2020; 35(8):1723–31.

Sperm Counts Are Falling Worldwide

For

Garima Srivastava

The deterioration of semen quality was first reported in 1974 by Nelson and Bunge. The topic has sparked plenty of controversy around the globe since Carlsen et al. published their review in 1992 about the decreasing quality of semen in the past 50 years [1].

It divided the scientific community for and against the topic for a long time without any firm conclusion.

Looking at the evidence published so far I am convinced that there has been a temporal and spatial decline in the sperm counts worldwide.

In the Carlsen review, linear regression analysis of mean sperm concentration weighted by the number of subjects in each publication showed a significant decrease in mean sperm concentration between 1940 and 1990 from 113×106/ml to 66×106/ml. They also found a significant decrease in mean seminal volume from 3.40 ml to 2.75 ml during the same period, indicating an even more pronounced decrease in total sperm count.

However, this paper was challenged based on methodological errors, i.e. using only the linear regression method. It was also deemed to suffer from spatial, temporal and several confounding biases.

Bahadur et al. re-evaluated the 61 papers included in Carlsen's report in 1996 using linear and quadratic modelling procedures to decipher the 'demographic contribution' and the 'time contribution' as factors in the sperm count decline [2]. Their study showed that the global linear decline in sperm count between 1938 and 1988 is largely accounted for by the early USA data (1938–1974) and not by the 'European' or the 'Asia/Africa/South America' data. The quadratic model importantly indicated that sperm count in the USA decreases asymptomatically towards a limiting value. They claimed this latter observation would not have been indicted by the linear regression used in Carlsen's study.

Swan et al. reanalysed the worldwide data using the multiple regression model in 1997 [3]. This showed an even steeper decline in sperm density in the United States (1938–1988) and in Europe (1971–1990) than that reported by Carlsen et al. but no decline in non-western countries, where data are sparse and are available only since 1978. When regional differences are considered, the data do not support either a 'hockey stick' (spline) or an upwardly curving (quadratic) function, as has been suggested by Bahadur et al.

It was concluded by Swan that the decline in sperm density reported by Carlsen et al. is not likely to be an artefact of bias, confounding, or statistical analysis.

By this time, the declining sperm parameters were believed to be a public health concern. This led to numerous good quality studies across the globe utilising a robust methodology to clear the confusion around this issue.

For example in 2017, Levine published a systematic review and meta-regression analysis trends in sperm counts as measured by sperm concentration (SC) and total sperm count (TSC), and their modification by fertility and geographic group [4]. This rigorous and comprehensive analysis finds that SC declined 52.4% between 1973 and 2011 among unselected men from Western countries, with no evidence of a 'levelling off' in recent years.

Mishra et al. analysed data for 6466 fertile and 7020 infertile men between 1979 and 2016 in India and concluded that semen parameters in Indian men have declined with time and the deterioration is quantitatively higher in the infertile group [5].

Similar attempts to report the declining trend of sperm concentrations in African population between 1965 and 2015 were carried out. Sengupta et al. concluded that a time-dependent decline of sperm concentration and an overall 72.6% decrease in mean sperm concentration was noted in the past 50 years in Africa [6].

Plentiful evaluations of laboratory semen records have indicated a decrease in semen quality as reported from Belgium, Canada, Finland, France, Greece, Norway, Scotland, the USA and the UK, while no variations have been reported from regions such as Denmark and Australia. However, this is still unconvincing considering the global temporal trends.

It has been speculated that changing lifestyle and environmental factors may be the endocrine disruptors that can deteriorate sperm quality. The pesticides, heavy metals, plastics, organic solvents, etc which are a part of everyday consumables may cause oxidative stress and degeneration of the sperm and surrounding cells. With technological progress, excessive use of Wi-Fi, laptops, mobile phones (radiofrequency-electromagnetic radiation) etc might result in the disruption of the hypothalamic-pituitary axis resulting in the decrease in the sperm parameters.

Besides these environmental factors, oestrogens which are a part of the human food chain can act on the male foetus during pregnancy and can be responsible for a spectrum of additional, male reproductive tract disorders including hypospadias and cryptorchidism along with low semen parameters.

To conclude, rather than debating whether sperm counts are declining or not, I think the need of the hour is for researchers, epidemiologists and public health workers to concentrate on the possible factors that are causing these very evident changes in the semen.

The aim should be to modify public health policies and environmental factors to reverse these changes, so that future generations do not have to rely heavily on ART procedures for male factor subfertility or face childlessness.

References

1. Carlsen E, Giwercman A, Keiding N, Skakkebaek NE. Evidence for decreasing quality of semen during past 50 years. *Obstet Gynecol Surv*. 1992;48(3):200–2.

2. Bahadur G, Ling KLE, Katz M. Statistical modelling reveals demography and time are the main contributing factors in global sperm count changes between 1938 and 1996. *Hum Reprod*. 1996;11(12):2635–9.

3. Swan SH, Elkin EF, Fenster L. Have sperm densities declined? A reanalysis of global trend data. *Environ Health Perspect*. 1997;105(11):1228–32.

4. Levine H, Jørgensen N, Martino-Andrade A, et al. Temporal trends in sperm count: a systematic review and meta-regression analysis. *Hum Reprod Update*. 2017;23 (6):646–59.

5. Mishra P, Negi MPS, Srivastava M, et al. Decline in seminal quality in Indian men over the last 37 years. *Reprod Biol Endocrinol*. 2018;16:103. https://doi.org/10 .1186/s12958-018-0425-z.

6. Sengupta P, Dutta S, Krajewska-Kulak E. The disappearing sperms: analysis of reports published between 1980 and 2015. *Am J Men's Health*. 2017;11(4):1279–1304.

Sperm Counts Are Falling Worldwide

Against

Allan Pacey

As an undergraduate, I was taught that correlation does not imply causation. It is a lesson that has served me well, and I would argue has served reproductive medicine well in recent years too. Thankfully, we now recognise the importance of randomised controlled trials, the value of quality evidence, the role of bias, randomisation and sampling error and of course the power of meta-analysis in making sense of similar studies conducted around the world. However, it has long been recognised that meta-analyses are only as good as the quality of data they include, and a meta-analysis of poor quality studies is almost meaningless. So, whilst we now understand this concept when evaluating one drug against the other (or the usefulness of an IVF add-on against standard treatment), it is alarming that we seem to have so spectacularly forgotten the concept when it comes to the debate about whether or not sperm counts are falling worldwide.

The debate began in 1992 when the *British Medical Journal* published a meta-analysis claiming to show that sperm concentration had apparently fallen worldwide over the previous 50 years [1]. Although a landmark study in many ways, it was highly criticised because of what was thought to be significant methodological failings. These included: (i) concern about the statistical methods used and whether a linear regression was the appropriate statistical approach; (ii) the population of men represented in each of the studies (e.g. patients vs. healthy volunteers vs. men attending for vasectomy), and whether they were really comparable; (iii) the fact that most studies were from the global north with relatively few from low and middle-income countries; and (iv) the fact that the studies included had used a wide array of different laboratory techniques to measure the sperm count they reported. The latter was the most important issue for me, and in a paper in 2013 entitled 'Are sperm counts declining? Or did we just change of spectacles?' [2], I made the point that because laboratory methods for counting sperm had altered so much since the 1930s, it was virtually impossible to compare studies that had used different techniques in the same meta-analysis and conclude anything from it: it was comparing apples and oranges. We knew, and the World Health Organization endorsed, that the only robust way to measure sperm concentration reliably was to use the technique of haemocytometry. Other (less reliable) methods tend to over-estimate the true value. Therefore it is not difficult to see how if laboratories had slowly switched to the haemocytometry method over time, that the apparent sperm concentration reported over the past 50 years would decline simply as a result of the gradual change in technique.

Therefore, for many observers, this criticism was felt to be largely resolved by the publication of a new meta-analysis which included only those studies which had measured sperm count by the technique of haemocytometry [3]. This analysis also showed a decline in sperm concentration over time, although one not as stark as the previous one [1]. 'Voila!' was cried, 'the issue is solved'. But whilst the 2017 analysis [3] was certainly a step forward, and addressed one of the central criticisms of the 1992 one [1], our knowledge of sperm counting techniques had moved on.

In between the publication of the two meta-analyses, it became clear that the choice of haemocytometry as a sperm counting technique, was by itself not the only important factor in obtaining an accurate result. For example, work by the European Society for Human Reproduction and Embryology showed that in 24 training courses held between 1995 and 1999, the variation in the results by individual users could decrease significantly in response to training [4]. Therefore, once again, it is easy to see how an apparent decline of sperm concentration over time, even when using the single method of haemocytometer, might reduce further simply because of increased levels of training (and recognition that that training was important). Therefore, whilst the 2017 analysis [3] was certainly a step forward, to my mind it is still not conclusive proof that a decline in sperm counts over time is anything other than changes in the methodology of the way we count sperm.

I appreciate that to those readers without such a fastidious interest in sperm counting, my arguments may seem very petty or nit-picky. But, as the American Cosmologist Carl Sagan said, 'Extraordinary claims require extraordinary evidence' and for me, the data presented in the two meta-analyses [1, 3] are simply not examples of extraordinary evidence. Rather they are a mish mash of data that was never collected with the purpose of answering the question about a possible decline in sperm counts over time. As such, in my opinion, they are both deeply flawed. Surely if the question is one worth answering, then what science needs are well-designed prospective studies where data on sperm counts are collected from representative large sample of young men over many years by standardised methodology with appropriate levels of training and quality control in place at the start. Slowly, we would then build up a picture of whether the sperm count of young men is changing over time or not. But, wait, hasn't that already been done? Data on sperm counts from over 5000 young men being assessed for military service were collected in Denmark over 19 years between 1996 and 2010 [5]. And guess what? It found no significant change. I rest my case.

References

1. Carlsen E, Giwercman A, Keiding N, Skakkebaek NE. Evidence for decreasing quality of semen during past 50 years. *Br Med J.* 1992;305:609–13.

2. Pacey AA. Are sperm counts declining? Or did we just change of spectacles? *Asian J Androl.* 2013;15:187–90.

3. Levine H, Jørgensen N, Martino-Andrade A, et al. Temporal trends in sperm count: a systematic review and met-regression analysis. *Hum Reprod Update.* 2017;23:646–59.

4. Björndahl L, Barratt CL, Fraser LR, Kvist U, Mortimer D. ESHRE basic semen analysis courses 1995–1999: immediate beneficial effects of standardized training. *Hum Reprod.* 2002;17:1299–305.

5. Bonde JP, Ramlau-Hansen CH, Olsen J. Trends in sperm counts: the saga continues. *Epidemiology.* 2011;22:617–19.

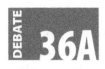

36A

There Is Value in Examining Sperm DNA Fragmentation

For

Lesley Haddock and Sheena EM Lewis

For over a decade it has been abundantly clear that semen analysis is unfit for purpose. In contrast, sperm DNA fragmentation testing has been reported in a plethora of studies as a robust biomarker for male infertility and yet it has not been adopted in routine male workups. Why?

One of the obstacles impeding routine adoption is the unfounded insistence that the four commonly used tests: (i) terminal deoxynucleotidyl transferase (TdT) dUTP nick-end labelling (TUNEL); (ii) the sperm chromatin structure assay (SCSA); (iii) sperm chromatin dispersion (SCD) or Halo test; and (iv) the single cell gel electrophoresis assay or Comet assay) should provide the same clinical thresholds and second, that they should be available for use in house. Both these objections miss the point of the tests. First, different tests measure different types of DNA from single-strand to double-strand breaks and from endogenous damage to induced damage. Second, the measurements differ from each of the tests. For example, the Comet is a quantitative test measuring the damage in individual sperm whereas in TUNEL, SCSA and Halo, the value is an all or nothing measure of the portion of damaged sperm in the semen sample. In summary, data from the four sperm DNA tests are not interchangeable [1]. To refute the second objection, these tests have an advanced molecular basis so they require specialised equipment and skilled scientists and need to be outsourced; just as is universally accepted in other molecular tests such as pre-implantation genetic diagnosis.

Is it ethical to continue using outdated semen analysis tools that result in a useless diagnosis of idiopathic infertility in 30% of men? Is it ethical to take that diagnosis to treat these men with a static and modestly successful technology; usually at their own considerable expense? Over 75% of men with idiopathic infertility have sperm DNA damage, when measured by the Comet assay. Other tests also detect sperm DNA damage in high proportions of men with normozoospermia. Classifying male factor by semen analyses alone can provide a misleading message leading to a less successful treatment.

Neglect of sperm DNA quality also raises an important issue when reviewing all the literature on 'male infertility'. As so many men are misdiagnosed, studies that classify men with normozoospermia into couples with 'female only factors' are confused and inaccurate. Currently, couples with normal semen analyses are repeatedly offered only IVF following failure. In one large study [2] of women having up to nine cycles of IVF, the live birth rate decreases with every cycle. One explanation for this is that those couples who were unsuccessful, had a major male factor in terms of poor sperm quality. Prospective studies of ART outcomes for IVF compared with ICSI for couples with idiopathic infertility are urgently needed. In such studies, the end points of studies using semen analysis or sperm DNA damage should always be live birth rates. The clinical focus on fertilisation or its failure as an important end point is not acceptable to couples. Recent surveys present compelling evidence that couples want to know their chances of having a baby; rather than those early proxy markers of success offered by clinics.

Until recently clinical dictum has been that female age over-rides all other factors. By what mechanism and by how much? Our group [3] has reported that the strength of the proportion of sperm with high DNA damage (high Comet score: HCS) is just as important as female age. We have shown that it would take ten years of additional female age to negate the benefit of using the HCS score to predict a live birth in IVF. The insignificant impact of anti-Müllerian hormone levels on live birth in this study adds to our hypothesis that is not the woman's ovarian reserve that is critical, but rather the lesser ability of older eggs to repair DNA damage. These data also show that older eggs can be equally successful if used with good quality sperm DNA. In ICSI, female age and sperm DNA quality, although less than in IVF, both have significant impact on live births so both should be included together in clinical decisions.

We have reported that both the average Comet score and the scores for proportions of sperm with high (HCS) or low (LCS) DNA damage are useful in diagnosing male infertility. These both provide additional discriminatory information for the prediction of IVF and ICSI live births. Using average DNA damage across a sample, there is no relationship with ICSI outcome. However, using the new Comet HCS parameter there is a strong correlation between sperm DNA quality and both IVF and ICSI live births.

Unlike sperm numbers, sperm quality can often be improved in the next spermatogenic cycle by minor surgical intervention or removal of lifestyle hazards. However, antioxidant supplements have not led to the benefits once promised. The recently updated Cochrane meta-analysis on antioxidants [4] for male subfertility concluded that antioxidants increased pregnancy and live birth rates. However, this was based on only seven studies with 1245 live births and 11 trials with 105 pregnancies. This weak deduction can be explained by the recent knowledge that not all sperm DNA damage is due to oxidative stress. A substantial amount of sperm DNA damage (in the form of double-stranded breaks that vary from man to man) occurs during spermatogenesis in the testis as a result of topoisomerase or endonuclease dysfunction. This type of DNA damage is more harmful due to the causation of genomic instability in the developing embryo and is a potent inducer of mutations and chromosomal abnormalities. Further, as double-strand broken ends are difficult to locate, they are less likely to be repaired by the oocyte post-fertilisation, and there is no complementary strand template from which to copy.

A further value of sperm DNA quality is its usefulness as a diagnostic tool for miscarriage [5]. Sperm DNA damage is significantly correlated with an increased risk of miscarriage following natural conceptions and following both IVF and ICSI. This is not surprising, since the sperm and egg make equal contributions to the genome of the resulting embryo and thus either could be responsible for fatal flaws in embryonic development, resulting in miscarriage. This is true for sporadic and recurrent miscarriage following both spontaneous and assisted conception.

A final area in which evaluation of sperm DNA damage may be beneficial is as a diagnostic tool prior to testicular biopsy. The rapid adoption by urologists of this invasive procedure for couples with ICSI failure needs prior semen testing to predict if testicular sperm are of better quality. This requires evidence that the damage in the ejaculate has low levels of double-stranded damage that occurred during spermatogenesis. Current research in our group with urologists is to establish such a biomarker using double-stranded DNA damage only.

For all the evidence set out above, this author believes that **there is value in examining sperm DNA fragmentation.**

References

1. Simon L, Zini A, Dyachenko A, et al. A systematic review and meta-analysis to determine the effect of sperm DNA damage on in vitro fertilization and intracytoplasmic sperm injection outcome. *Asian J Androl.* 2017;19(1):80–90.

2. Smith ADAC, Tilling K, Nelson SM, Lawlor DA. Live-birth rate associated with repeat in vitro fertilization treatment cycles. *JAMA.* 2015;314:2654–62.

3. Nicopoullos J, Vicens-Morton A, Lewis SEM. Novel use of COMET parameters of sperm DNA damage may increase its utility to diagnose male infertility and predict live births following both IVF and ICSI. *Hum Reprod.* 2019;34(10):1915–23.

4. Smits RM, Mackenzie-Proctor R, Yazdani A, et al. Antioxidants for male subfertility. *Cochrane Database Syst Rev.* March 2019. https://doi.org/10.1002/14651858 .CD007411.pub4.

5. Robinson L, Gallos ID, Conner SJ, et al. The effect of sperm DNA fragmentation on miscarriage rates: a systematic review and meta-analysis. *Hum Rep.* 2012;27:2908–17.

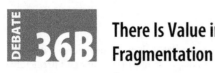

36B There Is Value in Examining Sperm DNA Fragmentation

Against

Armand Zini and Wael Almajed

One of the contemporary challenges in treating infertility is to identify those couples that will likely fail to conceive naturally or after assisted reproduction and will require more extensive interventions to achieve conception. The conventional sperm parameters (sperm concentration, motility, and morphology) provide us with information on the functionality of the seminiferous tubules and the reproductive tract. However, a major drawback of semen analysis is that conventional sperm parameters are crude indicators of male fertility potential and the reference ranges for these parameters were set based on a population of fertile couples who succeeded in achieving a natural conception [1]. Moreover, these same parameters are not useful in predicting reproductive outcomes with assisted reproductive technologies. As such, there is a real need to identify markers that can accurately assess male fertility potential and help predict reproductive outcomes with assisted reproductive technologies.

In the past two decades, there has been a growing interest in understanding the organisation and genomic integrity of human spermatozoa. Numerous tests of sperm chromatin and DNA damage have been developed with the hope that these assays may be useful in predicting natural conception and reproductive outcomes with assisted reproduction. These tests have provided us with a better understanding of sperm chromatin architecture and function but their use as specialised biomarkers in the evaluation of the infertile man has not been widely adopted.

The etiology of human sperm DNA damage is believed to be multifactorial. Human sperm DNA damage may be caused by primary defects in spermatogenesis (e.g. genetic or developmental abnormalities) or caused by extrinsic factors leading to testicular or post-testicular injury (e.g. gonadotoxins, hyperthermia, oxidants, endocrine abnormalities) [2]. It has been suggested that protamine deficiency (with consequent aberrant chromatin remodelling), reactive oxygen species and abortive apoptosis may be responsible for sperm DNA damage. Investigators have proposed a two-step model to explain the development of sperm DNA damage [3]. Based on this model, testicular spermatozoa with poor chromatin compaction due to incomplete replacement of histones by protamines (a result of defective spermiogenesis – 1st step) can sustain DNA damage because they are more susceptible to oxidative injury (2nd step).

The growing interest in measuring sperm DNA damage as a marker of sperm quality stems, in part, from the findings of several studies showing that infertile men have substantially higher levels of sperm chromatin and DNA damage than fertile men [2]. These studies have also shown that specific clinical parameters (e.g. advanced paternal age, varicocele, gonadotoxin exposure, genital tract infection, spinal cord injury and febrile illness) are associated with a higher prevalence of a positive or abnormal sperm DNA test. Prospective studies of couples with unknown fertility status indicate that sperm DNA damage is associated with a lower probability of conception (odds ratio = ~7) and a prolonged time to pregnancy. These studies also reveal that sperm DNA testing is a better predictor of pregnancy than conventional sperm parameters in this context. Taken together, the data suggest that it may be reasonable to test couples with unknown fertility status when the men present with clinical characteristics predisposing them to sperm DNA damage (e.g. prior exposure to gonadotoxins or advanced paternal age).

Although the use of sperm DNA fragmentation tests in clinical practice appears promising, testing has not gained wide approval and remains controversial. One of the major concerns regarding these tests is that there are multiple assays of sperm DNA damage and no standardised protocol for many of these assays. Indeed, there are differences in sperm chromatin decondensation protocol, enzyme and slide kit supplier and method of DNA damage detection that call into question the reliability of the test. Another drawback of the DNA fragmentation tests is that they need to be performed by highly trained technologists in a specialised laboratory. The very limited information on the precision of the assays due to a lack of reproducibility studies (intra- and inter-laboratory) is another important weakness. Finally, the fact that the clinical thresholds for many of these tests have not been formally validated is also an important shortcoming. Ultimately, these very important limitations seriously undermine the clinical value of these tests.

Several studies, including systematic reviews and meta-analyses, have examined the relationship between sperm DNA test results and reproductive outcomes after ARTs. Many of these studies have shown that sperm DNA damage is associated with lower intrauterine insemination (IUI) and conventional in vitro fertilization (IVF) pregnancy rates (odds ratio = ~1.5) but not with intracytoplasmic sperm injection (ICSI) pregnancy rates [2]. Moreover, studies have shown that sperm DNA damage may be associated with higher risk of pregnancy loss after IVF and ICSI. However, other reviews have shown that sperm DNA damage and ART outcomes are not significantly associated and have questioned the value of sperm DNA tests in this context [4]. As such, the widespread clinical application of sperm DNA tests in predicting IUI and IVF pregnancy has not been firmly established despite an already large number of clinical studies (40–50 relevant studies), because most studies are retrospective, relatively small (each study has reported on roughly 100–200 ART cycles), the study characteristics are heterogeneous and the precision of the different assays remains uncertain [5]. Another hurdle to the clinical acceptance of DNA damage tests is that they do not yield a result that has an associated applicable intervention (other than use of testicular sperm with ICSI) indicating that these tests may not be cost-effective and may entail delaying management of infertile couples.

In conclusion, the clinical value of sperm DNA tests as indicators of male fertility potential remains questionable. Several concerns regarding these tests have been raised including the standardisation of the assay protocols, and, the reproducibility and validation of the assays. As such, before these tests become widely accepted in clinical practice, standardisation of the assay protocols and large-scale prospective studies are needed to assess the clinical value of these tests in predicting natural pregnancy rates and ART outcomes.

References

1. Cooper TG, Noonan E, von Eckardstein S, et al. World Health Organization reference values for human semen characteristics. *Hum Reprod Update.* 2010;May–June;16 (3):231–45.

2. Zini A, Sigman M. Are tests of sperm DNA damage clinically useful? Pros and cons. *J Androl.* 2009 May–June;30(3):219–29.

3. De Iuliis GN, Thomson LK, Mitchell LA, et al. DNA damage in human spermatozoa is highly correlated with the efficiency of chromatin remodeling and the formation of 8-hydroxy-2'-deoxyguanosine, a marker of oxidative stress. *Biol Reprod.* 2009 Sept;81(3):517–24.

4. Cissen M, van Wely M, Scholten I, et al. Measuring sperm DNA fragmentation and clinical outcomes of medically assisted reproduction: a systematic review and meta-analysis. *PLoS ONE.* 2016;11(11): e0165125.

5. Practice Committee of the American Society for Reproductive Medicine. The clinical utility of sperm DNA integrity testing: a guideline. *Fertil Steril.* 2013;99 (3):673–7.

Testicular Sperm Should Be Considered for Repeated ICSI Failed Implantation Cases in Men with High Sperm DNA Damage

For

Lesley Haddock and Sheena EM Lewis

For couples with repeated intracytoplasmic sperm injection (ICSI) failure, there is currently no further treatment option for men wishing to father their own biological child. The only treatment offered is donor sperm; this is not an acceptable choice for many couples, leaving them saddened and dissatisfied with the lack of progress on this expensive journey. Over the past decade, a new option of retrieving sperm from the testis has been explored and early results look promising in terms of both better sperm quality and better treatment outcomes for participating couples. The key difference between ejaculated and testicular sperm is their DNA integrity. Large meta-analyses [1] conclude that sperm DNA damage is consistently associated with poor ART outcomes from fertilisation to live birth and miscarriage. Much of that damage is due to oxidative attack in the epididymis, despite it being the natural route for sperm to take as they mature. Many studies have reported that testicular and epididymal sperm have less DNA damage in those men with high damage in their ejaculated sperm. This is indicated on two levels: in the proportions of sperm with damaged DNA and also in the amount of damage inflicted on individual sperm. Such oxidative attack is often caused by varicoceles or genital infections and clinical interventions to reduce such stress should be undertaken to avoid biopsies where possible. Other causes of oxidative stress include smoking, obesity, exposure to occupational toxins and poor diet and effects can be lessened by healthier lifestyle choices. However, when none of these solutions lead to natural or assisted conception, testicular biopsies should be considered.

The decision to pursue this invasive route comes at the end of the couple's journey, when all other attempts to treat male infertility have failed. They will have had several failed ICSI cycles and possibly IVF cycles too, if they presented with normozoospermia. They will have tried every supplement for sperm and egg improvement that their clinics recommended. They will probably have had embryo quality tested by pre-implantation genetic diagnosis. If they have been well advised, they will have consulted with a urologist and been checked for infections or varicocele and had advanced sperm function tests including oxidative stress tests and DNA fragmentation. The cost-effectiveness of this approach is abysmal. The only apparent option left is donor sperm and this is not what they want. The male partner usually wants his own biological child, so the couple will opt for one last ICSI using testicular sperm, if it is offered.

Testicular sperm have markedly less DNA damage than ejaculated sperm in the same men [2]. This holds true both for men with normozoospermia and oligozoospermia, who have high DNA damage in their ejaculates. Testi-ICSI resulted in higher clinical pregnancy and live birth rates and lower miscarriage rates [3]. PICSI or IMSI as alternatives to Testi-ICSI are much less effective [4].

ICSI with testicular sperm, retrieved by an invasive surgical procedure, should NOT be offered to men with untested sperm DNA as evidence of benefit is ambivalent. In order to ensure that testicular sperm are indeed of better genomic quality than their ejaculate counterparts, diagnostic testing is required to avoid invasive biopsy unless indicated. This must be of a biomarker of testicular DNA quality that is also present in the ejaculate. Recent studies have reported just such a biomarker: a second type of sperm DNA damage that originates during spermatogenesis in the stem cells of the testis [4, 5], as a result of topoisomerase or endonuclease dysfunction. This is double-strand DNA breakage (DSB) and is detected by a neutral Comet assay. It is hypothesised that DSB has more adverse consequences than single-strand breaks (SSB) due to being more challenging to repair by the oocyte post-fertilisation and damage may not be prevented by antioxidants. The oocyte has more difficulty locating complimentary ends from double-strand breaks and has no template for repair. This leads to greater genomic instability in the developing embryo and results in failed implantation or spontaneous pregnancy loss. DSB is also present in disease conditions such as cancer [2].

A DSB test would be an ideal biomarker to separate the damage occurring in the epididymis from that in the testis. If DSB damage were found in the ejaculate, there would be no benefit in an invasive biopsy. In contrast, if the damage were primarily SSB, as detected by most DNA tests, then a testicular biopsy would be indicated as a way of retrieving sperm with better quality DNA.

To date, a major confounding factor in assessing the benefits of Testi-ICSI with conventional ICSI is female age. The latest HFEA data (www.hfea.gov.uk) show that live birth rates decrease from 21.8% in women aged between 35–37 years to 15.5% by 38–39 years and even more dramatically to 8.9% between 40–42 years. Most studies do not take this key factor into consideration and compare previous ICSI outcomes with their Testi-ISCI outcomes several years later as if female age remained unchanged even though these women are usually >40 years. Hence, conclusions can be skewed.

In conclusion, when careful diagnosis has been made and all other interventions have failed, ICSI with testicular sperm should be offered. Prospective live birth outcome studies with younger women are urgently needed to evaluate if this is a worthwhile approach. These data will become available over the next decade, particularly if current trends continue and expand to offer Testi-ICSI earlier in couple's fertility journeys, to men presenting with oligospermia in addition to those following repeated failed ICSI.

References

1. Simon L, Emery BR, Carrell DT, et al. Review: Diagnosis and impact of sperm DNA alterations in assisted reproduction. *Best Pract Res Clin Obstet.* 2017;44:38–56.

2. Bradley CK, McArthur SJ, Gee AJ, et al. Intervention improves assisted conception intracytoplasmic sperm injection outcomes for patients with high levels of sperm DNA fragmentation: a retrospective analysis. *Andrology.* 2016;4:903–10.

3. Esteves SC, Roque M, Bradley CK, Carrido, N. Reproductive outcomes of testicular versus ejaculated sperm for intracytoplasmic sperm injection among men with high levels of DNA fragmentation in semen: systematic review and meta-analysis. *Fertil Steril.* 2017;108:456–67.

4. Ribas-Maynou J, Benet J. Single and double strand sperm DNA damage: different reproductive effects on male fertility. *Genes.* 2019;10(2):105.

5. Kumar K, Lewis S, Vinci S, et al. Evaluation of sperm DNA quality in men presenting with testicular cancer and lymphoma using alkaline and neutral Comet assays. *Andrology.* 2018 Jan;6(1):230–5.

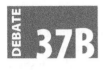

Testicular Sperm Should Be Considered for Repeated ICSI Failed Implantation Cases in Men with High DNA Damage

Against

Ashok Agarwal

Sperm DNA Damage and Male Infertility

Utilising ejaculated sperm with an elevated sperm DNA fragmentation (SDF) has been found to result in poor intracytoplasmic sperm injection (ICSI) outcomes. Ejaculated sperm from the epididymis is more prone to DNA damage, due to the oxidative stress associated with epididymal transit as described by Esteves et al. [1], who found a DNA fragmentation index (DFI) of 8.3% in testicular sperm vs. 40.7% in ejaculated sperm. Similar findings were reported by Greco et al. [2].

With this knowledge many clinicians are increasingly inclined to perform ICSI with testicular sperm in patients with failed implantation and high levels of DNA damage. However, no randomised controlled trials have documented the benefit of using testicular compared to ejaculated sperm [3]. In contrast, despite the lower SDF in testicular sperm, Moskovtsev et al. [4] showed that testicular sperm have 2–3 fold higher aneuploidy rates than ejaculated samples. These results have been contested, though, in a recent study in which the rates of aneuploidy in testicular sperm were not higher than ejaculated sperm. However, it is important to recognise that the studies concerning aneuploidy have small samples and are inconclusive.

Evidence on Testicular vs. Ejaculated Sperm

A meta-analysis conducted by Abhyankar et al. [5] included five cohort studies using testicular and ejaculated sperm from men with cryptozoospermia. Despite the need for extra centrifugation, in this case, the authors showed no difference in fertilisation or pregnancy rates with ICSI, when comparing testicular and ejaculated sperm.

Greco et al. [2] selected 18 couples who had undergone two unsuccessful ICSI attempts, using ejaculated spermatozoa and performed another ICSI cycle using testicular sperm. In this study, all male partners had >15% of ejaculated spermatozoa with damaged DNA. Although implantation and clinical pregnancy rates were reported to favour testicular sperm, the study population was small and the SDF cut-off value of >15% is controversial, not to mention that live birth rate was not reported.

A contemporary retrospective study performed by Alharbi et al. [6] examined the results of ICSI cycles using testicular sperm harvested by testicular sperm aspiration (TESA) in 52 non-azoospermic males and compared them with the results using ejaculated sperm in a cohort of men in the same clinic, all with elevated SDF >15%. They failed to report any significant improvement in clinical pregnancy rates per embryo transfer, miscarriage rate and live birth rate with testicular sperm independent of the SDF level.

Rafael F Ambar, MD helped with the literature review and in the writing of this article.

A systematic review evaluated ICSI outcomes using fresh ejaculated spermatozoa vs. surgically extracted spermatozoa from the testes in patients with abnormal semen parameters but without azoospermia. Only four articles met the inclusion criteria and each study used different study populations, ovarian stimulation protocols and SDF assays; therefore a proper analysis was not feasible [7].

Limitation of Sperm DNA Damage Evaluation Techniques

There is large variability among the tests used to determine DNA damage. TUNEL and Comet are direct assays that measure DNA fragmentation, while SCSA is an indirect assay and SCD evaluates chromatin maturity. Furthermore, testicular sperm differs from ejaculated sperm in their DNA and surface markers, as well as remodelling of histone/protamine complex which further complicates matters. Because of these shortcomings, sperm DNA fragmentation index assessment has yet to be standardised in testicular sperm [3].

Expert Opinion

Many investigators have published their results showing the benefit of using testicular sperm instead of ejaculated sperm. However, it is important to look at these studies critically and have a broad understanding of the issue at hand.

First, adequate clinical management of sperm DNA fragmentation has to be considered, rather than used as a justification for an impulsive switch to a potentially harmful surgical sperm retrieval. The control of exogenous factors such the use of medication, obesity and smoking combined with an increase of ejaculation frequency and use of appropriate antioxidants can help reduce DNA fragmentation.

Furthermore, the possibility of higher aneuploidy rates and the fact that DNA fragmentation tests are not standardised in testicular sperm should not be ignored.

It is important to emphasise that the majority of articles published on the use of testicular sperm in patients with high SDF consist of small cohorts or case series, comparing different populations of men regarding their seminal status (cryptozoospermia, severe oligozoospermia, moderate oligozoospermia, and even normozoospermia) and number of failed ICSI cycles. Additionally, several of these studies lack an adequate control group, and more importantly many do not report live birth rates.

Finally, it is important to keep in mind the fact that using testicular sperm involves surgery which by itself can have complications, including testicular haematoma, wound infection, post-operative pain, and damage to testosterone producing tissue, and together with anaesthesia, can significantly increase the cost and risks of the invasive procedure.

Given these factors, despite recent publications advocating the use of testicular sperm in non-azoospermic men with repeated failed ICSI cycles and high DNA fragmentation, many of these studies have methodological bias and high heterogeneity; therefore, there remains a lack of convincing evidence to support this approach at this time.

References

1. Esteves SC, Sánchez-Martin F, Sánchez-Martin P, et al. Comparison of reproductive outcome in oligozoospermic men with high sperm DNA fragmentation undergoing intracytoplasmic sperm injection with ejaculated and testicular sperm. *Fertil Steril*. 2015;104(6):1398–405.

2. Greco E, Scarselli F, Iacobelli M, et al. Efficient treatment of infertility due to

sperm DNA damage by ICSI with testicular spermatozoa. *Hum Reprod.* 2005;20 (1):226–30.

3. Halpern JA, Schlegel PN. Should a couple with failed in vitro fertilization/ intracytoplasmic sperm injection and increased sperm DNA fragmentation use testicular sperm for the next cycle? *Eur Urol Focus.* 2018;4(3):299–300.

4. Moskovtsev SI, Alladin N, Lo KC, et al. A comparison of ejaculated and testicular spermatozoa aneuploidy rates in patients with high sperm DNA damage. *Syst Biol Reprod Med.* 2012;58(3):142–8.

5. Abhyankar N, Kathrins M, Niederberger C. Use of testicular versus ejaculated sperm for intracytoplasmic sperm injection among men with cryptozoospermia: a meta-analysis. *Fertil Steril.* 2016;105 (6):1469–75.e1.

6. Alharbi M, Almarzouq A, Zini A. Sperm retrieval and intracytoplasmic sperm injection outcomes with testicular sperm aspiration in men with severe oligozoospermia and cryptozoospermia. *Can Urol Assoc J.* 2021;15(5):E272–5.

7. Awaga HA, Bosdou JK, Goulis DG, et al. Testicular versus ejaculated spermatozoa for ICSI in patients without azoospermia: A systematic review. *Reprod Biomed. Online,* 2018;37(5):573–80.

38A

DEBATE

Genome Editing Should Be Allowed for the Prevention of Life-Threatening Genetic Diseases

For

Kevin Smith

While far-future dystopian outcomes are frequently posited by opponents of genome editing, these scenarios are of little relevance to practical reproductive medicine. The more interesting question is this: Should we go ahead with genome editing now? I shall argue that the answer is yes, we ought to proceed without undue delay.

With current technology (most notably clusters of regularly interspaced short palindromic repeats [CRISPR]), genome editing has the potential to prevent life-threatening genetic diseases. The main arguments commonly raised against going ahead are threefold:

1. Current technology should be used instead of genome editing.
2. Genome editing technology is presently too dangerous.
3. Allowing genome editing will lead to misuse of the technology.

In my view these objections do not amount to strong grounds against genome editing. I shall consider each in turn.

1. Current Technology Instead? –– Pre-implantation genetic diagnosis (PGD) is the only current technology able to detect genetic problems in embryos. As such, PGD is highly valuable as a means to avoid genetic disorders; however, it is a limited tool, in several respects. First, it can only be used for well-characterised monogenic disorders. Second, its modus operandi is the identification of problematic embryos, meaning it is constrained by the supply of embryos from the prospective parents. Thus, PGD is intrinsically unsuited to polygenic conditions, or to more than one genetic disorder, because unfeasibly large numbers of embryos would be required in order to find one 'disease-free' embryo. Finally, even in some monogenic cases PGD is of no use. This applies if both prospective parents are either homozygous for a recessive disease-causing allele, or one of them is homozygous for a dominant disease-causing allele.

Genome editing could be used at present to prevent specific monogenic disorders. Instead of simply identifying problematic embryos for rejection (as per PGD), CRISPR offers the prospect of actually correcting deleterious genetic sequences within the embryo [1]. Genome editing could first be attempted with monogenic conditions in parents for whom PGD would not work; and then, as the technology improves through such work, it could be extended to other genetic disorders. Its use to deal with polygenic and multiple disorders lies further in the future, but this goal will only be attainable once the production of genome-edited children gets underway.

2. Too Dangerous? –– The main safety concerns are mosaicism and mutation. These effects were found to occur at relatively high frequency in the early days of genome editing. However, the accuracy of CRISPR has been radically improved through extensive experimental work, with several recent experiments showing very low levels of CRISPR-induced damage in cells, embryos and animals (see for examples, refs. [2] and [3]).

While the risk of harm from CRISPR cannot be zero, it would be wrong to assume that a new mutation in the child's genome would inevitably have an effect on their health. Given the structure and functionality of the human genome, it is clear that a single CRISPR-induced mutation would have only a small likelihood of leading to the child manifesting a genetic disorder. And some context is required: In natural reproduction, each embryo is expected to harbour around 70 new mutations. The majority of these mutations do not cause disease, and an additional CRISPR-induced mutation (should it somehow escape genetic screening) would add only a very small extra risk of disease.

An ethically acceptable genome editing attempt would incorporate appropriate genetic testing, including preliminary assay work carried out using cells from the prospective parents. Subsequently, embryos generated following genome editing would be subject to deep sequencing to identify and reject any problematic embryos.

Recently (November 2018), the field was shocked by the announcement of the World's first gene-edited babies, by the now-disgraced scientist He Jiankui. This notorious experiment has been broadly condemned for its flawed scientific design and execution [4]. It was replete with multiple ethical failings, and it is possible that the gene-edited children so-produced may have been harmed. However, it would be short-sighted to assume – as many commentators have – that this episode represents a knockdown argument against genome editing. The reality is that this was an aberrant experiment by a rogue scientist, and it can tell us little about the safety of the technology. By contrast, scientifically sound low-risk genome editing approaches can be conceived that would permit the use of CRISPR to prevent serious human disease.

3. Misuse? –– A frequently expressed fear is that genome editing will end up being used for ethically questionable applications, with the spectre of eugenics foremost in the common imagination. Concerns centre on the generation of so-called designer babies, and the concomitant emergence of a society in which genetically-enhanced individuals and their descendants have a grossly unfair advantage over everyone else. On this view, a 'slippery slope' is perceived that would lead inexorably from the use of genome editing for medically valuable purposes to its disastrous misuse.

While the general concept of a slippery slope is intuitively attractive to many laypeople and media commentators, the concept lacks a logical basis: why should the initial use of genome editing inexorably lead to disaster? I suggest that the onus resides with the proponents of this slippery slope to establish a plausible and strong link between the legitimate use of genome editing and the feared dystopian future. I know of no such case having been made effectively.

Of course, possible future downsides of genome editing can be envisioned, and it would be complacent to assume the obverse – that genome editing technology will inexorably lead to a utopia. However, history demonstrates that progress in medical technology has indubitably produced major net benefits for humanity, and there is every reason to believe that as genome editing technology evolves, major medical benefits will accrue to future generations. The posited downsides lie far in the future; their likelihood and extent is highly uncertain, and technological or legislative solutions may well emerge to avoid them. To eschew the use of genome editing today based on the putative downsides of tomorrow would be to rule out a highly promising means of avoiding serious genetic diseases. Such a stance appears both unwise and unethical [5].

Conclusions

Genome editing has the potential to revolutionise reproductive medicine. While not risk-free, CRISPR is now sufficiently advanced to allow well-conceived protocols designed to prevent specific monogenic disorders. No principled reasons exist to support a risk-averse 'precautionary' delay in the use of genome editing for this purpose. A permanent or long-term prohibition on its use would be antithetical to medical progress. The sooner we start editing the genome, the sooner will future children reap the benefits. And once the genome editing revolution is underway, we can look forward to the technology advancing apace, with future generations benefitting from a reduced burden of genetic disease.

References

1. Ranisch R. Germline genome editing versus preimplantation genetic diagnosis: is there a case in favour of germline interventions? *Bioethics*. 2020;34(1):60–9.

2. Carey K, Ryu J, Uh K, et al. Frequency of off-targeting in genome edited pigs produced via direct injection of the CRISPR/Cas9 system into developing embryos. *BMC Biotechnol*. 2019;19:24.

3. Doman J, Raguram A, Newby GA, Liu DR. Evaluation and minimization of Cas9-independent off-target DNA editing by cytosine base editors. *Nature Biotechnol*. 2020;38(5):620–8.

4. Davies B. The technical risks of human gene editing. *Hum Reprod*. 2019;34(11):2104–11.

5. Smith K. Time to start intervening in the human germline? A utilitarian perspective. *Bioethics*. 2020 34(1):90–104.

Genome Editing Should Be Allowed for the Prevention of Life-Threatening Genetic Diseases

Against

Kirsten Riggan and Megan Allyse

Arguments against the use of germline genome editing (GGE) frequently centre on deontological debates about 'designer babies' or human nature. While important, there is a more fundamental reason to be opposed to GGE, namely violations to the principle of health equality and distributive justice. Here, we will argue from a more consequentialist framework:

1. GGE Does Not Meet the Ethical Requirements of Clinical Research and Translation –– The first ethical priority of any clinical research is that the target therapy must be (a) necessary; (b) safe; and (c) effective. With the exception of a few rare scenarios, GGE does not address an unmet medical need given the availability of IVF with pre-implantation genetic testing (PGT) for genetic disease prevention. Further, there are significant technological challenges, including on and off-target effects, incomplete bi-allelic correction, and embryo mosaicism [1–3]. Current methods of genetic analysis do not allow for full assessment of the embryonic genome prior to implantation, nor do we know the pleiotropic effects of many genes implicated in human disease. For instance, the attempt of a scientific team in China in 2018 to confer protection against HIV infection by disabling the *CCR5* gene, was not only unsuccessful – the existing data suggest significant mosaicism – but the edits in question may make the resulting offspring more susceptible to other viral infections. In a reproductive context where unintended effects may have an unknown and potentially lifelong impact on the health of resulting offspring, it is appropriate to be sceptical about the application of clusters of regularly interspaced short palindromic repeats (CRISPR) to human embryos. Real persons will have to live with its successes and failures; it is for this reason that proponents of a child's right to an open future object to many applications of GGE [4].

2. GGE Will Exacerbate Existing Disparities in Access to Research and Health Care –– While many gene editing techniques are relatively inexpensive, assisted reproduction is not. This raises concerns about the potential for exploitation of vulnerable persons during the research phase and financial inaccessibility in clinical translation. While, theoretically, GGE might become more affordable if widely adopted, free market principles do not apply to many medical technologies. IVF has been commercially available for almost 40 years but remains prohibitively expensive, even in a private sector model. With the exception of some nations that provide state support for IVF services, most jurisdictions show significant socioeconomic and racial disparities in access to assisted reproduction. Adding risky, new, and experimental procedures such as GGE to this process would only exacerbate this trend.

Global access to genome editing is likely to be unequal – not simply in terms of development status, regulations on assisted reproduction, and existing medical/scientific infrastructure – but as a result of the unique cultural and religious contexts of each nation. Several major world religions have prohibitions against assisted reproduction. Even if proven to be safe and effective, certain people groups will most likely be excluded of its benefits due to its inherently controversial nature. This in turn may have profound societal consequences, whereby geography and socioeconomic status dictates the presence of genetic disease. Similar phenomena are observed with disparate access to genetic technologies: certain racial and socioeconomic groups experience greater morbidity and mortality, especially in the United States [5].

3. GGE Will Exacerbate the Stigmatisation and Marginalisation of Those Living with Health Conditions –– Proponents of GGE often reply to the possibility of a 'slippery slope' in the use of GGE by arguing that it should and will be reserved for the prevention of 'life-threatening' or 'severe' conditions. However, after many years of debate, there is still no consensus on how to categorise 'severe' or 'life-threatening.' Is a life-threatening condition one that is lethal in early childhood, such as Tay-Sachs, or not until late in life, such as Huntington's or Alzheimer's disease? Should we use GGE to reduce disease risk, such as the highly penetrant gene mutations implicated in breast or colon cancer? As the British Human Fertilization and Embryology Authority learned when they approved PGT for BRCA 1 and 2 mutations in 2006, the prevention of even relatively well-known and seemingly uncontroversial diseases and conditions is not universally accepted.

Further, promoting the use of GGE for certain diseases or conditions sends a message to individuals and their families who live with that condition that theirs is a life that should not exist (i.e. the expressivist objection). Indeed, one critique of the 2018 China experiments to proactively prevent HIV infection was the implication that persons should not be born with even the *potential* to contract HIV, contributing to the already significant discrimination in that country towards persons who are HIV-positive. Advocates also point out that even conditions that cause significant health differentials do not necessarily equate to a life that is not worth living, and warn against the fallacy of equating the condition with the whole person (i.e. synecdoche model of disability). The rich lives lived, even with a genetic disease, are worth preserving. Given the predominantly medical model of disability in the medical/scientific community, persons living with genetic conditions, even life-threatening ones, are right to be concerned that the use of GGE will lead to their erasure, rather than their benefit [2].

4. GGE Diverts Significant Resources Away from Effective Solutions to Broader Public Health Concerns –– Finally, the intense scientific focus on GGE as a disease cure detracts from investment in research lines and treatments that have a broader public health impact. We are beginning to see the results of the persistence of the scientific and medical community and patient advocates to develop effective treatments for previously insurmountable genetic diseases. This includes life-extending therapies for cystic fibrosis and spinal muscle atrophy type I. Early clinical trials examining somatic gene editing for sickle cell disease and β-thalassaemia also hold significant promise. As these therapies advance, there will be less impetus for GGE as a curative treatment. Focusing research efforts and investing in treatments that serve existing patients, rather than theoretical ones, is more consistent with utilitarian public health commitments to human health and well-being.

While gene editing remains an essential research tool, GGE is not appropriate for clinical translation and the significant resources necessary to get it there should be directed towards more fruitful avenues.

References

1. Davies B. The technical risks of human gene editing. *Hum Reprod.* 2019;34 (11):2104–11.

2. Ormond KE, Bombard Y, Bonham VL, et al. The clinical application of gene editing: ethical and social issues. *Per Med.* 2019;16(4):337–50.

3. Ledford H. CRISPR gene editing in human embryos wreaks chromosomal mayhem. *Nature.* 2020;583(7814):17–18.

4. Mintz RL, Loike JD, Fischbach RL. Will CRISPR germline engineering close the door to an open future? *Sci Engin Ethics.* 2019;25(5):1409–23.

5. Smith CE, Fullerton SM, Dookeran KA, et al. Using genetic technologies to reduce, rather than widen, health disparities. *Health Aff (Millwood).* 2016;35(8):1367–73.

PGT-A Should Be Offered for Recurrent Implantation Failure

For

Gon Shoham and Zeev Shoham

In order to discuss the benefits of pre-implantation genetic testing for aneuploidies (PGT-A) for recurrent implantation failure (RIF), we first need to define this condition. However, despite extensive research and due to numerous contributing factors, there is not yet a single agreed-upon definition.

It is well-established that the major cause of pregnancy loss is chromosomal aneuploidy. Sato et al. showed that even though PGT-A could not improve the live birth rate per patient, it reduced the overall incidence of pregnancy loss in patients with repeated implantation failure (RIF) [1]. Pirtea et al. had a different perspective, suggesting that true RIF is rare for those patients with the ability to produce euploid blastocysts. In analysing 4515 patients, 94.9% of them achieved clinical pregnancy in up to three consecutive transfers of frozen single euploid embryos [2].

PGT-A has continuously improved, with fertility specialists utilising new techniques such as next generation sequencing (NGS), which has allowed mosaicism to be detected with greater sensitivity and categorising once-healthy transferable embryos as 'abnormal'. Munné et al. demonstrated that the implantation potential was different for various types of mosaic embryos. In a recent study involving 2654 PGT-A cycles with euploid embryo transfers, of which 253 PGT-A embryo-transfer cycles were characterised as mosaic and 10 PGT-A cycles had fully abnormal embryos transferred, Munné et al. observed a significant difference in ongoing implantation rates between embryos with high ($>40\%$) and low (20–40%) rates of abnormal cells (27% vs. 50%, $p < 0.025$) in the biopsied trophectoderm samples analysed [3]. When taking the leap from the bench to the bedside, a survey was conducted by Patrizio et al. in 2019 among 125 IVF centres that performed PGT-A, in aggregate performing 135,800 IVF cycles annually. Seventy percent of respondents performed PGT-A for RIF; this indication was second only to advanced maternal age as the leading indication. Overall, only 20% of the IVF centres that utilised PGS/PGT-A reported the transfer of chromosomally 'abnormal' embryos, whether mosaic or aneuploid. The most interesting finding of this survey, however, was the remarkably high ongoing pregnancy and live birth rates (combined 49.3%) after transfers of allegedly chromosomally 'abnormal' embryos and the equally impressive low miscarriage rate of only 9.3% [4].

These research observations contribute to the hypothesis that what we consider RIF is, in fact, a cluster of conditions that we have not yet succeeded in discerning. Nonetheless, a crude categorisation would include patients with mechanical/structural/endometrial conditions, patients with abnormal embryos that cause implantation failure and finally, those with unexplained RIF. With PGT-A, the resolution of embryo quality assessment is continuously growing. This technique can provide a powerful prognostic marker in patients with RIF.

In addition, when evaluating the benefits of such procedures, we must also consider their safety, efficacy and cost-effectiveness.

Regarding safety, it has been shown that a trophectoderm biopsy does not impair the implantation potential of the embryo. Moreover, new techniques such as in vivo blastocyst recovery by uterine lavage offer minimally invasive nonsurgical, strategies to recover embryos from fertile women, with reduced risk during embryo retrieval [5].

There is no doubt that PGT-A comes with an additional financial cost. Nonetheless, as with all new technologies, the price may decrease over time. Moreover, successful implantation following PGT-A may actually reduce the total cost of infertility care and save total office visit time. An additional cost that should not be overlooked is the emotional burden. Using PGT-A can reduce futile transfers, potentially shortening the time to achieve a successful pregnancy, with fewer clinical pregnancy losses.

Fertility specialists, who have their patients' best interests in mind, would discontinue performing PGT-A for RIF if they would not see benefit in the process; thus, when we consider the large and diverse community of survey participants, we should be able to trust in the wisdom of the crowd. This finding is in line with the recent ESHRE guidelines published in March 2020, which state that although PGT-A remains heavily debated in clinical practice, RIF is considered an indication for PGT-A.

We are living in the era of big data, and artificial intelligence, whose influence and application arrived late to the field of medicine, now spreads like wildfire and is considered the next frontier in medical research. The abundant, quality data that was gathered following PGT-A cycles will fuel the algorithms that will assist future infertility specialists, even though there are already proven benefits and recommendations for utilizing PGT-A for RIF. We should continue to document every aspect of treatment, publishing new research, and with the power of unsupervised machine learning algorithms, we could cluster patients by characteristics, conditions and outcomes and support the claim that, indeed, true RIF is rare.

References

1.   Sato T, Sugiura-Ogasawara M, Ozawa F, et al. Preimplantation genetic testing for aneuploidy: a comparison of live birth rates in patients with recurrent pregnancy loss due to embryonic aneuploidy or recurrent implantation failure. *Hum Reprod.* 2019;34 (12):2340–8.

2.   Pirtea P, De Ziegler D, Marin D, et al. The rate of true recurrent implantation failure (RIF) is low: results of three successive frozen euploid single embryo transfers (SET). *Fertil Steril.* 2019;112(3, Supplement):e438–9.

3.   Munné S, Spinella F, Grifo J, et al. Clinical outcomes after the transfer of blastocysts characterized as mosaic by high resolution Next Generation Sequencing- further insights. *Eur J Med Genet.* 2020;63 (2):103741.

4.   Patrizio P, Shoham G, Shoham Z, Leong M, Barad DH, Gleicher N. Worldwide live births following the transfer of chromosomally 'Abnormal' embryos after PGT/A: results of a worldwide web-based survey. *J Assist Reprod Genet.* 2019;36 (8):1599–607.

5.   Munné S, Nakajima ST, Najmabadi S, et al. First PGT-A using human in vivo blastocysts recovered by uterine lavage: comparison with matched IVF embryo controls. *Hum Reprod.* 2020;35(1):70–80.

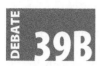
39B PGT-A Should Be Offered for Recurrent Implantation Failure

Against

N Ellissa Baskind

Where recurrent implantation failure (RIF) has been experienced following in vitro fertilisation (IVF), various modifications to treatment have been suggested; one of these is preimplantation genetic testing for aneuploidies (PGT-A) previously known as preimplantation genetic screening (PGS). When it was first implemented in the 1990s it was regarded as a revolutionary technique with the hope that it would reduce the risk of aneuploidy related miscarriages and improve IVF success by selecting only euploid embryos for transfer, a concept particularly beneficial to patients experiencing RIF. However, initial studies using early technologies failed to demonstrate a benefit in live birth rates, either with polar body or single blastomere testing, and in fact a large influential trial in the Netherlands concluded that PGS using fluorescence in situ hybridisation reduced live birth rates. More advanced technology is now available and next generation DNA sequencing (NGS) of a trophoectoderm blastocyst biopsy is routinely used and has been thought to be the panacea for embryo selection. In certain countries, universal PGT-A screening is recommended, not just for the RIF population but also for all IVF cycles. Yet testing remains controversial, and the Human Fertilisation and Embryology Authority (UK) have recently classified PGT-A as red as part of their 'add on' traffic light system and conclude that there is no evidence to show that it is effective or safe.

Here we will discuss the limitations of PGT-A and argue why it should not be used universally or offered for RIF.

The first question to consider is the accuracy of PGT-A and whether the biopsied cells are truly representative of the chromosomal status of the embryo. Certainly, there is a great deal of speculation surrounding the older techniques using single polar body analysis, but even with the trophoectoderm blastocyst biopsy of 5–7 cells there is a concern that these cannot reliably reflect the entire embryo. Trophoectoderm derived placentas have been shown to include pockets of aneuploid cells, with a normal euploid foetus. Furthermore, there is evidence that abnormal embryos self-correct beyond the blastocyst stage. Overall using statistics from a non-selection study, the data has been extrapolated to demonstrate a false-positive rate of around 10%, which would result in the equivalent of 6.8% of viable embryos being discarded [1]. Thus, PGT-A may lead to the disposal of large numbers of perfectly normal embryos, which for women in their 40s and cancer patients with limited oocytes may have devastating consequences. Moreover, there are multiple reported cases of embryos that have been transferred that have been allegedly aneuploid according to PGT-A, which have resulted in live births of chromosomally euploid children [2].

Blastomeres divide at very high rates, particularly in the trophoectoderm, increasing the risk for mitotic errors and mosaic aneuploidy. Mosaicism occurs in around 20% of all embryos. There is evolving evidence that the abnormal cells in a mosaic embryo grow at slower rates and are preferentially excluded from the embryo during development, suggesting that the few aneuploid cells identified in a mosaic blastocyst trophoectoderm biopsy has little bearing on the ploidy status of the resulting foetus. Indeed, mosaicism may persist throughout pregnancy and has been identified in chorionic villus samples. The transfer of embryos with ≤50% abnormal cells has resulted in euploid babies with implantation and delivery rates compared with embryos defined as euploid. Even when embryos with >50% abnormal cells were transferred, healthy pregnancies have resulted, albeit at a lower rate comparatively [3]. This is concerning, as many clinics use arbitrary thresholds for transferring mosaic embryos without any scientific basis. It is also important to consider the reverse; that is, of the blastomeres sampled, it is not possible to be certain that if these are all euploid, there are not aneuploid cells also within the trophoectoderm that have simply not been biopsied, resulting in false-negatives, hence prenatal testing is strongly recommended.

The final question to consider is whether PGT-A for RIF or used universally makes a difference to the overall outcome of IVF. The ESHRE-funded randomised control ESTEEM trial found that PGT-A made no difference to live birth rates following biopsy of the first or second polar body using array comparative genomic hybridisation analysis, although it may be associated with fewer miscarriages and greater efficiency of embryo transfers [4]. Notably this trial used older techniques. The more recent global multicentre STAR trial, which is one of the largest randomised control trials undertaken to date and utilised NGS of a blastocyst biopsy, included women with ≤2 prior failed IVF cycles. This study failed to demonstrate any statistically significant improvement in ongoing pregnancy rates when comparing those who had had PGT-A with controls, and furthermore there were no significant differences between miscarriage rates [5]. A multicentre retrospective pilot study specifically looked at the use of PGT-A for patients with recurrent pregnancy loss and RIF and again failed to demonstrate that PGT-A improved the live birth rate per patient. Whilst it did have the advantage of reducing the number of embryo transfers required to achieve a similar number live births compared with those not undergoing PGT-A, it is important to consider the accuracy of the analysis as described above, and whether the discarded embryos were falsely positive for aneuploidy.

In conclusion, embryos are inherently fragile structures, and the biopsy process provides an additional stress that may negatively impact the outcome. The cost of PGT-A remains high and for couples with RIF, who are one of the most vulnerable cohorts of patients, there is a duty to provide clear counselling that PGT-A is not the panacea to their treatment.

PGT-A using current technologies generates false-positive results, and identifies mosaic embryos. This results in the erroneous discarding of euploid embryos. For PGT-A to be a valid test, it needs to be minimally invasive, and accurate with results that are straightforward to interpret, and with a low cost.

References

1. Scott RT Jr, Ferry K, Su J, Tao X, Scott K, Treff NR. Comprehensive chromosome screening is highly predictive of the reproductive potential of human embryos: a prospective, blinded, nonselection study. *Fertil Steril.* 2012;97:870–75.

2. Patrizio P, Shoham G, Shoham Z, Leong M, Barad DH, Gleicher N. Worldwide live births following the transfer of

chromosomally 'Abnormal' embryos after PGT/A: results of a worldwide web-based survey. *J Assist Reprod Genet.* 2019;36:1599–607.

3. Spinella F, Fiorentino F, Biricik A, et al. Extent of chromosomal mosaicism influences the clinical outcome of in vitro fertilization treatments. *Fertil Steril.* 2018;109:77–83.

4. Verpoest W, Staessen C, Bossuyt PM, et al. Preimplantation genetic testing for

aneuploidy by microarray analysis of polar bodies in advanced maternal age: a randomized clinical trial. *Hum Reprod.* 2018;33:1767–76.

5. Munné S, Kaplan B, Frattarelli JL, et al. Preimplantation genetic testing for aneuploidy versus morphology as selection criteria for single frozen-thawed embryo transfer in good-prognosis patients: a multicenter randomized clinical trial. *Fertil Steril.* 2019;112:1071–9.

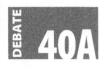

PGT-A Should Be Offered for All Women

For

Elizabeth Burt

Aneuploidy represents a major factor contributing to failed IVF treatment and PGT-A offers embryo screening beyond morphological selection criteria. Traditionally PGT-A has been reserved for women with recurrent implantation failure and miscarriage, but we argue that this technology should be accessible and offered to all undergoing IVF treatment as standard practice.

Reproductive choice is paramount, with the patient's wellbeing at the forefront of our minds. Whilst it has been demonstrated that PGT-A does not improve cumulative live birth rates per treatment cycle started (data cited by those against the routine use of PGT-A), with equivocal live birth rates demonstrated in those with and without the use of this technology, the same paper showed a reduction in miscarriage rate (7 vs. 14%) and the need for fewer embryo transfers in those who had PGT-A to achieve the same result [1]. Whilst the ultimate treatment aim is of course a baby, this needs to be balanced with the potential detrimental impact of treatment which may be secondary to numerous treatment cycles, miscarriage, multiple pregnancy and long-term embryo storage. The burden of treatment may lead to physical, psychological and financial sequela and therefore offering a treatment which may mitigate these, which is both clinically beneficial and cost-effective, is surely a wise move.

The era of embryo biopsy has evolved and, with the use of blastocyst trophectoderm biopsy, original safety concerns of cleavage cell biopsy have been superseded, with the former demonstrating equivalent reproductive potential as a non-biopsied blastocyst [2]. Extended embryo culture and blastocyst biopsy delivers the opportunity for embryo selection on two occasions and, compared to routine IVF, PGT-A trophectoderm biopsy is associated with enhanced implantation rates and live birth rates [3].

To date, in order to circumvent the risk of aneuploidy, double embryo transfer, with the aim of a singleton pregnancy, has been advocated in many clinical scenarios and also many, without indication, will request a double embryo transfer as they believe this will optimise their chances of success. This practice will leave patients vulnerable to the biggest risk of IVF, multiple pregnancy and the potential deleterious health repercussions to mother and babies. With the knowledge that selective transfer of a euploid embryo leads to greater success rates above standard IVF, which is applicable across maternal age groups, confidence in applying a gold standard elective single-embryo transfer (eSET) protocol after PGT-A for all should be promoted [4].

With the advent of new techniques, so does the sphere of clinical indications for its use grow. As well as subfertility, PGT-A may be offered to those undergoing IVF for fertility preservation. The results of PGT-A will allow an informed decision with regard to fertility planning and the option of multiple cycles in order to increase the yield of euploid embryos.

The psychological effects of IVF should never be underestimated and may stem from numerous sources. Failed cycles of IVF, disruption to family, work and social life are just the tip of the iceberg and the application of PGT-A, with the aim of reducing the time to pregnancy, may help alleviate this. Furthermore, miscarriage is a traumatic experience which takes a significant physical and psychological toll and therefore the ability to reduce the likelihood of miscarriages should be welcomed. A risk of PGT-A, which increases with age, is having no euploid embryo to transfer. On balance, although devastating news, one may argue that this is psychologically better than false hope of each doomed treatment cycle.

PGT-A comes at a price and at present is only available in the private sector in the UK. On balance, compared to several treatment cycles, using PGT-A may be cost-effective for many, making the IVF journey more efficient. From a health initiative and wider economic standpoint there may be a financial incentive in the provision of PGT-A by the NHS. Although the primary motivation for the reduction of multiple pregnancy is the prevention of adverse health complications, a drive for eSET will also be financially beneficial as care for twins costs the NHS three times more than that of singletons. In the same vein if miscarriage rates can be reduced, with the transfer of euploid embryos, there will also be a cost saving implication [5].

PGT-A and its use remains a contentious issue within the world of reproductive medicine. PGT-A is a valuable adjuvant to IVF; however, caution should be exercised, and PGT-A should not be 'sold' as the miracle test. Patients should be counselled that the chance of success per embryo transferred is dependent on many factors and a euploid embryo does not guarantee a baby. The uptake of this cutting-edge technology will not be 100%, but offers a choice conferring many advantages.

References

1. Verpoest W, Staessen C, Bossuyt PM, et al. Preimplantation genetic testing for aneuploidy by microarray analysis of polar bodies in advanced maternal age: a randomized clinical trial. *Hum Reprod.* 2018;33(9):1767–76.

2. Scott RT, Upham KM, Forman EJ, Zhao T, Treff NR. Cleavage-stage biopsy significantly impairs human embryonic implantation potential while blastocyst biopsy does not: a randomized and paired clinical trial. *Fertil Steril.* 2013;100 (3):624–30.

3. Dahdouh EM, Balayla J, García-Velasco JA. Comprehensive chromosome screening improves embryo selection: a meta-analysis. *Fertil Steril.* 2015;104(6):1503–12.

4. Maxwell SM, Grifo JA. Should every embryo undergo preimplantation genetic testing for aneuploidy? A review of the modern approach to in vitro fertilization. *Best Pract Res Clin Obstet Gynaecol.* 2018;53:38–47.

5. Sacchi L, Albani E, Cesana A, et al. Preimplantation genetic testing for aneuploidy improves clinical, gestational, and neonatal outcomes in advanced maternal age patients without compromising cumulative live-birth rate. *J Assist Reprod Genet.* 2019;36 (12):2493–504.

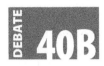

PGT-A Should Be Offered for All Women

Against

Susan P Willman

Aneuploidy is a major source of adverse pregnancy outcome. For this reason, universal prenatal screening is recommended by the American College of Obstetricians and Gynecologists. Aneuploidy is also understood to be a large factor in implantation failure in IVF. Should universal screening be performed for IVF? The goal of genetic screening of embryos would be to maximise the birth of a healthy child through improved embryo selection. Yet there are several differences between screening in pregnancy and screening in IVF. Prenatal genetic screening meets the appropriate criteria as a screen: it is non-invasive and cost-effective; the screening cut-offs of the various tests have been clinically evaluated and thresholds set to minimise false-negatives. More importantly, if there is a positive screen, accurate diagnostic testing can be performed for verification which helps determine what threshold is acceptable for a false-positive result.

Does pre-implantation genetic testing-A (PGT-A) meet the criteria for a screening test? Trophectoderm (TE) biopsy of an expanded blastocyst with vitrification is the present paradigm for PGT-A. A prospective clinical trial of a two-embryo fresh transfer pairing one TE-biopsied embryo with one non-biopsied embryo demonstrated no adverse effect on implantation [1], but long-term effects have not been studied. While reassuring, minimising embryo manipulation is desirable and its risks must be balanced with the benefits. Cryopreservation with vitrification for future frozen embryo transfer (FET) is now an accepted approach to improve endometrial receptivity for implantation and to reduce ovarian hyperstimulation syndrome. Pregnancies from FET also have a lower risk of preterm delivery, lower risk of intrauterine growth restriction (IUGR) and higher birth weight than fresh transfer.

The real conundrum of PGT-A at present is the genetic testing platform: its predictability of outcome, reproducibility and cost. Predictability is best evaluated by demonstrating a tolerable low false-positive predictive value (PPV) and an acceptable false-negative predictive value (NPV).

Some may argue that only a zero false-positive rate is tolerable. While it is of course undesirable to discard any embryos that could possibly be abnormal, this is done all the time with IVF out of necessity. Decisions must be made on disposition of embryos based on visual evidence of fertilisation, embryo development and embryo grade. But presently there is no consensus on PPV and NPV thresholds because they are largely undescribed.

New technologies for PGT have advanced swiftly and with the same rapid pace; these new technologies have been widely applied before adequate clinical validations have been performed. FISH was the first platform used for PGT which over time was replaced by aCGH, qPCR, SNP and most recently NGS. All genetic testing platforms, however are not alike. A nonselection study using SNP-based technology was performed in 2012 demonstrating NPV to be 96% and PPV of 41% [2]. There have not been appropriate assessments of other platforms for PPV and NPV. What is a tolerable NPV and what is an acceptable PPV? Which platform results in the most predictable clinical outcome?

Looking for answers in clinical trials is a 2015 meta-analysis of comprehensive chromosome screening. Three randomized controlled trials (RCT) ($n = 659$) and eight observational studies (OS) ($n = 2993$) showed an improved sustained implantation rate [3]. The three RCTs were single-site studies limited to a homogenous and good prognosis patient population, whereas the OS had a more heterogenous population and included day 3 and day 5 biopsies. The platforms used were qPCR and aCGH. Over time, with many single-site studies reporting high success rates with PGT-A, there has been increased use of PGT-A despite lack of robust clinical trials. With every published study showing a beneficial outcome, well-designed or not, there is the inference that the results can be duplicated and this may not be the case.

NGS was advanced with the positive attributes of greater sensitivity, higher throughput, and lower cost. (The lower cost has yet to be passed on to patients.) With the greater sensitivity of NGS came the unanticipated nuance of mosaicism. Mosaic results introduced uncertainty, confusion and lack of confidence in the testing in the clinical community. But even more detrimental was the public perception that PGT-A was a diagnostic test, creating unrealistic expectations. The problem was lack of knowledge of the true NPV and PPV for these variable test results.

The first prospective RCT using NGS was a multicentre international study [4]. IVF clinics were selected for participation based on high reported clinical pregnancy rates and expertise in blastocyst culture and TE biopsy. The study design was drafted before the impact of mosaicism was recognised. Women aged 25–40 with two expanded blastocysts were randomised to either PGT-A or no biopsy followed by vitrification ($n = 661$) and FET. Mosaic embryos were considered abnormal and not transferred. The ongoing pregnancy rate per embryo transfer was equivalent in the treatment and control group but in the subgroup of women aged 35–40, there was an improvement of OPR (51–37%).

Why didn't PGT-A in the younger patients result in an improved outcome? One explanation could be that mosaicism is not influenced by age with a reported incidence in the 30% range. Since the proportion of euploid embryos declines with age but the mosaic rate is constant, the proportion of mosaic embryos with a euploid cell line will decrease from 26.6% for women <35 years to 10.5% for women >42 years [5]. Given this, PGT-A may demonstrate a greater clinical benefit when aneuploidy has a greater prevalence and the PGT result is not clouded by a mosaic result.

While it is a compelling argument that aneuploidy in the embryo is a primary cause of implantation failure, it is a more complex situation than simply chromosome copy number. Not all mosaicism is alike. Mosaicism may be reflective of physiologic incompetence in that the embryo has deceased capacity for normal mitosis. Euploid embryos miscarry and so, too, euploid embryos might not implant. As an analogy, prenatal screening does not rely on NIPT alone. Maternal serum markers and ultrasound evaluation of fetal anatomy are equally important to evaluate fetal health. Embryo assessment in IVF should look for a similar paradigm using genetic information along with other embryo assessments and other clinical parameters. With genetic reports, a rank order giving information of the statistical confidence of the result (which is available with one SNP platform) rather than a 'normal/not normal' result would be more useful. While PGT-A still is a potential valuable screening tool, it's benefit is not yet well-established enough to offer to all patients. As the practice committees for ASRM and SART conclude, more studies are needed to better define the risks, benefits and cost-effectiveness of universal screening.

References

1. Scott R, Upham K, Forman E, Zhao T, Treff N. Cleavage-stage biopsy significantly impairs human embryonic implantation potential while blastocyst biopsy does not: a randomized and paired clinical trial. *Fertil Steril*. 2013;100(3):24–63.

2. Scott R, Ferry K, Su J, et al. Comprehensive chromosome screening is highly predictive of the reproductive potential of human embryos: a prospective, blinded, nonselection study. *Fertil Steril*. 2012;97 (4):870–75.

3. Dadouh E, Balayla J, Garcia-Velasco A. Comprehensive chromosome screening improves embryo selection: a meta-analysis. *Fertil Steril*. 2015;104(6):1504–12.

4. Munne A, Kaplan B, Frattarelli J, et al. Preimplantation genetic testing for aneuploidy versus morphology as selection criteria for single frozen-thawed embryos transfer in good prognosis patients: a multicenter randomized clinical trial. *Fertil Steril*. 2019;112(6):1072–8.

5. Munne S, Wells D. Detection of mosaicism at blastocyst stage with use of high-resolution next-generation sequencing. *Fertil Steril*. 2017;107(5):1085–91.

41A AMH Is a Better Predictor of Ovarian Response Than AFC

For

Antonio La Marca and Valentina Grisendi

In medically assisted reproduction, markers of ovarian reserve are largely used as predictors of ovarian response with the aim to individualise ovarian stimulation therapy and to counsel patients on reproductive outcome. For several years, serum anti-müllerian hormone (AMH) and ultrasound antral follicle count (AFC) have shown to be the most accurate markers and to be highly correlated.

In 2002, the first prospective study on AMH predictive ability was published [1]. The study reported a high correlation between AMH and the number of oocytes retrieved (R = 0.57, p < 0.01) and a good discriminating potential for predicting poor ovarian response (ROC$_{AUC}$ 0.85). In the same study, AMH was compared to AFC and serum day 3 follicle stimulating hormone (FSH). AFC revealed a similar predictive ability to AMH, while FSH showed a worse predictive performance.

Subsequently, a large number of studies confirmed the first reports. More recently, two meta-analysis studied the predictive ability of AMH and AFC on poor response [2] and on hyper-response [3]. The predictive accuracy of markers was high for poor response (area under the curve (AUC) 0.78 and 0.76 for AMH and AFC, respectively) and for excessive response (in the multivariable models the added value to the AUC of AMH or AFC on female age resulted in 0.81). None of markers showed added value to female age in prediction of ongoing pregnancy rate in poor responder patients.

In the first years, doubts regarding reliability of AMH dosage were raised. Only two manual immunoassays were available for the analyses but these kits produced heterogeneous results, not repeatable among different laboratories and not comparable among studies. The reliability of the last manual AMH gen II assay was even shaken by the reporting of complement interference. This generated contrast in the serum concentrations measured and very low reliability. Recently, to overcome these limitations and to improve quality of AMH measurements, the first fully automated AMH electrochemiluminescent immunoassays (Elecsys® AMH assay by Roche Diagnostics and Access assay by Beckman Coulter) were developed, which promise to give more robust results with minimal inter-laboratory variation.

Regarding AFC, the main limitation is the intra- and inter-observer variability. Although a systematic method of measuring and counting antral follicles in routine practice was described, the low repeatability is still a problem. First of all, the different ultrasound equipment used doesn't guarantee the same resolution; second, there is always the risk to incorrectly counting of follicles, especially in the very high counts; third, the presence of a functional ovarian cyst may affect the count. The introduction of three-dimensional (3D) technique brings about significant advantages over the two-dimensional ultrasound. It permits accurate volume measurements and, applying the software for automated follicular count (SonoAVC), it is possible to automatically identify the antral follicles present in a given ovarian volume. Unfortunately 3D technique is more time-consuming and today not largely available, so that it has not yet become the gold standard to perform AFC.

A recent prospective multicentric study, undertaken in seven infertility centres on 451 healthy patients, compared the automated AMH with AFC. It showed that AMH measured by automated Elecsys assay doesn't have significant variation in distribution between centres, although there is significant variation in AFC, also after adjusting for age. The study confirmed that there is a strong positive correlation between AMH and AFC (Spearman's rho = 0.68, P < .001), but Spearman's rho varied among centres from 0.49 to 0.87 [4]. Thus, there are emerging data suggesting that AMH is a more reproducible measure of the ovarian reserve than AFC.

To better define if one of the above-mentioned markers has a better predictive ability than the other when ovarian response to FSH is the primary outcome, it is very useful to look at data coming from the post-hoc analysis of some trials such as the MERIT and MEGASET studies. Indeed the authors found that AMH was more strongly correlated to oocyte yield than AFC in both trial populations. Assessment of the relative capacity of AMH and AFC for predicting oocyte yield demonstrated a firm superiority of AMH (AMH: R^2 = 0.29 and 0.23; AFC: R^2 = 0.07 and 0.07 for MERIT and MEGASET trial, respectively) [5]. Besides these retrospective analyses, only one RCT has been specifically designed to compare AMH and AFC as predictive biomarkers [6]. In the Xpect trial, AMH resulted in the only significant predictive factor of the number of oocytes retrieved and of an excessive ovarian response, while for AFC, an association with the number of retrieved oocytes was not shown [6].

In conclusion, the demonstration of AMH's major predictive value in one trial and two trials post-hoc analyses lay a first solid foundation for the supremacy of this marker. Other studies are needed, but we think that AMH dosing with new automated assays could only confirm these results.

References

1. van Rooij IA, Broekmans FJ, te Velde ER, et al. Serum anti-Müllerian hormone levels: a novel measure of ovarian reserve. *Hum Reprod.* 2002;17(12):3065–71.

2. Broer SL, van Disseldorp J, Broeze KA, et al. Added value of ovarian reserve testing on patient characteristics in the prediction of ovarian response and ongoing pregnancy: an individual patient data approach. *Hum Reprod Update.* 2013;19 (1):26–36.

3. Broer SL, Dólleman M, van Disseldorp J, et al. Prediction of an excessive response in in vitro fertilization from patient characteristics and ovarian reserve tests and comparison in subgroups: an individual patient data meta-analysis. *Fertil Steril.* 2013;100(2):420–9.e7.

4. Anderson RA, Anckaert E, Bosch E, et al. Prospective study into the value of the automated elecsys antimüllerian hormone assay for the assessment of the ovarian growing follicle pool. *Fertil Steril.* 2015;103 (4):1074–80.e4.

5. Nelson SM, Klein BM, Arce JC. Comparison of antimüllerian hormone levels and antral follicle count as predictor of ovarian response to controlled ovarian stimulation in good-prognosis patients at individual fertility clinics in two multicenter trials. *Fertil Steril.* 2015;103 (4):923–30.e1.

6. Andersen AN, Witjes H, Gordon K, Mannaerts B. Predictive factors of ovarian response and clinical outcome after IVF/ ICSI following a rFSH/GnRH antagonist protocol with or without oral contraceptive pre-treatment. *Hum Reprod.* 2011;26:3413–23.

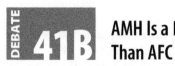

41B AMH Is a Better Predictor of Ovarian Response Than AFC

Against

Frank Broekmans

Let us be honest with each other. Prediction of ovarian response to ovarian hyperstimulation for IVF/ICSI is considered an important action with the purpose of optimising safety of ART. Yet, it is only meaningful to prior identify the high/excessive responder if there is an effective change in the usual management which clearly reduces the risk for this potential high responder to become an OHSS patient. Today, the uptake of GnRH antagonist co-medicated stimulation cycles and with the GnRH agonist trigger, reduced hCG trigger dosage and freeze-all as toolbox parts to manage the actual high responder, ovarian reserve testing may well be redundant. But okay, the task was to argue about whether these tests are equally effective in response prediction.

The antral follicle count (AFC) at transvaginal ultrasound or the anti-müllerian hormone (AMH) serum level will estimate the number of antral follicles present at a given time point in both ovaries, and thereby the likely response of the ovaries when applying regular stimulation FSH dosages. Test characteristic studies revealed that the AFC has a slightly higher intra-individual fluctuation than AMH, both within and between cycles, while test to test (operator and assay) variation have appeared to be at an equally low level for either test. This suggests AMH may be the better cycle-independent parameter to predict ovarian response.

However, predictive performance studies with regards to the response categories Low and High have revealed accuracy levels to be highly similar for the two tests [1] (Table 41B.1). In contrast, a more recent position paper using pharma initiated RCT data, suggested superiority for AMH in predicting ovarian response over the AFC. This work may have disqualified itself by the fact that AMH was assessed in a central laboratory for all study sites, while description of the methods to assess the AFC was remarkably absent. Any comparison with true meaning for daily practice has thereby become a fairy tale [2]. Therefore, until demonstrated differently, AMH and the AFC are equally capable in ovarian response prediction.

It is then the right time to ask the most important question: which test serves best the purpose of response testing, which is: FSH dosage adjustments in order to prevent OHSS in predicted high responders? The answer needs to be established in direct comparisons of real-life application of both tests in dosage individualisation. It should however be noted that the precision of the FSH stimulation drug in terms of pharmaco-kinetics and pharmaco-dynamics may fail the desired mark. Both the interindividual variation in FSH serum levels as well as the between cycle variation in ovarian response using a standard dosage of 150 IU recombinant FSH daily appeared unpleasantly high [3]. This implies that the 'art' of FSH dosage adjustment for response optimisation may lie close to what is currently known as gambling.

Anyhow, the desired direct randomised comparison of the two tests has been studied only in a single study, where for each test stratification of the test result led to the assignment to a stimulation dosage (375, 225 or 150 IU daily of rec FSH). Overall, no

Table 41B.1. Areas under the curves of prediction models of age and ovarian reserve tests for the forecasting an excessive response. Data were derived from 10 studies where all three ORTs were applied. In the univariable analysis it is shown that both AMH and AFC have a comparably high accuracy. In the multivariable models the added value to the AUC of an ORT on female age is similar for AFC and AMH. Moreover, adding any of the two ORTs yields a significant rise in the AUC [1].

	Three-test study group (N= 1,023)			
	AUC	95% CI	P value	N
Univariable analysis				
Age	0.61	0.54 – 0.68	NA	1023
FSH	0.66	0.60 – 0.73	0.071	1023
AFC	0.79	0.74 – 0.85	<0.001	1023
AMH	0.81	0.76 – 0.87	<0.001	1023
Multivariable analysis				
Age & FSH	0.68	0.62 – 0.75	<0.001	1023
Age & AFC	0.81	0.76 – 0.87	<0.001	1023
Age & AMH	0.81	0.76 – 0.87	<0.001	1023
Age & AMH & AFC	0.85	0.80 – 0.90	<0.001	1023
Age & AMH & AFC & FSH	0.85	0.80 – 0.90	<0.001	1023
AMH & AFC	0.85	0.80 – 0.90	<0.001	1023

difference in desired ovarian response level, cancellation rate, pregnancy rate, or OHSS rate was noted [4]. As this study was underpowered to identify potentially meaningful differences in several parameters, the urge was expressed for additional RCTs of larger size. I truly hope some scientific group has picked up this task.

Further information comes from indirect comparisons: a study where AMH was added to a conventional dosage regimen based on age, antral follicle count (AFC) and BMI, appeared not to improve the rate of desired ovarian response, defined as 5–12 oocytes, nor decreased the rate of OHSS or poor ovarian response cycles [5]. Also, trials using either AMH or the AFC as part of a dosage picking algorithm, compared to standard dosing without prior testing, have clearly come to comparable results: no impact on the live birth prospects, but improvement in the safety profiles [6], (Figure 41B.1). As such, if OR testing is applied for the main relevant purpose, high responder management, using AFC or AMH as the tool alongside other predictive markers such as female age, and bodyweight, leads to equivalent results.

So, AFC and AMH produce comparable levels of predictive accuracy in high response prediction and offer the same utility level when used for FSH dosage adjustments with the purpose of creating a normal instead of a high response, with OHSS risk reduction as the result. Of course, we may still think about the value of prior low response prediction, equally effective when using AMH and the AFC, as we have seen. This prediction may possibly be meaningful in the sense that a predicted low responder with indeed a low response in the first attempt may be counselled for further refraining from treatment. But as this is only true for older women, 'measuring' age and looking at the first cycle response as the 'ovarian response test' may be highly sufficient [7].

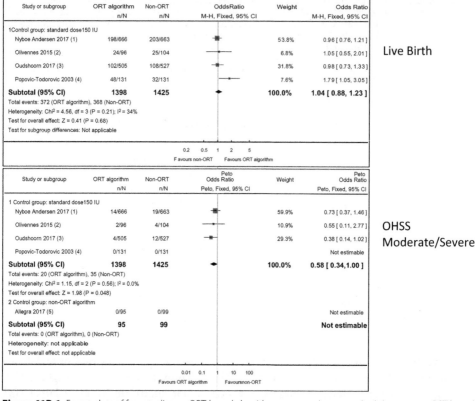

Figure 41B.1 Forest plots of four studies on ORT-based algorithm compared to a standard dose or non-ORT based algorithm based FSH dosing [6]. Outcome live birth or ongoing pregnancy in the upper panel. Outcome moderate or severe OHSS in the lower panel. The overall effects on live birth are not different, while the rate of moderate to severe OHSS is reduced by almost 50%. (1) Algorithm using AMH vs. 150 IU. (2) CONSORT algorithm using AFC vs. 150 IU. (3) AFC (3 categories) vs. 150 IU. (4) Algorithm using AFC vs. 150 IU. (5) Algorithm using AMH vs. algorithm using age only.

Areas under the curves of prediction models of age and ovarian reserve tests for the forecasting an **excessive response**. Data were derived from ten studies where all three ORTs were applied. In the univariable analysis it is shown that both AMH and AFC have a comparably high accuracy. In the multivariable models the added value to the AUC of an ORT on female age is similar for AFC and AMH. Moreover, adding any of the two ORTs yields a significant rise in the AUC [1].

References

1. Broer SL, van Disseldorp J, Broeze KA, et al. Added value of ovarian reserve testing on patient characteristics in the prediction of ovarian response and ongoing pregnancy: an individual patient data approach. *Hum Reprod Update.* 2013;19(1): 26–36.

2. Iiodromiti S, Anderson RA, Nelson SM. Technical and performance characteristics of anti-mullerian hormone and antral follicle count as biomarkers of ovarian response. *Hum Reprod Update.* 2015;21(6): 698–710.

3. Oudshoorn SC, van Tilborg TC, Hamdine O, et al. Ovarian response to controlled

ovarian hyperstimulation: what does serum FSH say? *Hum Reprod.* 2017;32(8): 1701–9.

4 Lan VT, Linh NK, Tuong HM, Wong PC, Howles CM. Anti-mullerian hormone versus antral follicle count for defining the starting dose of FSH. *Reprod Biomed Online.* 2013;27(4): 390–9.

5. Magnusson A, Nilsson L, Olerod G, Thurin-Kjellberg A, Bergh C. The addition of anti-mullerian hormone in an algorithm for individualized hormone dosage did not improve the prediction of ovarian response – a randomized, controlled trial. *Hum Reprod.* 2017;32(4): 811–19.

6. Lensen SF, Wilkinson J, Leijdekkers JA, et al. Individualised gonadotropin dose selection using markers of ovarian reserve for women undergoing in vitro fertilisation plus intracytoplasmic sperm injection (IVF/ICSI). *Cochrane Database Syst Rev.* 2018;2018(2).

7. Leijdekkers JA, Eijkemans MJC, van Tilborg TC, et al. Cumulative live birth rates in low-prognosis women. *Hum Reprod.* 2019;34(6): 1030–41.

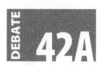

Pituitary Suppression Using GnRH Agonist for IVF Is Outdated

For

Efstratios Kolibianakis

In 1984, at the time of gonadotrophin-releasing hormone (GnRH) analogue introduction in ovarian stimulation for IVF, both agonists and antagonists were available. GnRH antagonists should have been naturally the analogue of choice to suppress premature luteinising hormone (LH) surge, since they were associated with distinct advantages compared to GnRH agonists. These included rapid initiation and reversibility of action, no flare-up effect, no ovarian cyst formation and no hypo-estrogenic side-effects. However, the main reason behind the so-called GnRH-agonist era, i.e. the exclusive use of GnRH agonists in ovarian stimulation until 2000, was the lack of safety of GnRH antagonists. At that point in time, GnRH antagonists were associated with allergic reactions which rendered them unsuitable for clinical use.

Although these safety problems were absent in the third generation of GnRH antagonists, introduced in clinical practice in the early 2000s, adoption of antagonists was rather slow, despite being a more patient-friendly protocol, associated with a shortened duration of stimulation and less gonadotrophin consumption. This was largely due to conflicting early meta-analyses regarding the comparative efficacy of the two analogues. It took more than a decade for the scientific community to accept that there was no difference in the probability of live birth between the two GnRH analogues [1].

Despite the confirmation of equal efficacy to GnRH agonists, the main reason behind the shift from GnRH agonists to GnRH antagonists was ironically based on the same factor that prohibited their utilisation back in 1984, their safety profile. Since their introduction, there was unanimous acceptance that the use of GnRH antagonists was associated with a decreased probability of the most fearful complication of ovarian stimulation for IVF, ovarian hyperstimulation syndrome (OHSS) [1]. Moreover, a few years after their introduction, it became clear that by replacing hCG with GnRH agonist for triggering final oocyte maturation, the incidence of OHSS became virtually zero [2]. This is a unique feature of a GnRH antagonist protocol that is especially important not only for high responders, but also for patients who unexpectedly show a high ovarian response to gonadotrophins. In these patients, the use of GnRH agonists limits dramatically the options for maintaining safety and efficacy, something completely feasible with GnRH antagonists [3].

Currently, an equal probability of live birth to GnRH agonists, combined with a vastly superior safety and patient friendly profile, allows us to recognise beyond doubt which GnRH analogue should be the first choice in ovarian stimulation for IVF. Nevertheless, GnRH agonist use for suppressing premature LH surge is still practised by a proportion of clinicians. This is explained by their reluctance to change long-standing stimulation habits, fuelled by false arguments that occasionally appear in the published literature.

An effort to currently justify the use of GnRH agonists, at least for the general population, is based on the argument of higher ongoing pregnancy rates (3.2%) with GnRH agonists suggested by a recent meta-analysis [4]. That meta-analysis was characterised by several problems such as inclusion of studies with asymmetric co-interventions,

216

misclassification of eligible studies, questionable methodological rigidity, lack of prospective registration, lack of application of basic meta-analysis principles in some of the estimates produced and more importantly by the questionable choice of using surrogate outcome measures instead of live birth per woman [5].

Nevertheless, even if we momentarily accept the presence of a small difference (3.2%) in ongoing pregnancy rate in favour of GnRH agonists, balancing this difference with a concomitantly increased probability of OHSS, as the authors of that meta-analysis have suggested [4], is at least problematic. This is due to the fact that in this way, patients' safety and treatment efficacy are being treated as if of equal importance. Obviously, not achieving pregnancy after IVF is a totally different situation than being admitted to the intensive care unit due to development of severe OHSS. Even if we assume that patients are willing to take a risk for their own health, medicine should not be practised according to questionable or irrational patient wishes. The crucial issue is not what patients prefer but what physicians are ethically entitled to do, by adhering to evidence-based medicine.

In summary, both GnRH analogues are characterised by a similar probability of live birth, while eliminating OHSS by GnRH-agonist triggering and freezing of all embryos is only feasible in GnRH-antagonist cycles. This advantage has driven utilisation of the antagonist protocol in the general population, to allow management of an unexpected high

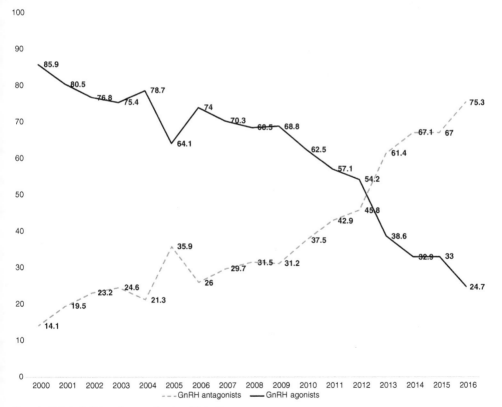

Figure 42A.1 GnRH analogue utilisation (%) in Germany.
(Based on data from the German IVF Registry)

ovarian response by ensuring maximum safety and efficacy. Moreover, GnRH antagonists remain the analogue of choice in specific patient groups such as oocyte donors, women seeking fertility preservation and certainly women with PCOS.

It comes as no surprise that taking all the advantages of GnRH-antagonists into account, recent clinical development programmes in ovarian stimulation for IVF have been exclusively performed in GnRH-antagonist protocols. Moreover, based on data from the German Registry (2001–2016), the use of GnRH antagonists in every day practice shows an impressive clear trend for replacing GnRH agonists as the analogue of choice for suppressing the premature LH rise, essentially leading to the end of the GnRH agonist era (Figure 42A.1).

References

1. Al-Inany HG, Youssef MA, Aboulghar M, et al. Gonadotrophin-releasing hormone antagonists for assisted reproductive technology. *Cochrane Database Syst Rev.* 2011;CD001750.

2. Tarlatzis B, Bosdou J. Elimination of OHSS by GnRH agonist and freezing embryos. In: Rizk B, Gerris J (eds). *Complications and Outcomes of Assisted Reproduction.* Cambridge: Cambridge University Press, 2017, pp. 149–63.

3. Bosdou JK, Venetis CA, Tarlatzis BC, et al. Higher probability of live-birth in high, but not normal, responders after first frozen-embryo transfer in a freeze-only cycle strategy compared to fresh-embryo transfer: a meta-analysis. *Hum Reprod.* 2019;34:491–505.

4. Lambalk CB, Banga FR, Huirne JA, et al. GnRH antagonist versus long agonist protocols in IVF: a systematic review and meta-analysis accounting for patient type. *Hum Reprod Update.* 2017;23:560–5.

5. Kolibianakis EM, Griesinger G, Venetis CA. GnRH antagonists vs. long GnRH agonists in IVF: significant flaws in a meta-analysis lead to invalid conclusions. *Hum Reprod Update.* 2018;24:242–3.

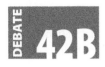

42B Pituitary Suppression Using GnRH Agonist for IVF Is Outdated

Against

Cornelis B Lambalk

What is the principle? The aim of the treatment with either the agonist or the antagonist is to prevent premature luteinisation. And the idea that immediate blockade with a GnRH antagonist should be simple, safe and versatile compared to the complex road the agonist has to take via desensitisation is highly valid and understandable. So do both drugs do what they promise and to the same extent? The answer is no, as elegantly demonstrated in an analysis by Kolibianakis showing that daily agonist yielded less than 1% of cycles with premature LH secretion against 8% with antagonist [1]. Remarkably many LH rises occurred before the antagonist treatment was even started.

Let's now turn to answer the question of whether the antagonist benefits the principal clinical goal, namely, the improvement of the final outcome: more chance to have a baby? Well, the answer is we don't really know. If we consider, which is quite usual in our field, a difference of 5% live births as clinically relevant, then no single study ever done was sufficiently powered to find this out. So in order to come close to an answer, systematic reviews are of great help. The most recent one could not trace a significant difference in live birth rates [2]. However, there was insufficient power since many studies included in the analyses did not report live birth rate. But if ongoing pregnancy, which increases power tremendously, and can be considered as a highly reliable surrogate measure for live birth, was evaluated then the antagonist resulted in a 3.6% significantly lower outcome [3].

So at first sight these two observations are not very convincing to advocate for the general use of the antagonist.

However, from the beginning it appeared that in many of the RCTs there was an indication that the OHSS rate, one of the most feared side-effects of ovarian hyperstimulation for ART, was lower with the antagonist and this was indeed convincingly confirmed as significant in systematic reviews. It should be of note however that OHSS was almost never the primary endpoint for which the studies were powered, and it was often poorly defined. As such, recently the only study comparing agonist versus antagonist with OHSS as the endpoint was published [4]. This study showed a significant reduction of OHSS with the use of the antagonist.

The balance was made up. The discussion about the mode of prevention of a premature LH surge during hormonal ovarian hyperstimulation for IVF/ICSI seems to have been settled with the endorsement by the field of the ESHRE guideline 2019 for ovarian stimulation [5].

Based on the underpowered statement of no differences in live birth rates and the reduction in occurrence of the most important side-effect, OHSS, general use of the antagonist received a green light.

However, should we disregard the fact that there is one baby less born in 28 cycles against prevention of one severe OHSS in 40 cycles with the use of an antagonist? Or in other words a 3.6% lower chance of a baby against the reduction of the chance to experience OHSS from 4% to 2%?

Let's ask the patient: In a discrete choice analysis study it was shown that patients were willing to undergo the presumed less patient-friendly agonist scenario if it would lead to a 2.5% higher chance of pregnancy [6].

So if we would ask the patient and follow her choice then long agonist treatment would most likely prevail.

But obviously we as physicians have our own responsibility and prevention of an important dangerous side-effect is, even when rarely occurring, important. This could justify the antagonist option when based on a fully shared decision basis with the optimally informed patient.

Of note: the use of the antagonist will not completely eradicate OHSS. One potential danger of proclaiming antagonist use because it prevents OHSS is that doctors assume that use of antagonist safeguards against any OHSS which is not the case. It should be realised that the higher rate of OHSS with agonist is not caused by the agonist but by ill-adjusted dosing of gonadotropins (LH/FSH for stimulation and the need for hCG triggering). Antagonist use in the stimulatory phase of the ART cycle allows the use of a GnRH agonist for triggering of final maturation instead of the long-acting hCG which helps to further reduce occurrence of OHSS. However, even with this scenario severe OHSS has been reported.

In general, this option, a GnRH agonist-induced ovulation trigger in the context of OHSS prevention should be considered as advantageous and extends the hormonal armament for ART.

Another feature that should be taken into account is the complex nature of timing of the ART procedure with antagonist use which depends on the start of natural menstruation. In comparison is the planning convenience of the long agonist protocol based on firmly settled pituitary desensitisation. Unfortunately, timing antagonist cycles with a hormonal contraceptives has shown to be detrimental and is discouraged.

A novel aspect to be considered is in fact the lack of sufficient randomised studies with the only relevant endpoint for the patient, namely the cumulative live birth rate that takes into account the fate of subsequently thawed and transferred cryopreserved embryos. This is exactly what Toftager et al. [4] studied in a trial adequately powered for OHSS as the primary endpoint. They reported no difference in cumulative live birth rates.

But is it really settled? I would say no. It should be admitted that a well-conducted large RCT study of first cycle data in a general IVF population showed a non-significantly lower pregnancy rate in antagonist cycles, but contributed to the overall significantly lower ongoing pregnancy rate in the most recent meta-analysis [2].

So, with regard to general expected normal responder ART patients, we should expect a higher pregnancy rate in the first cycle at the cost of OHSS risk going from 2% to 4%. Furthermore considering the details from the study by Toftager [4] on CLBR there could be merit in fine-tuning the stimulation protocol in favour of agonist for older women and the antagonist for overweight patients.

The finding of no differences in pregnancy rates of any type and the undisputed lowering of OHSS in patients with PCOS are strong arguments to avoid the long GnRH agonist protocol for prevention of premature luteinisation. To summarise: the advice is to share the decision to choose either the long agonist protocol or the antagonist protocol with the optimally informed ART patient.

So to conclude this debate: There are enough reasons to state that: 'Pituitary suppression using a GnRH agonist for IVF' is NOT outdated.

References

1. Kolibianakis EM, Venetis CA, Kalogeropoulou L, Papanikolaou E, Tarlatzis BC. Fixed versus flexible gonadotropin releasing hormone antagonist administration in in vitro fertilization: a randomized controlled trial. *Fertil Steril.* 2011;95:558–62.

2. Lambalk CB, Banga FR, Huirne JA, et al. GnRH antagonist versus long agonist protocols in IVF: a systematic review and meta-analysis accounting for patient type. *Hum Reprod Update.* 2017 Sept 1;23 (5):560–79.

3. Braakhekke M, Kamphuis EI, Dancet EA, Mol F, van der Veen F, Mol BW. Ongoing pregnancy qualifies best as the primary outcome measure of choice in trials in reproductive medicine: an opinion paper. *Fertil Steril.* 2014 May;101(5):1203–4.

4. Toftager M, Bogstad J, Bryndorf T, et al. Risk of severe ovarian hyperstimulation syndrome in GnRH antagonist versus GnRH agonist protocol: RCT including 1050 first IVF/ICSI cycles. *Hum Reprod.* 2016;31:1253–64.

5. Bosch E, Broer S, Griesinger G, et al. ESHRE guideline: ovarian stimulation for IVF/ICSI. *Hum Reprod Open.* 2020 May 1;2020(2).

6. van den Wijngaard L, van Wely M, Dancet EA, et al. Patients' preferences for gonadotrophin-releasing hormone analogs in in vitro fertilization. *Gynecol Obstet Invest.* 2014;78:16–21.

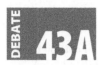

43A The Maximum Effective Dose of FSH for Ovarian Stimulation in IVF Is 300 IU

For

Sarah Lensen

Background

During an IVF cycle, daily doses of gonadotropin follicle-stimulating hormone (FSH) are used to induce multifollicular development in the ovaries. A low (or poor) ovarian response has been classified as the retrieval of three or fewer oocytes, and is associated with a higher probability of cycle cancellation, a reduced number of available embryos to transfer, and a lower probability of pregnancy and live birth. Conversely, a hyper (or high) response is often defined as the retrieval of more than 15 or 20 oocytes and is associated with an exponential increase in the risk of ovarian hyperstimulation syndrome (OHSS), and an increase in the risk of cycle cancellation. Severe OHSS is a rare but serious condition, with the potential to cause thromboembolic phenomena, multiple organ failure and death. Generally, production of between 5 and 15 oocytes is considered a normal response, and is correlated with the highest chance of pregnancy and live birth [1]. Therefore, the aim of most stimulation protocols is to produce a normal ovarian response.

The number of oocytes retrieved depends on both the ovarian reserve of the woman and the dose of FSH applied, however, individual women's responses vary. Ovarian reserve can be predicted by factors such as a women's age, and more recently by more sophisticated measures such as antral follicle count and anti-müllerian hormone (AMH). Research has demonstrated that AMH correlates with ovarian response to stimulation; women with lower AMH levels generally produce a fewer number of oocytes. It has also been demonstrated that, up to certain limits, increasing the dose of FSH increases the number of oocytes produced. It has therefore become common to tailor the FSH dose to each woman based on their predicted response, for example, increasing the dose in women expected to be low-responders (e.g. low AMH). As this discussion centres around the *maximal* effective dose, only anticipated low-responders are considered within scope (anticipated normal and high-responders are not discussed).

Evidence from Randomised Controlled Trials

As with all aspects of health care, wherever possible, we should look to evidence from randomised controlled trials to guide our clinical practice. A total of five trials are available in anticipated low-responders (women with low AMH or AFC counts), as summarised in a Cochrane review [2].

Two trials compared 300 and 450 IU to 150 IU. These higher doses of FSH resulted in higher oocyte yields, more women with a normal response, lower cancellation rates and more women with at least one embryo available to transfer. However, there was insufficient evidence to determine whether increasing FSH dose impacts on probability of pregnancy or live birth, as most studies were small and reported results had wide confidence intervals. However, in one study, a higher dose of 450 IU appeared to *reduce* the probability of pregnancy compared to 150 IU.

Three trials compared high doses against each other (e.g. 600 vs. 450 IU). At this end of the spectrum, comparing high doses to even higher doses, does not appear to impact on the probability of any outcomes, although confidence intervals are wide and consistent with moderate effects in either direction.

No case of OHSS was reported in any trial, which may be expected in a predicted low-responder cohort. Administering higher FSH doses is also associated with increased costs. In one trial, the cost of higher doses was associated with an average increased cost of €1099 per women [3]. It is based on this evidence that ESHRE guidelines do not recommend exceeding 300 IU [4].

Discussion and Interpretation

Among anticipated low-responders, FSH doses of 300 and 450 IU appeared to increase the probability of upstream outcomes but this did not appear to translate into effects on clinical outcomes, namely live birth and pregnancy. This could be due to several reasons. First, the included trials may not have been large enough to have sufficient statistical power to detect effects on clinical outcomes, which tend to be more difficult to detect than more common outcomes (having at least one embryo) or continuous outcomes (e.g. number of oocytes). Second, as these trials seldom measure cumulative pregnancy rates, it is not clear whether increasing FSH dose might lead to higher number of embryos which may be frozen, and ultimately lead to a higher pregnancy and live birth rate, per complete IVF cycle. Both of these points suggest that there is an unobserved but true effect from dosing more than 300 IU on the outcome of pregnancy and live birth. Indeed, it does not (necessarily) follow that any effect on ovarian response should translate to improvement in clinical outcomes. The observation that the optimal number of oocytes retrieved which lead to a higher probability of live birth [1], demonstrates only that the sort of women who tend to yield between 5 and 15 oocytes, have a higher probability of conception. It may be some prognostic factor about these women that gives them a higher probability of conceiving – rather than the oocyte yield per se. For example, if a woman has four oocytes collected in her first cycle, she will not necessarily stand a greater chance of live birth if she has an increased number of oocytes retrieved in her second cycle (which may or may not be achieved by increasing her FSH dose).

Lastly, it has been suggested that increased FSH dose, and the consequent increased oestrogen production in the ovaries, may have a detrimental impact on oocyte quality and endometrial receptivity, and therefore implantation. In one study, increasing doses of FSH led to increased oocyte yield but simultaneously reduced the fertilisation rate, resulting in fewer blastocysts per oocyte [5]. This reinforces the need for caution in using surrogate outcomes, such as number of oocytes, in place of clinically important outcomes, such as live birth.

Conclusion

Current evidence does not provide a clear justification for increasing FSH dose above 300 IU. Although higher doses may increase the number of oocytes retrieved and other upstream outcomes, there is no evidence that this translates to any impact on clinical outcomes, such as pregnancy live birth. This is especially so given that increasing FSH dose is associated with increased costs, which are often borne by the patient.

References

1   Sunkara SK, Rittenberg V, Raine-Fenning N, Bhattacharya S, Zamora J, Coomarasamy A. Association between the number of eggs and live birth in IVF treatment: an analysis of 400 135 treatment cycles. *Hum Reprod.* 2011;26:1768–74.

2. Lensen SF, Wilkinson J, Mol BWJ, La MA, Torrance H, Broekmans FJ. Individualised gonadotropin dose selection using markers of ovarian reserve for women undergoing IVF/ICSI. *Cochrane Database of Syst Rev.* 2018.

3. Van Tilborg TC, Torrance HL, Oudshoorn SC, et al. Individualized versus standard FSH dosing in women starting IVF/ICSI: an RCT. Part 1: the predicted poor responder. *Hum Reprod.* 2017;32 (12):2496–505.

4. ESHRE Reproductive Endocrinology Guideline Group. Ovarian stimulation for IVF/ICSI. Guideline of the European Society of Human Reproduction and Embryology. 2019.

5. Arce JC, Andersen AN, Fernandez-Sanchez M, et al. Ovarian response to recombinant human follicle-stimulating hormone: a randomized, antimullerian hormone-stratified, dose response trial in women undergoing in vitro fertilization/intracytoplasmic sperm injection. *Fertil Steril.* 2014;102(6):1633–40.

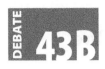

43B The Maximum Effective Dose of FSH for Ovarian Stimulation in IVF Is 300 IU

Against

Georgios Lainas

The first IVF child was the result of one oocyte, derived from a natural cycle IVF. Sir Robert Edwards suggested that natural cycle IVF is not an efficient therapy protocol for infertile couples.

The introduction of ovarian stimulation and LH suppression protocols have been of paramount importance, as they resulted in a higher number of oocytes retrieved and consequently an increase in pregnancy rates.

The dose regimen of gonadotropins administered during ovarian stimulation has been linked to the number of oocytes retrieved. However, the response of each individual to exogenous FSH varies. In the absence of data, the gonadotropin dose administered is based on experience, rather than on good comparative studies and therefore is characterised by high variability. In current clinical practice the dosage of gonadotropins administered ranges from 100 IU per day up to 600 IU or more.

Ovarian response has been established as the most important predictor of pregnancy outcome in an IVF cycle, along with female age. Several interventions have been proposed in order to increase oocyte yield, especially in the population of poor responders.

Is the Number of Oocytes Retrieved Associated with the Dose of Gonadotropin?

Up to a certain limit, an increase in the FSH dose may increase the number of growing follicles and the resulting oocyte yield. This is mainly of interest in poor responders. The majority of previously published RCTs in predicted poor responders, have shown that an increased gonadotrophin dose does not increase pregnancy rates.

Nonetheless, most of the previously published RCTs were underpowered to assess live birth and suffered methodological weaknesses [1].

Therefore, it is still unclear whether women with a predicted poor response who are undergoing IVF/ICSI, might benefit from a higher gonadotrophin dose.

In addition, in women with a predicted poor response (0–7 oocytes), a low dose of FSH (150 IU) was associated with a significantly higher risk of cancellation due to poor or unexpected poor response, when compared to higher gonadotropin dose (450 IU) [1].

Furthermore, the relative risks for cycle cancellation and live birth did not differ significantly when a 450 or 600 IU dose of recombinant FSH were compared to 300 IU. Most importantly, the higher dose is associated with a statistically significant higher number of oocytes retrieved [2].

It can be deduced that if increased FSH dosing has a positive effect on the number of oocytes retrieved, this could be translated into a higher number of embryos available for freezing.

Is the Number of Oocytes Associated with Cumulative Live Birth Rate?

The association of the number of oocytes retrieved with live birth rate in IVF/ICSI cycles is well-documented. Recent large-scale observational data, including transfer of fresh and frozen thawed embryos, demonstrated the linear increase of cumulative live birth rate with the number of oocytes derived from one stimulation cycle [3].

Considering the substantial progress in the cryopreservation techniques and the increasing use of embryo freezing, cumulative LBR is considered the most appropriate measure of success in IVF [4].

The large majority of the existing studies included in the recent meta-analysis on gonadotropin dose [2] do not account for the cumulative LBR and therefore, do not assess the potential benefit of the transfer of supernumerary frozen embryos. The recent guideline on ovarian stimulation which produced recommendations on the optimal gonadotropin dose are based on the same meta-analysis [2].

The results of the only study comparing different gonadotropin doses and reporting cumulative live birth rate as outcome should be interpreted with caution [5]. This is due to the extremely low Live birth rates reported after transfer of frozen thawed embryos, compared with fresh embryo-transfer (23.7% vs. 69.8), implying a potential issue of cryopreservation techniques.

Do Higher Gonadotrophin Doses Affect Oocyte or Embryo Quality?

Studies in animal models demonstrated a potential negative effect of high gonadotropin dose on oocyte quality and aneuploidy rate. However, research in humans has not detected the same effect [6].

Data from a large cohort suggested a linear increase in the number of blastocysts, euploid embryos and cumulative live birth rate with the number of oocytes retrieved [3].

Is Higher Gonadotropin Dose Associated with a Higher Cost?

A higher FSH dosing may be associated with greater cost in terms of price of FSH medication increasing the cost of ART treatment. On the other hand, if tailoring the dose of FSH is proven to be associated with an increase in ovarian response, an increase in cumulative live birth rate and a decrease in number of cancelled cycles, then this strategy could be proven more cost-effective.

Conclusion

There is evidence to suggest that higher gonadotropin dose might be associated with higher number of oocytes retrieved. The potential association of the higher number of oocytes and cumulative live birth rates, in particular in poor responders, needs to be further investigated in well-designed randomised trials. Nevertheless, the gonadotropin regimen should be administered with caution, taking into account patient safety and efficacy, until further evidence could justify the use of higher gonadotropin dose during ovarian stimulation in poor responders.

References

1. van Tilborg TC, Torrance HI, Oudshoorn SC, et al. Individualized versus standard FSH dosing in women starting IVF/ICSI: an RCT. Part 1: the predicted poor responder. *Hum Reprod.* 2017;32:2496–505.

2. Lensen SF, Wilkinson J, Leijdekkers JA, et al. Individualised gonadotropin dose selection using markers of ovarian reserve for women undergoing in vitro fertilisation plus intracytoplasmic sperm injection (IVF/ICSI). *Cochrane Database Syst Rev.* 2018;2:CD012693.

3. Polyzos NP, Drakopoulos P, Parra J, et al. Cumulative live birth rates according to the number of oocytes retrieved after the first ovarian stimulation for in vitro fertilization/intracytoplasmic sperm injection: a multicenter multinational analysis including approximately 15,000 women. *Fertil Steril.* 2018;110:661–70.e661.

4. Wong KM, van Wely M, Moi F, et al. Fresh versus frozen embryo transfers in assisted reproduction. *Cochrane Database Syst Rev.* 2017;3:CD011184.

5. Oudshoorn SC, van Tilborg TC, Eijkemans MJC, et al. Individualized versus standard FSH dosing in women starting IVF/ICSI: an RCT. Part 2: the predicted hyper responder. *Hum Reprod.* 2017;32:2506–14.

6. Labarta E, Bosch E, Alama P, et al. Moderate ovarian stimulation does not increase the incidence of human embryo chromosomal abnormalities in in vitro fertilization cycles. *J Clin Endocrinol Metab.* 2012;97:E1987–94.

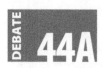

There Is No Place for Natural and Mild Stimulation IVF

For

Raj Mathur

Introduction

The first IVF baby was a result of IVF carried out in a natural cycle, but rapid advances in clinical pharmacology and medicine subsequently enabled the near-universal use of exogenous gonadotropin stimulation with control of the endogenous luteinising hormone (LH) surge. This greatly increases the number of eggs available for assisted conception, and the number of embryos from which a choice can be made for transfer. The net effect of this and other advances, evident in mandatory national databases such as that of the UK Human Fertilisation and Embryology Authority (HFEA), has been a steady increase in the likelihood of having a baby after a cycle of IVF, year-on-year since the start of data collection.

Like any medical treatment, ovarian stimulation is associated with side-effects, some widely recognised (such as ovarian hyperstimulation syndrome (OHSS) and impaired endometrial receptivity) and others largely theoretical (increased embryo aneuploidy rates). Understandable concern about these has led to persistent interest in 'natural' and 'mild' approaches to IVF. I shall consider below why these approaches have no significant place in modern practice.

One problem when assessing the evidence around these interventions is the lack of precise definition as to the meaning of 'mild' ovarian stimulation. 'Natural' IVF has been defined as IVF carried out with oocytes collected from a woman's ovaries in a spontaneous menstrual cycle without any medication. There is little doubt that carrying out 'natural' IVF requires precise monitoring, specific clinical expertise and great dedication from clinics and patients alike. Equally, there is little doubt that the likelihood of success with this treatment is very poor, with HFEA data revealing that no oocytes were collected in 44.2% and no embryos were available for transfer in 57.1% of natural IVF cycles in the UK over a 20-year period, yielding a live birth rate of 4.7% per cycle [1]. It is sometimes argued that the psychological burden of treatment with 'natural' IVF is lower than that with standard treatment, but the impact of repeated failure cannot be ignored. Clinicians must have strong reasons to offer a treatment that would fall under the category of 'very poor prognosis', defined by the ASRM Ethics Committee as 'treatment for which the odds of achieving a live birth are very low but not non-existent (1% to <5% per cycle).'

Despite attempts at standardisation, the definition of 'mild' IVF remains problematic. A representative definition from the literature is, 'The method when [follicle-stimulating hormone] (FSH) or [human menopausal gonadotrophin] (HMG) is administered at lower doses, and/or for a shorter duration in a [gonadotrophin-releasing hormone] (GnRH) antagonist co-treated cycle, or when oral compounds (anti-estrogens, or aromatase inhibitors) are used, either alone or in combination with gonadotrophins. [Human chorionic gonadotropin] (HCG) injection and luteal support are also administered. The aim is to collect between two and seven oocytes' [2]. There are inherent problems in defining a treatment through a comparison with an undefined standard (lower than what?) and the intent of treatment, rather than the treatment *per se*. I suspect that most modern practitioners use GnRH antagonist cycles with a 150 iu starting dose and achieve seven oocytes in a proportion of their patients. Are these physicians unknowingly practising mild IVF? I am reminded of Molière's hero who was surprised to learn that he had been 'speaking prose all his life'.

Definitions aside, the central point remains that 'mild' IVF by intentionally limiting the number of oocytes available, is not likely to improve the chance of having a baby. Analysis of large databases confirms that increasing numbers of eggs collected are associated with an increased likelihood of live birth per cycle, the outcome of greatest clinical and health economic importance. When one looks at cumulative live birth rates, the difference is even more obvious [3]. This is not to say that there are no problems with increasing egg numbers – the risk of ovarian hyperstimulation syndrome (OHSS) rises with egg numbers above 20 – but to make the simple point that if you choose to get fewer eggs from your patient you are likely harming her chance of having a baby.

Could there be specific patient groups where the mild approach has value? In women with a very high ovarian reserve and a concomitant high OHSS risk, modern standard regimes use GnRH antagonist, FSH dose no higher than 150 iu and agonist trigger. Elective freeze-all of embryos in this population is associated with excellent live birth rates, while minimising the risk of OHSS. There seems little reason to adopt a milder approach and reduce the cumulative live birth rate. In potential poor responders, mild ovarian stimulation provides fewer eggs and a higher cancellation rate [4]. Importantly, the incidence of aneuploid blastocyst embryos is not increased by exogenous gonadotropins [5].

It is self-evident that individuals and couples with subfertility seek assisted conception with the primary aim of having a healthy child. Hence, the first criterion in choosing fertility treatment has to be the likelihood of a live birth per unit of treatment or course of treatment. 'Natural' and 'mild' IVF are not as efficient as conventional IVF in achieving this outcome. If conventional IVF were shown to be associated with unacceptable or excessive risk, then a case could possibly be made for a role for these less effective alternatives. In the absence of such evidence, there is no role for 'natural' or 'mild' stimulation in modern reproductive medicine.

References

1. Sunkara SK, LaMarca A, Polyzos NP, et al. Live birth and perinatal outcomes following stimulated and unstimulated IVF: analysis of over two decades of a nationwide data. *Hum Reprod*. 2016;31 (10):2261–7.

2. Nargund G, Fauser BCJM, Macklon NS, et al. The ISMAAR proposal on terminology for ovarian stimulation for IVF. *Hum Reprod*. 2007;22(11):2801–4.

3. Polyzos NP, Drakopoulos P, Parra J, et al. Cumulative live birth rates according to the number of oocytes retrieved after the first ovarian stimulation for in vitro fertilization/intracytoplasmic sperm injection: a multicentre multinational analysis including 15,000 women. *Fert Steril*. 2018;4:662–9.

4. Van Tilborg TC, Torrance HL, Oudshoorn SC, et al. Individualized versus standard FSH dosing in women starting IVF/ICSI: an RCT. Part 1: The predicted poor responder. *Hum Reprod*. 2017;32 (12):2496–505.

5. Hong KH, Franasiak JM, Weiner MM, et al. Embryonic aneuploidy rates are equivalent in natural cycles and gonadotropin-stimulated cycles. *Fertil Steril*. 2019;112:670–6.

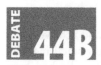

44B There Is No Place for Natural and Mild Stimulation IVF

Against

Ippokratis Sarris

In the age of personalised and precision medicine, the call for individualised treatment is now more apparent than ever before. The 'one size fits all' prescriptive approach to ovarian stimulation may well result in good outcomes for the majority of couples undergoing IVF, however, for certain cohorts of patients this method may result in suboptimal responses and therefore outcomes.

This debate must begin by clarifying the disparities in the definition of natural and mild stimulation. In 2007, the Rotterdam-based International Society for Mild Approaches in Assisted Reproduction (ISMAAR) Group convened to agree on a consensus on terminology for ovarian stimulation (OS) for IVF [1]. The group proposed a concise and simplified revised nomenclature for different approaches to OS for IVF. A natural cycle for IVF was defined as IVF carried out during a spontaneous menstrual cycle without gonadotropin support, aiming to collect the naturally selected single oocyte of the cycle. Mild ovarian stimulation (mOS) incorporates the use of follicle stimulating hormone (FSH) or human menopausal gonadotropin (HMG) administered at lower doses and/or for a shorter duration in a GnRH antagonist co-treated cycle **or** when oral compounds (anti-estrogens, or aromatase inhibitors) are used, either alone or in combination with gonadotropins. The intention of mild stimulation is the collection of 2–7 oocytes.

For clinicians, optimal IVF entails establishing the balance between achieving optimal ovarian stimulation with the best treatment outcomes whilst minimising complications, namely severe ovarian hyperstimulation syndrome (OHSS) and/or multiple pregnancies. For patients, however, what constitutes the best treatment outcomes may vary significantly. One couple may be attracted to the 'one and done' approach to IVF, generating all the embryos they may ever require for their desired family number within one cycle of oocyte stimulation and retrieval, whereas another couple may only be comfortable with the idea of creating one potential embryo at a time for a multitude of reasons (which may include ethical or religious beliefs).

Therefore, understanding the wishes of a couple is paramount prior to planning a cycle and natural or mild stimulation is a useful tool to have available in order to achieve this, as it may often be the best way to align with a couple's needs.

Typically, there are a number of factors that one would use to define IVF success. The remainder of this debate will focus on why natural or mild stimulation may well represent the strategy to achieve these successes for certain cases.

Safety – Primum Non Nocere

Regardless of one's desire to achieve the wishes of our patients, namely a healthy live birth, if this is at the expense of a patient's health, then arguably one cannot conclude that the treatment was a success. In this current age of ART, where the objective is to become an OHSS free clinic, natural or mild stimulation surely has a place in our practice. In addition, achieving a singleton term healthy birth whilst also minimising maternal complications should be the goal, first and foremost.

SART database analysis of more than 256,000 cycles have demonstrated that the retrieval of more than 15 eggs increases the risk of OHSS, without further improving live birth rate in fresh transfers [2].

HFEA data obtained from cycles performed between 1991 and 2008, also linked excessive ovarian response with higher obstetric complications [3]. Pregnancies resulting from cycles where more than 15 eggs were collected, were shown to have higher rates of pre-term birth as well as low birth weight, compared to pregnancies where only 4–15 oocytes were retrieved. The complex origin of implantation and placentation may well therefore be detrimentally impacted by excessive ovarian stimulation and should not be underestimated when planning fresh treatment cycles.

Proponents of conventional ovarian stimulation will argue that replacing hCG with GnRH agonist triggers in antagonist cycles and adopting a freeze all policy will eliminate the morbidity associated with OHSS. However, there are still cases reported where, despite this strategy having been employed, women still experience severe OHSS. Furthermore, there may well be yet undiscovered epigenetic sequelae of aggressive stimulation of oocytes on quality and function, as well as long term patient health.

There is also a subgroup of patients who may not mount the necessary response to an agonist trigger, resulting in suboptimal numbers, maturation and quality of oocytes retrieved. Women previously taking long-term hormonal contraception, younger women with low BMIs at risk of potential hypothalamic hypogonadism and those with very low endogenous serum LH levels on the day of LH trigger are at increased risk for a suboptimal GnRH-agonist trigger response.

Freeze-all strategy often goes against the wishes of the patient who may prefer a fresh transfer. Additionally, the 'time to live birth' and cost implications of such a strategy, forced upon by avoidable iatrogenic aggressive stimulation, has not been properly evaluated.

Mandating a freeze-all strategy due to excessive ovarian stimulation may exacerbate the findings of increased risk of large for gestational age babies as well as hypertensive disorders of pregnancy seen with frozen embryo transfer cycles. Emerging data has highlighted the absence of the corpus luteum resulting from medicated HRT cycles being implicated in a higher risk of pre-eclampsia.

Other challenges associated with overstimulated ovaries, and typically not seen in mild stimulation cycles, include a greater risk of bleeding during oocyte retrieval, longer operative times requiring greater sedation, pain as well as the risk of ovarian torsion.

Oocyte/Embryo Quality – mOS vs. cOS

Initial studies pointed to the possibility that more aggressive ovarian stimulation might lead to a larger number of abnormal oocytes.

An often quoted study by Baart et al. (2007) [4], compared mild (mOS) versus conventional (cOS) ovarian stimulation in the context of the number of chromosomally normal embryos generated from the cycle. Although mOS produced a significantly lower number of oocytes and therefore embryos, both regimens appeared to result in a similar number of chromosomally normal embryos. The group concluded that increasingly higher gonado-trophin dosages resulted in an increased rate of meiotic segregation errors and therefore aneuploid embryos. Embryos, however, were biopsied and diagnosed by the older method of fluorescent in-situ hybridisation (FISH).

It is true to say, however, that subsequent data challenge this finding. The latest meta-analysis looking at 28 studies reporting data on 291,752 cycles found no reliable evidence to suggest that more aggressive ovarian stimulation increases aneuploidy rates in embryos to a significant degree [5].

Pregnancy and Live Birth Outcomes

There have not been many studies that have examined pregnancy or live birth rates in mOS vs. cOS. Due to the high levels of heterogeneity within these studies in terms of inclusion criteria, numbers of oocytes/embryos transferred as well as day of transfer, it is difficult to pool the data in meta-analyses or systematic reviews.

It is becoming increasingly clear from the data that higher numbers of oocytes result in a higher chance of cumulative live birth. A European multi-centre study in 2018 retrospectively evaluated the impact of ovarian response on cumulative live birth rates, and found that cumulative rates continued to improve with increasing egg numbers, reaching 70% when more than 25 eggs were retrieved [6].

SART data collected from 2014 to 2015, and published in 2019 showed that odds of clinical pregnancy in the first fresh IVF cycle were 8% higher for each additional fertilised oocyte collected up to nine, and then declined by 9% for every additional fertilised oocyte thereafter [7].

However, one has to also consider the cohort of patients who no matter how much gonadotrophin is administered, the response remains either expectedly low or unexpectedly low on several occasions. Data has shown that for poor responders, natural, natural modified and mild stimulation cycles are associated with a similar pregnancy rate, and possibly a higher livebirth rate [8], when compared to conventional high dose ovarian stimulation [9].

Indeed, administering high dose stimulation in an attempt to generate the maximal number of oocytes in patients who may already have high levels of resting FSH, could exacerbate the asynchrony of follicular growth rate and endometrial proliferation, potentially affecting the crucial window of implantation in a fresh IVF cycle.

This has led to the ARSM guidance from 2018 stating that, 'In patients who are classified as poor responders and pursuing IVF, strong consideration should be given to a mild ovarian-stimulation protocol (low-dose gonadotropins with or without oral agents) due to lower costs and comparable low pregnancy rates compared with traditional IVF stimulation protocols' [9].

Patient Views

From a patient's perspective, mild stimulation may be perceived as being more patient friendly. Patients respond positively to the idea of having to take less amounts of drugs for a shorter period of time, trying to keep the intervention as natural as possible, whilst still achieving the desired outcome.

As medical practitioners, we must respect the ethical views and religious beliefs of our patients. Many will not want to create surplus embryos which will be ultimately either discarded or stored away, cryopreserved in time, never to be used. We should not under-estimate the psychological distress some couples feel about having to decide what to do with surplus viable embryos once their family is complete.

Cost

Although the cost-effectiveness of mild stimulation versus conventional stimulation can be debated, perhaps in low resource countries low-cost IVF coupled with mild stimulation protocols to keep the drug cost down may provide an opportunity to couples who otherwise may not be afforded the chance to have treatment.

One could also argue that especially for those women with very low ovarian reserve, high stimulation has no place as it currently has not been shown to offer an added benefit and only increases the cost.

Conclusion

During the evolution of IVF, inefficiencies of in-vitro culture systems were overcome by the generation and transfer of excess embryos to result in a gradual increase in treatment success outcome. As we see continual improvements in lab technology, the drive towards elective single embryo transfer demonstrates that less is sometimes enough. If we take this adage one step further, reducing treatment burden by milder forms of ovarian stimulation without compromising success rates should be the objective that we should all be working towards.

The question is not if natural and mild stimulation IVF protocols are better than conventional, but if there is no place for these at all. There is no doubt that in many patient groups conventional stimulation will be the preferred choice, as for them the greater the number of oocytes retrieved the better the potential cumulative pregnancy outcome may be. However, this is not precision medicine and we should not treat all of our patients the same. We must acknowledge that mild ovarian stimulation does still have a place at our clinics and should form part of our available protocols when considering treatment options for our patients. Dismissing these protocols from the armoury of our medical practice is a mistake, as it is clear that for some (albeit not all) these strategies are suitable and perhaps even preferable. Therefore, the statement that 'There is no place for natural and mild stimulation IVF' is simply wrong.

References

1. Nargund G, Fauser BCJM, Macklon NS, et al. The ISMAAR proposal on terminology for ovarian stimulation for IVF. *Hum Reprod.* 2007;22:2801–4.

2. Yeh JS, Steward RG, Dude AM, et al. Pregnancy rates in donor oocyte cycles compared to similar autologous in vitro fertilization cycles: an analysis of 26,457 fresh cycles from the Society for Assisted Reproductive Technology. *Fertil Steril.* 2014;101:967–73.

3. Sunkara S, La Marca A, Seed PT, et al. Increased risk of preterm birth and low birthweight with very high number of oocytes following IVF: an analysis of 65,868 singleton live birth outcomes. *Hum Reprod.* 2015;30(6):1473–80.

4. Baart EB, Martini E, Eijkemans MJ, et al. Milder ovarian stimulation for in-vitro fertilization reduces aneuploidy in the human preimplantation embryo: a randomized controlled trial. *Hum Reprod.* 2007;22:980–8.

5. Vermey BG, Chua SJ, Zafarmand MH, et al. Is there an association between oocyte number and embryo quality? A systematic review and meta-analysis. *RBMO*. 2019;39:751–63.

6. Polyzos NP, Drakopoulos P, Parra J, et al. Cumulative live birth rates according to the number of oocytes retrieved after the first ovarian stimulation for in vitro fertilization/intracytoplasmic sperm injection: a multicenter multinational analysis including ~15,000 women. *Fertil Steril*. 2018;110:661–70.

7. Smeltzer S, Acharya K, Truong T, et al. Clinical pregnancy (CP) and live birth (LB) increase significantly with each additional fertilized oocyte up to 9 and CP and LB declines after that: an analysis of 15,803 first fresh in vitro fertilization (IVF) cycles from the SART registry. *Fertil Steril*. 2019;112:520–6.

8. Lainas TG, Sfontouris IA, Venetis CA, et al. Live birth rates after modified natural cycle compared with high-dose FSH stimulation using GnRH antagonists in poor responders *Human Reprod*. 2015;30:2321–30.

9. Practice Committee of the American Society for Reproductive Medicine. Comparison of pregnancy rates for poor responders using IVF with mild ovarian stimulation versus conventional IVF: a guideline. *Fertil Steril*. 2018;109(6):993–9.

DEBATE 45A

Metformin Is an Effective Treatment for Infertility Associated with Anovulatory PCOS

For

Stefano Palomba

One of the most interesting debates of the reproductive medicine regards the use of metformin as a fertility drug for women with polycystic ovary syndrome (PCOS). Metformin is a drug widely recommended in the clinical practice for the treatment of women with PCOS for its heterogeneous effects on metabolism with particular regard for preventing/treating the complications associated to insulin-resistance. The mechanism of action is partially unclear, even if it is known that metformin reduces gastrointestinal absorption of glucose uptake, inhibits hepatic glucose production, and increases tissue insulin-stimulated glucose uptake. The popularity of metformin is due to a good safety profile and low costs. Metformin is related to an increased risk of gastrointestinal side-effects; however, their absolute incidence is low particularly using the slow-release formulations, and severe complications are anecdotal in young women without renal disease. Notwithstanding few pharmacoeconomic studies have assessed the costs of different treatments for inducing ovulation in women with PCOS, the treatment with metformin is very cheap especially when compared with gonadotropins, letrozole and laparoscopic ovarian drilling (LOD).

A recent meta-analysis of 41 randomised controlled trials (RCTs) comparing metformin to placebo, no treatment, or combination with or compared with clomiphene citrate (CC), letrozole and LOD as strategy for treating subfertility in women with PCOS concluded that metformin improves up to 2.5-fold the pregnancy/live birth rates in comparison with placebo or no treatment, and up to 10% and 200%, respectively, the live birth and pregnancy rates in women who receive CC [1]. The beneficial effect of metformin on fertility seems to be modulated positively by baseline insulin levels [2].

The efficacy of metformin as first-line treatment for anovulatory infertility in women with PCOS is still debated. When metformin is compared to CC, the efficacy of one drug over the other is discriminated by obesity. In fact, metformin is more effective than CC in non-obese patients but less effective in the presence of obesity [1]. In particular, in non-obese women with PCOS the treatment with CC is associated with a live birth rate of 26%, which may increase from 26% to 50% using metformin [1]. Moreover, recent data suggest to consider letrozole as gold standard therapy for ovulation induction in women with PCOS in consideration of the increased likelihood of live birth of 40–60% (vs. CC) and of the reduced side-effects (including multiple pregnancies) [2]. Thus, new interesting unsolved questions should regard the efficacy of metformin in comparison with letrozole as first-line treatment, the efficacy of metformin plus CC and of metformin plus letrozole associations vs. letrozole in naïve-therapy patients and as second-line treatments. At the moment, the little evidence available demonstrate that there is no difference in live birth rates between metformin and metformin plus letrozole [3] and that letrozole is probably more effective than metformin plus CC combination in terms of ovulations and clinical pregnancies [4].

Of limited clinical relevance are the findings showing no difference between metformin and LOD or metformin plus LOD in women with PCOS. On the other hand, metformin improves the live-birth and pregnancy rate of about two-fold reducing the risk of hyperstimulation and of cycle cancellation when given in patients who receive gonadotropins for ovulation induction [5]. When metformin is administrated in patients with PCOS scheduled for multiple ovulation induction with gonadotropins for in vitro fertilisation (IVF) or intracytosplamic sperm injection (ICSI) cycles, the risk of ovarian hyperstimulation syndrome (OHSS) reduces by 80% and the miscarriage rate improves by about 50%.

In conclusion, the use of metformin should be suggested in all anovulatory women with PCOS before a specific infertility work-up in order to restore the normal menstrual cycle, especially in case of glucose intolerance and/or obesity. This strategy is safe, cheap and effective. The insulin sensitising drug should be not stopped during the administration of other drugs for the potential beneficial metabolic and obstetric effects when given before pregnancy. In the case of diagnosed anovulatory infertility, CC is probably more effective in terms of time-to-pregnancy and, thus, it should be added for no more six cycles, as many international guidelines recommend. In patients under metformin who are candidates for letrozole, the insulin sensitising drug did not reduce the efficacy of the aromatase inhibitor. Finally, the use of metformin should be considered in patients with PCOS with high risk of hyper-response to gonadotropins who are undergoing controlled ovarian stimulation because it may reduce the incidence of hyper-response, cancellation and OHSS rate.

References

1. Sharpe A, Morley LC, Tang T, Norman RJ, Balen AH. Metformin for ovulation induction (excluding gonadotrophins) in women with polycystic ovary syndrome. *Cochrane Database Syst Rev.* 2019;12: CD013505.

2. Wang R, Li W, Bordewijk EM, et al. Reproductive Medicine Network; International Ovulation Induction IPDMA Collaboration. First-line ovulation induction for polycystic ovary syndrome: an individual participant data meta-analysis. *Hum Reprod Update.* 2019;25 (6):717–32.

3. Liu C, Feng G, Huang W, et al. Comparison of clomiphene citrate and letrozole for ovulation induction in women with polycystic ovary syndrome: a prospective randomized trial. *Gynecol Endocrinol.* 2017;33(11):872–6.

4. Rezk M, Shaheen AE, Saif El-Nasr I. Clomiphene citrate combined with metformin versus letrozole for induction of ovulation in clomiphene-resistant polycystic ovary syndrome: a randomized clinical trial. *Gynecol. Endocrinol.* 2018;34 (4):298–300.

5. Palomba S, Falbo A, La Sala GB. Metformin and gonadotropins for ovulation induction in patients with polycystic ovary syndrome: a systematic review with meta-analysis of randomized controlled trials. *Reprod Biol Endocrinol.* 2014;12:3.

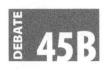

Metformin Is an Effective Treatment for Infertility Associated with Anovulatory PCOS

Against

Arnold M Mahesan

The role of metformin in polycystic ovary syndrome (PCOS) is a subject that has been oft debated over the years. Metformin was initially conceived as having potential utility in PCOS due to its role as an insulin sensitiser. Since it was unknown to what extent hyperinsulinaemia influences the pathogenesis of the ovulatory disorder in PCOS, it was reasonable to assess any role of metformin. Early studies were encouraging, but it has since become clear that metformin alone is not an effective treatment for infertility associated with anovulatory PCOS.

Insulin resistance is known to be a common feature in PCOS, independent of obesity. Metformin lowers blood glucose in hyperglycaemic individuals but has no effect on glucose levels in normal subjects. It has no effect on weight gain and may be associated with modest weight loss. It has an unclear mechanism of action but does reduce absorption of glucose from the GI tract, inhibits hepatic gluconeogenesis and increases insulin sensitivity in the periphery. In PCOS women, metformin has also been shown to improve menstrual regularity, to contribute to a reduction in circulating androgens, and potentially to contribute to weight loss. Notably, many studies that used metformin to treat women with PCOS did not establish whether insulin resistance was present and this heterogeneity has made it difficult to assess the benefit of metformin in different subgroups.

Many studies show an increased ovulation rate with metformin alone compared with placebo, but metformin alone should not be used as first line because oral ovulation induction agents like clomiphene citrate (CC) and letrozole are much more effective at increasing ovulation rates, and pregnancy and live birth rates, in women with PCOS [1].

Studies are conflicting on whether pregnancy rate is improved with metformin alone compared with placebo, though a meta-analysis did suggest improvement in clinical pregnancy rate [2]. However, a large randomised controlled trial showed higher ovulation and live birth for CC or combination CC and metformin compared with metformin alone. The difference in pregnancy rates between the CC and combination CC and metformin arms was not significant. Of note, this population was obese (BMI > 34, androgenised (>75% clinically hirsute) and insulin resistant (mean HOMA-IR > 5) [3].

A meta-analysis on CC vs. metformin of 14 trials pooled four studies to demonstrate metformin had a lower live birth rate than CC. When stratified by weight, studies conflict on the superiority of CC to metformin. However, at higher BMIs >30, metformin alone was clearly associated with lower live birth than CC alone [4].

When comparing the combination of metformin + CC for ovulation induction, it is clearly superior to metformin alone for all relevant outcomes including ovulation, clinical pregnancy rate, and live birth rate. However, metformin in combination with CC for ovulation induction has shown limited evidence for an increase in live birth rates compared with CC alone.

Metformin may play a role as an adjunct in CC resistance. CC resistance, which has been defined as failure to conceive after six cycles of CC 150 mg/day, failure of 'follicular development' after two cycles of CC 150 mg/day, absence of 'ovarian response' after three cycles of CC 150 mg/day, failure to ovulate or conceive after at least three consecutive cycles of CC 150 mg/day, and failure to ovulate in response to a 5-day course of CC 150 mg/day with no minimum number of cycles mentioned. The literature clearly demonstrates a statistically significantly increased rate of ovulation and/or pregnancy rate with addition of metformin with CC compared with CC alone.

However, metformin in conjunction with gonadotropins does not improve ovulation or pregnancy rates. Further, in IVF cycles, adjuvant treatment with metformin does not improve pregnancy or live birth rates, but it appears to decrease risk of OHSS.

Regarding the postulate that metformin may help decrease miscarriage risk in PCOS, pre-pregnancy use of metformin in decreasing miscarriage risk in non-ART pregnancies has no difference in outcomes. No increase in rate of miscarriage was observed when metformin was stopped at initiation of pregnancy [1].

Metformin alone is not an effective treatment for anovulatory PCOS. Other ovulatory agents such as CC have been shown to be superior. Metformin as an adjunct may have benefit in CC resistance but not in gonadotropin cycles of IVF. Notably, good data does not exist for letrozole compared against metformin, but letrozole compared with CC in PCOS shows letrozole is superior and should be the medication of choice [5].

References

1. Penzias A, Bendikson K, Butts S, et al. Role of metformin for ovulation induction in infertile patients with polycystic ovary syndrome (PCOS): a guideline. *Fertil Steril.* 2017;108(3):426–41.

2. Tang T, Lord JM, Norman RJ, Yasmin E, Balen AH. Insulin-sensitising drugs (metformin, rosiglitazone, pioglitazone, D-chiro-inositol) for women with polycystic ovary syndrome, oligo amenorrhoea and subfertility. *Cochrane Database Syst Rev.* 2012.

3. Legro RS, Barnhart HX, Schlaff WD, et al. Clomiphene, metformin, or both for infertility in the polycystic ovary syndrome. *N Engl J Med.* 2007;356(6):551–66.

4. Siebert TI, Viola MI, Steyn DW, Kruger TF. Is metformin indicated as primary ovulation induction agent in women with PCOS? A systematic review and meta-analysis. *Gynecol Obstet Invest.* 2012;73 (4):304–13.

5. Legro RS, Brzyski RG, Diamond MP, et al. Letrozole versus clomiphene for infertility in the polycystic ovary syndrome. *N Engl J Med.* 2014;371(2):119–29.

46A Laparoscopic Ovarian Drilling Should Be Performed for CC-Resistant PCOS

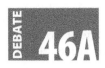

For

Ellen Greenblatt

'To an REI nothing looks like a scalpel.'

Polycystic ovarian syndrome (PCOS) is prevalent, with an incidence of 5–13% depending on ethnic background. A common clinical presentations of PCOS is infertility secondary to ovulatory dysfunction. Initially, treatment of infertility in PCOS women was surgical, specifically laparotomy and ovarian wedge resection (OWR). Although highly successful in inducing regular ovulatory cycles, OWR fell into disfavour due to the complications of ovarian damage and pelvic adhesions coupled with the development of clomiphene citrate (CC), which led to the transition from surgery to medical treatment.

First line management of anovulation/oligo-ovulation in infertile women with PCOS is lifestyle modification and medical therapy with oral agents to induce ovulation. These include selective oestrogen receptor modulators (CC and tamoxifen) and more recently aromatase inhibitors (i.e. letrozole). However approximately 20% of PCOS women are resistant to oral ovulation induction and management becomes more complicated. Second line therapies include combinations of oral agents (CC and tamoxifen, CC and metformin) gonadotropins, laparoscopic ovarian drilling (LOD) or in vitro fertilisation (IVF). A recently published multidisciplinary, international guideline for the diagnosis and management of PCOS, including the management of infertility, confirms letrozole as the initial approach [1].

Following the growth of IVF in the 1980s and 1990s and its application to all forms of infertility, coupled with an increase in expertise with gonadotropins for ovulation induction and controlled ovarian stimulation (COS), many Reproductive endocrinology and infertility clinicians (REIs) no longer perform fertility enhancing surgery. This has led to infrequent consideration of LOD for women with PCOS who are resistant to oral agents. However just because an REI clinician does not perform surgery, does not mean that surgery is not an option.

In this essay I will argue FOR the consideration of LOD in women with PCOS who are resistant to CC ovulation induction.

Laparoscopic ovarian drilling, initially termed laparoscopic ovarian electrocautery, was first described in 1984 by Gjönnaess as a minimally invasive surgery, similar to OWR but with fewer complications, for CC resistant infertile women with PCOS [2]. Although the mechanism of action remains uncertain, it has been suggested that similar to OWR, destruction of ovarian stromal leads to a decreased ovarian androgen production, manifested as a decline in serum androgens and normalisation of LH and FSH concentrations noted in women who successfully ovulate after LOD. Since Gjonnaess' publication [2], many papers have examined ovulation rates, pregnancy rates, live birth rates, complications and cost-effectiveness as well as selection of candidates most likely to benefit from LOD.

Approximately 40–80% of CC resistant PCOS women will ovulate after LOD, either spontaneously or with the reintroduction of previously unsuccessful oral agents, 20–50% will conceive within 6–12 months and 30% will not respond to LOD.

Two recent Cochrane meta-analyses comparing second line medical therapies to LOD in infertile women with CC resistant PCOS have recently been published [3, 4].

Farquhar et al. [3] reviewed 25 randomised clinical trials (RCT) comparing LOD to other forms of medical management in CC resistant PCOS women. Primary outcomes were live birth rate and incidence of multiple pregnancy. The proportion of live births following LOD ranged from 24% to 44% versus 27% to 62% with other medical therapies, with overlapping confidence intervals (CI). However multiple pregnancies (MPR), mainly in studies comparing LOD to gonadotropin therapy, did differ with a higher MPR in cycles using gonadotropins. They also found that the cost of therapy was higher in gonadotropin cycles, cost-effectiveness may depend on what treatments are publicly funded versus private pay in a particular jurisdiction. They concluded that there is no difference between laparoscopic ovarian drilling (with or without medical ovulation induction) compared to ovulation induction with gonadotrophins for women with polycystic ovarian syndrome and CC resistance for the outcomes of pregnancy and ovulation after 12 months follow-up. Multiple pregnancy rates are reduced with ovarian drilling compared with other medical treatments [3].

Similarly, Bordewijk et al.'s Cochrane review of 38 RTC, came to the same conclusion. Although they found a possibly slightly lower LBR with LOD compared to medical therapy (42% LBR with medical therapy versus 28–40% with LOD), many studies were of poor quality and when considering only high quality RCTs, there was uncertainty about any difference between treatments. They did find that LOD was associated with a reduction in multiple pregnancies compared with gonadotropin therapy [4].

It is clear that there are several options for treating anovulatory infertility in women with PCOS who do not respond to CC or other first line oral ovulation induction. Although most REI MDs may feel more comfortable using and offering gonadotropins or even IVF (particularly if other subfertility factors exist), both of these treatments are costly, complicated and require extensive monitoring at a tertiary fertility centre. Inherent in these treatments are the risk of cycle cancellation due to excessive response (gonadotropins for ovulation induction) and ovarian hyperstimulation syndrome in COS for IVF. For women who live remote from such a clinic, or who do not have benefits that support these treatments or medications, and who live in a jurisdiction where surgery is covered through a public health system, LOD, in well-selected individuals, should not be dismissed. LOD may initiate ovulatory cycles and allow for conception without ongoing medical intervention or intensive monitoring. Furthermore, many studies have demonstrated ongoing ovulation after both OWR and LOD which may allow more than one successful pregnancy.

Of course, surgery should never be embarked upon without appropriate informed consent related to risks of anaesthesia and laparoscopy, including bleeding, infection, trauma, adhesions and lack of response in 30%. Although similar to any pelvic surgery, postoperative adhesions are a possible complication of LOD that require disclosure. Although second look laparoscopies performed after LOD have demonstrated adhesions in 35–100%, pregnancy rates parallel restoration of ovulatory cycles and not adhesion scores. Although concerns have been raised regarding the potential negative impact on ovarian reserve after LOD, this has not been confirmed.

In summary, LOD should be discussed, along with other second line treatment options, in women with PCOS who fail to ovulate with CC and/or other first line oral agents. For fertility clinicians who do not perform surgery, identifying and partnering with a minimally invasive surgeon who can offer this expertise, is advised.

References

1. Teede HJ, Misso ML, Costello MF, et al. International PCOS Network Recommendations from the international evidence-based guideline for the assessment and management of polycystic ovary syndrome *Hum Reprod.* 2018;33 (9):1602–18.

2. Gjönnaess H. Polycystic ovarian syndrome treated by ovarian electrocautery through the laparoscope. *Fertil Steril.* 1984;41:20–5.

3. Farquhar C, Brown J, Marjoribanks J. Laparoscopic drilling by diathermy or laser for ovulation induction in anovulatory polycystic ovary syndrome. *Cochrane Database Syst Rev.* 2012;23:CD001122.

4. Bordewijk EM, Ng KYB, Rakic L, et al. Laparoscopic ovarian drilling for ovulation induction in women with anovulatory polycystic ovary syndrome. *Cochrane Database Syst Rev.* 2020, 2. Art. No.: CD001122.

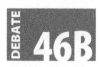

Laparoscopic Ovarian Drilling Should Be Performed for CC-Resistant PCOS

Against

Madelon van Wely

In the past clomiphene citrate (CC) used to be the preferred first-line treatment for ovulation induction in women with PCOS. Most guidelines nowadays advise using letrozole as it is more effective and seems to result in fewer multiple pregnancies, but as letrozole is off-label for this indication, CC is still commonly used as first-line treatment. Approximately 20% of the women who do not ovulate on CC are called CC-resistant. These women can undergo ovulation induction with letrozole, gonadotrophins or laparoscopic drilling before moving on to IVF.

Laparoscopic ovarian drilling is suggested as optional treatment in CC-resistant women with PCOS in all guidelines. The most recent International PCOS network guideline [1] state: 'There is no convincing evidence of inferiority of laparoscopic drilling over other common ovulation induction agents, there is no need for monitoring (because of mono-ovulation) and only a background risk of multiple pregnancy.' Whether an invasive procedure should be chosen above a less invasive and possibly more effective treatment is debated here. I will shortly describe the history of the procedure, the evidence on its effectiveness and safety and argue why LOD should not be considered a first-choice procedure in CC-resistant PCOS.

A Short History

Bilateral ovarian wedge resection by laparotomy, a procedure introduced by Stein and Leventhal in 1935, was the first effective treatment to restore ovulation in anovulatory women with polycystic ovary syndrome (PCOS). This procedure was abandoned due to an unacceptably high incidence of adhesion formation after the wedge resection when clomiphene citrate became available. In the 1980s new and less invasive ovarian drilling techniques were developed: laparoscopic laser surgery and laparoscopic electrocautery of the ovaries. Laparoscopic laser surgery has a shorter operating time and a diminished risk of adhesions, but the laser systems are expensive and require extensive and costly upkeep. In laparoscopic electrocautery the ovarian surface is cauterised with an electrode to create between three to eight holes in each ovary laparoscopic electrocautery of the ovaries. This ovarian drilling procedure is the most commonly used surgical treatment in patients with clomiphene citrate resistant polycystic ovary syndrome.

The mechanism of action of LOD is thought to be similar to that of ovarian wedge resection. By destroying a part of the ovarian tissue, less androgen and, consequently less oestrogen will be produced. The endocrine changes following the surgery are thought to restore the hormonal environment such that normal follicular development can occur. Furthermore some CC-resistant women will become sensitive to ovulation induction with CC after LOD. Consequently LOD is often followed up by ovulation induction with CC in case LOD did not result in ovulation.

The main complication of ovarian drilling is postoperative adhesion formation, although the incidence of severe adhesions appears to be low. Pelvic adhesions can result in fertility problems, abdominal pain and dyspareunia. There are also the associated risks and morbidity of laparoscopy under general anaesthesia, especially in obese women [2]. This is relevant as obesity is strongly associated with PCOS; depending on the geographic region the prevalence of obesity in women with PCOS ranges from 20 to 80%.

Evidence on Effectiveness and Safety

The Cochrane review on LOD with or without medical ovulation induction in women with CC-resistant PCOS has just been updated [3]. This updated review included 38 trials and 3326 women in the meta-analyses. The review found LOD may decrease live birth when compared with medical ovulation induction alone (odds ratio (OR) 0.71, 95% confidence interval (CI) 0.54–0.92; nine studies, 1015 women; I^2 = 0%; low-quality evidence). Overall the absolute risk difference of a live birth was 7% (95% CI –13 to –2) lower for LOD. The largest difference was found when LOD was compared to letrozole where LOD decreased the absolute risk of a live birth by 12% (95% CI –22 to –2). Restricting to RCTs that followed women for six months after LOD and six cycles of ovulation induction only, the results were found to be consistent with the main analysis. It was also observed that LOD probably reduces multiple pregnancy rates (Peto OR 0.34, 95% CI 0.18–0.66; 14 studies, 1161 women; I^2 = 2%; moderate-quality evidence). LOD decreased the absolute risk of multiple pregnancy by 3% (95% CI 1–6).

Economic studies suggest use of LOD before further medical treatment is cost-effective when compared to direct ovulation induction with gonadotrophins [3].

The incidence of de-novo adhesion formation at second look laparoscopy might occur in up to 50% of laparoscopic surgery cases but the clinical implications are unclear. Use of barrier agents might reduce the incidence of adhesions [4]. Long-term follow-up studies of women that had undergone LOD did not suggest morbidity.

Conclusion

LOD, with or without subsequent ovulation induction with CC, can restore ovulation in CC-resistant women with PCOS. This way LOD can partially prevent treatment with gonadotrophins and IVF and is consequently seen as less costly. LOD followed by CC however appears to be less effective in term of a live birth than gonadotrophins. LOD is particularly less effective when compared to letrozole. In view of the low cost of letrozole LOD can never be cost-effective. When we also consider the risks of the surgical procedure, particularly in view of the high obesity prevalence in these women, LOD should not be considered a first-choice procedure in CC-resistant PCOS.

References

1. Teede HJ, Misso ML, Costello MF, et al. Recommendations from the international evidence-based guideline for the assessment and management of polycystic ovary syndrome. *Hum Reprod.* 2018 Sept 1;33(9):1602–18.

2. Pouwels S, Buise MP, Twardowski P, Stepaniak PS, Proczko M. Obesity surgery and anesthesiology risks: a review of key concepts and related physiology. *Obes Surg.* 2019 Aug;29(8):2670–7.

3. Bordewijk EM, Ng KYB, Rakic L, et al. Laparoscopic ovarian drilling for ovulation induction in women with anovulatory polycystic ovary syndrome. *Cochrane Database Syst Rev.* 2020; 2, Art. No.: CD001122.

4. Ahmad G, Kim K, Thompson M, et al. Barrier agents for adhesion prevention after gynaecological surgery. *Cochrane Database Syst Rev.* 2015;4.

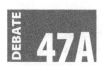

Asymptomatic Polycystic Ultrasound Appearance of the Ovary Is Favourable for IVF Outcome

For

Julio Ricardo Loret de Mola

The prevalence of polycystic ovary (PCO) morphological ultrasonographic criteria currently established by the 2003 Rotterdam Consensus Conference has been estimated as high as 33% in asymptomatic patients, and due to its lack of specificity, 21–63% of apparently normal women will meet this criterion as well. Consequently, the prevalence of 'ultrasound only PCO' (UPCO) patients in an IVF centre with infertility is approximately between 18–25%, representing a fairly large portion of couples treated with assisted reproductive technologies (ART). Recent advances in ultrasound technology have allowed such accurate identification of small antral follicles that this may have contributed to an artificial increase in the prevalence of polycystic ovary syndrome (PCOS) and PCO based on ultrasound criteria alone. To reduce the risk of over-diagnosing these patients, a new threshold of 24 follicles (sum of both ovaries) should be considered when using newer ultrasound equipment, and centres should be encouraged to identify their own thresholds, with a reassessment of the criteria as newer machines come to the market. An interesting and distinguishing feature of this patient population is a much higher anti-müllerian hormone (AMH) level than normal controls, suggestive of excessive secretion of AMH per follicle, which may be a reflection of an increased number of granulosa cells within each follicle or over-expression of AMH by each granulosa cell [1]. Furthermore, studies using color Doppler ultrasound have shown that women with PCO have a higher ovarian stromal blood flow velocity prior to commencement of gonadotrophin therapy than women with normal ovaries, and if measured before commencing gonadotrophin stimulation is predictive of a good ovarian response [2]. It has also been shown that women with 'UPCO' have higher serum vascular endothelial growth factor concentrations in the early follicular phase, compared to women with normal ovaries, which may explain the increased vascularity seen in this patient population as well as the improved in vitro fertilisation (IVF) outcomes. Ovarian blood flow plays an important role during ovulation, and animal studies have suggested that increased follicular vascularity may be a primary determinant of follicular dominance and that dominant follicles have an increased uptake of serum gonadotrophins. Increased ovarian stromal blood flow velocity may therefore be associated with an increased delivery of gonadotrophins to the target cells for stimulation of follicular growth resulting in the production of more oocytes which is associated with their improved response and therefore higher pregnancy rates. Another unique feature of these 'UPCO' patients is the significantly enlarged cohort of antral and recruitable follicles that increase the risk of cycle cancellation and/or ovarian hyperstimulation syndrome (OHSS). Therefore, in many respects these patients reflect a clinical phenotype that more closely resembles a 'high responder' than a patient with clinical PCOS when analysing their clinical response to controlled ovarian hyperstimulation (COH), complications, oocyte quality and IVF outcomes.

Finding the optimal IVF stimulation protocol for these patients, in order to decrease the OHSS risk, optimise follicular growth and oocyte quality is challenging. Few studies indeed have specifically addressed this key point. It has been suggested that women with 'UPCO' on a long duration suppression protocol, which sequentially combines an oral contraceptive pill (OCP) and then daily injections of a GnRH agonist, has shown improvements in the IVF outcome in terms of implantation and pregnancy rates in patients who previously experienced high responses or OHSS during COH, in comparison to the classic GnRH agonist protocol. However, more recent studies have not found a difference in the duration of stimulation, dose of gonadotrophins used, incidence of severe OHSS and pregnancy rates in 'UPCO' between GnRH agonist and antagonist COH protocols. However, GnRH agonist long protocols have shown higher responses than antagonist protocols regarding oestradiol levels on day of hCG and number of retrieved oocytes [3]. But given the lack of significant superiority for either a GnRH agonist or antagonist approach, and due to the increased risk for complications associated with COH in this patient population, strong consideration should be given to utilising protocols that use a GnRH agonist trigger for oocyte maturation and freeze-all approaches with postponement of embryo transfer [3].

The actual live birth outcomes are improved in this patient population. Engmann et al. [3] suggested that the odds of achieving a live birth, after undergoing up to three cycles of IVF treatment in women who have 'UPCO' are 82% higher than those of women with normal ovaries, requiring fewer ampules of gonadotrophins, producing more follicles and viable oocytes with similar fertilisation and miscarriage rates to those who have normal ovaries [4–6]. This is consistent with the findings of studies involving patients with 'UPCO' undergoing ovum donation. The reason why women with 'UPCO' undergoing IVF treatment with coexistent causes of infertility perform better than women with normal ovaries is probably because they produce more oocytes, but of comparable quality and fertilisation rates. Consequently, there is a wider choice of embryos to select for transfer in these patients, thereby resulting in a higher chance of conception. In addition, some reports have shown that these women have embryos with less fragmentation which cleave faster, cavitate earlier and had more cells at the blastocyst stage than embryos from women with tubal disease.

There are several implications to consider in women with 'UPCO'. The identification on transvaginal ultrasound of the polycystic ovarian morphology, and/or an elevated AMH without clinical manifestations of PCOS and who are undergoing IVF because of other coexistent infertility factors have a favourable prognosis for a live birth. Since these women exhibit an exaggerated response to gonadotrophin therapy regardless of COH protocol, the major problem remains the increased risk of OHSS. Since no COH protocol is superior to manage these patients, strong consideration should be given to protocols that reduce the risk of OHSS, use of GnRH antagonists for ovarian suppression, including those that trigger oocyte maturation with a GnRH agonist, with or without a 'freeze-all' approach [2]. Therefore, it is important that every patient undergoing IVF has a baseline ultrasound scan, antral follicle count and AMH levels, as well as assessment of ovarian morphology before commencing assisted reproductive technology treatments in order to assess risk and reduce complications.

References

1. Catteau-Jonard S, Bancquart J, Poncelet E, Lefebvre-Maunoury C, Robin G, Dewailly D. Polycystic ovaries at ultrasound: normal variant or silent polycystic ovary syndrome? *Ultrasound Obstet Gynecol.* 2012 Aug;40(2):223–9.

2. Mizrachi Y, Horowitz E, Farhi J, Raziel A, Weissman A. Ovarian stimulation for freeze-all IVF cycles: a systematic review.

Hum Reprod Update. 2020 Jan 1;26 (1):118–35.

3. Engmann L, Sladkevicius P, Agrawal R, et al. The pattern of changes in ovarian stromal and uterine artery blood flow velocities during IVF treatment and its relationship with outcome of the cycle. *Ultrasound Obstet Gynecol.* 1999 Jan;13 (1):26–33.

4. Kim YJ, Ku SY, Jee BC, et al. A comparative study on the outcomes of in vitro fertilization between women with polycystic ovary syndrome and those with sonographic polycystic ovary-only in

GnRH antagonist cycles. *Arch Gynecol Obstet.* 2010 Aug;282(2):199–205.

5. Engmann L, Maconochie N, Sladkevicius P, Bekir J, Campbell S, Tan SL. The outcome of in-vitro fertilization treatment in women with sonographic evidence of polycystic ovarian morphology. *Hum Reprod.* 1999 Jan;14(1):167–71.

6. Selçuk S, Özkaya E, Eser A, et al. Characteristics and outcomes of in vitro fertilization in different phenotypes of polycystic ovary syndrome. *Turk J Obstet Gynecol.* 2016 March; 13(1):1–6.

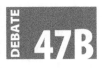

Asymptomatic Polycystic Ultrasound Appearance of the Ovary Is Favourable for IVF Outcome

Against

Lisa Webber

Polycystic ovaries in asymptomatic women have an increased number of antral follicles but otherwise behave the same as ovaries with normal counts. The dominant follicle grows in a similar number of days, ovulation occurs reliably and the luteal phase is normal. There is no excess androgen production to cause acne or drive unwanted hair growth. There are subtle differences though. The dynamics of follicle development right from the primordial follicle stage are not the same as in the morphologically normal ovary, with a higher proportion of pre-antral follicles at growing stages in the ovulatory PCO. Polycystic ovarian morphology is found in just over 20% of asymptomatic women – it is therefore not a pathological finding but a variation of normal, the product of the expression of different genes. It is analogous to eye colour which is also inherited and polygenic.

IVF success rates are influenced by ovarian response to stimulation and the number of mature eggs collected. So it might be thought that the high antral follicle count (AFC) of the PCO would be advantageous for outcome. A meta-analysis of IVF outcomes for women with PCOS published in 2006 does not support this view [1]. The number of eggs collected was higher than from women with normal ovaries, but the number that fertilised was the same, presumably because of an increased number of immature eggs collected from the PCOS group. Both pregnancy and live birth rates were the same in the two groups. There is not even a financial advantage for the PCOS group as the total dose of gonadotropin used was the same. These findings have been replicated in egg donors with PCOS and there is no reason to believe that the outcome for the asymptomatic PCO would be better.

So having established that there is no advantage to PCO morphology in the context of IVF, next we must consider whether there is a disadvantage. The obvious one is ovarian hyperstimulation syndrome (OHSS): second to multiple pregnancy, it is the commonest complication of IVF. The incidence will depend on the severity of the OHSS being considered and it tends to be under-reported. It causes ascites, pleural effusions, dysfunction of the liver and kidneys, and is a significant risk for venous thromboembolism and even death. Symptomatic OHSS may affect around 5% of cycles but severe OHSS requiring hospitalisation is uncommon, affecting 0.3% of cycles in Europe [2]. High AFC and high AMH are risk factors for over-response/OHSS [3] and the risk is probably 3–4 times that for women with normal ovaries. More egg collections are cancelled for over-response in women with PCOS compared to normal [4]. Cycle cancellation has a cost implication, let alone the distress caused to the woman and her partner or supporters.

Risk of OHSS can be reduced by using a gonadotropin releasing hormone (GnRH) antagonist to prevent the LH surge instead of a GnRH agonist protocol. Use of a GnRH agonist trigger for oocyte maturation in antagonist cycles instead of hCG further reduces the risk, and freezing all embryos prevents late onset OHSS, which occurs when pregnancy ensues. However, this is a more expensive strategy, because of the extra monitoring and embryology work required for the frozen embryo replacement cycle that follows. The delay to embryo transfer and more visits to the clinic may have an adverse psychological impact as well. If fresh embryo transfer is performed after a GnRH agonist trigger, the clinical pregnancy rate is compromised. Luteal phase support including LH activity (hCG or LH) can rescue the pregnancy rates, but this is at the cost of reduced OHSS prevention [3].

Any discussion about polycystic ultrasound appearance of the ovary must consider what is actually being described. The Rotterdam criteria describe an ovary as being polycystic if 12 or more antral follicles of 2–9 mm in diameter are present or the ovarian volume is greater than 10 ml. However, the international evidence-based guideline for the assessment and management of polycystic ovary syndrome 2018 [4] challenges these criteria, arguing that modern ultrasound technology has higher resolution, and that an ovary should only be considered polycystic if the antral follicle count is 20 or above and/or the ovarian volume is 10 ml or higher. Applying this cut off when examining ovaries with ultrasound of sufficient resolution may enable better targeting of women at risk of OHSS because of high antral follicle counts. The added benefit will be that many women will lose an unnecessary label that causes stigma and concern.

The polycystic ovary in the asymptomatic woman does have implications for IVF but none of them are favourable. There is no advantage to having higher than normal AFC or AMH and there are certainly disadvantages. The motion that polycystic ultrasound appearance of the ovary in the absence of PCOS is favourable for IVF outcome cannot be supported.

References

1. Heijnen EMEW, Eijkemans MJC, Hughes EG, et al. A meta-analysis of outcomes of conventional IVF in women with polycystic ovary syndrome. *Hum Reprod Update*. 2006;12(1):13–21.

2. De Geyter C, Calhaz-Jorge C, Kupka MS, et al. ART in Europe, 2015: results generated from European registries by ESHRE. *Hum Reprod Open*. 2020;1–17.

3. ESHRE Reproductive Endocrinology Guideline Group. Ovarian stimulation for IVF/ICSI: Guideline of the European Society of Human Reproduction and Embryology, 2019.

4. Teede H, Misso M, Costello M. International evidence-based guideline for the assessment and management of polycystic ovary syndrome. 2018. Monash University on behalf of the NHMR. Available from: monash.edu/medicine/sphpm/mchri/pcos.

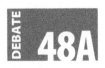

48A Ultrasound Monitoring Is Not Required for Letrozole Treatment

For

Ahmed Badawy

Aromatase enzyme is a microsomal cytochrome P450 hemoprotein-containing enzyme (the product of the CYP19 gene). It catalyses the production of oestrogens by conversion of androgens (androstenedione and testosterone) to estrone and estradiol in many tissues of the human body including the brain and ovaries.

Letrozole is an aromatase enzyme inhibitor that reduces oestrogen levels down to very low concentrations (up to 97–99% of its original serum level). This marked reduction of serum oestrogens, after letrozole administration early in the menstrual cycle, will blunt the oestrogen-negative feedback loop in the brain (in contrary to clomiphene citrate which depletes the oestrogen receptors). This will release the hypothalamic/pituitary axis from oestrogenic negative feedback and temporarily increase the gonadotropin secretion which will stimulate ovarian follicle growth. However, this FSH spurt does not continue as letrozole has a relatively short half-life (about 45 hours) and is cleared from the body rapidly. It has been reported that as soon as the dominant follicle grows in the ovary and oestrogen levels rise again, FSH will drop due to intact normal negative feedback and atresia of the smaller growing follicles will occur. A single dominant follicle will reach maturity, and mono-ovulation will take place. There is now a plethora of research that documented the value of aromatase inhibitors alone or with other medications to accomplish mono-follicular ovulation in anovulatory patients.

It had been postulated the letrozole might has added values in increasing the follicular sensitivity to FSH due to temporary increase in intraovarian androgens which will lead to upgrading FSH receptor expression and increasing IGF-1 in the follicular milieu. It is also noticed that endometrial growth is not affected by drop of serum oestrogen due to up-regulation of oestrogen receptors in the endometrium, leading to rapid endometrial growth and may be increased blood flow once oestrogen secretion is re-established.

The aim of ultrasound monitoring of stimulation cycles is to witness the number of growing follicles and subsequently to avoid multiple pregnancy and ovarian hyperstimulation syndrome (OHSS). Furthermore, the endometrial thickness is measured to be sure that is sufficient for the implantation process later. It is now clear that a major advantage of letrozole for ovulation induction is monofollicular ovulation in standard patients. Also, because negative effects on the endometrium are not present, minimal ultrasound monitoring is needed for endometrial thickness. This might encourage the gynaecologists, without complete admittance to ultrasound monitoring, to participate confidently in the management of anovulatory women.

The same hold true largely for polycystic ovary syndrome (PCOS) patients. Multiple follicular growth and subsequently ovarian hyperstimulation syndrome and undesirable multiple pregnancy can be noticeably avoided by the use of letrozole in ovulation induction due to the aforementioned mechanisms. Yet, in PCOS women there are many follicles in their ovaries which represent a cohort ready to respond to normal FSH levels. Hence, in some situations, multiple ovulation might occur especially with higher doses of letrozole

(7.5 mg) which leads to delayed clearance of the drug and subsequently prolonged FSH elevation compared with the low doses. Dose finding studies proved that a modest dose of letrozole, i.e. 5 mg, is effective and less likely to cause unwanted outcomes. In this particular group of women, PCOS women, to avoid multiple pregnancies or even OHSS with all fertility medications including aromatase inhibitors, minimal ultrasound monitoring is required, and the options of cycle cancellation must be presented to the patients if more than the target number of follicles develops.

To sum up, extensive ultrasound monitoring of the letrozole-induced cycles is not required for either the number of follicles or endometrial thickness when a standard dose of 2.5 or 5 mg is used based on our previous experience and many research studies but at least minimal monitoring is mandatory for the particular group of women with PCOS especially when higher doses of letrozole are required.

Further Reading

Al-Omari WR, Sulaiman WR, Al-Hadithi N. Comparison of two AIs in women with clomiphene-resistant polycystic ovary syndrome. *Int J Gynecol Obstet.* 2004;853:289–91.

Cole PA, Robinson CH. Mechanism and inhibition of cytochrome P-450 aromatase. *J Med Chem.* 1990;33:2933–44.

Mitwally MFM, Casper RF. Use of an AI for induction of ovulation in patients with an inadequate response to clomiphene citrate. *Fertil Steril.* 2000;75:305–9.

Roberts V, Meunier H, Vaughan J, et al. Production and regulation of inhibin subunits in pituitary gonadotrophs. *Endocrinology.* 1989;124:552–4.

Rosenfeld CR, Roy T, Cox BE. Mechanisms modulating estrogen-induced uterine vasodilation. *Vascul Pharmacol.* 2002;382:115–25.

Weil S, Vendola K, Zhou J, Bondy CA. Androgen and follicle-stimulating hormone interactions in primate ovarian follicle development. *J Clin Endocrinol Metab.* 1999;848:2951–6.

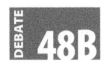

Ultrasound Monitoring Is Not Required for Letrozole Treatment

Against

Mohamed F Mitwally

Since first reports in the literature by Mitwally and Casper over the last two decades, the aromatase inhibitor, letrozole has been found as a useful and safe agent for ovulation induction in anovulatory women, e.g. in PCOS (polycystic ovary syndrome), ovarian superovulation in ovulatory women, unexplained infertility, and in conjunction with gonadotropins to achieve better ovarian response during assisted reproduction [1–5].

This debate discusses whether ultrasound is not required during letrozole treatment alone, as an agent for ovarian stimulation. I am against not using ultrasound monitoring during letrozole treatment.

I think ultrasound is required in patients undergoing letrozole treatment, at two points: a baseline ultrasound when starting administration and a follow-up ultrasound a few days after finishing letrozole administration.

A baseline ultrasound is recommended for two reasons:

1. The first reason is to rule out contraindications for starting letrozole; a relatively common contraindication is the presence of significant ovarian cyst(s) and a less common one but more serious, is to avoid starting letrozole treatment when early pregnancy bleeding may be mistaken for menstrual cycle bleeding.
2. The second reason is to decide on the regimen of letrozole treatment (starting day, dose and duration). This is an empiric topic. Several letrozole treatment regimens have been reported including starting on different days in the menstrual cycle (as early as menstrual cycle day one and as late as cycle day five). Letrozole has been given for a variable number of days (as short as one day single dose administration and as long as extended regimens for more than one week). Letrozole has been administered as the same daily dose or in variable doses on different treatment days, e.g. step-up of increasing doses [1–4].

Unfortunately, the ideal letrozole regimen has not been determined yet. However, I think there is no such one size that fits all. I believe in modifying the letrozole regimen, basing it on the underlying ovulatory disorder and the aim of treatment whether mono-ovulation or multiple follicular development. My recommendations (not supported with adequate studies) are to start letrozole earlier in the menstrual cycle, preferably no later than the first five days of the menstrual cycle, administer it in an extended regimen up to three weeks when no response is achieved, e.g. resistant PCOS, but to shorten treatment duration and dose (four days or less) when ovarian reserve is low. Low ovarian reserve is usually associated with fast growing follicle(s) that will result in ovulation that too early in the menstrual cycle will not give enough time for adequate endometrial development (and possible inadequate oocyte cytoplasmic development). So starting letrozole early in the menstrual cycle and for shorter duration in those patients with low ovarian reserve may be advisable. When multiple follicular development is desired, using the letrozole in step-up doses starting as early as possible in the menstrual cycle may be more likely to achieve the goal.

It is obvious that without ultrasound mentoring, it will not be possible to fine-tune the letrozole regimen to suit individual patients. However, whether such fine-tuning can result in better treatment outcomes is still undetermined and needs further studies.

A follow-up ultrasound is recommended for four reasons:

1. The first reason is to determine the response to letrozole treatment including: whether a mature follicle is growing in anovulatory women and whether multiple follicular development is achieved in ovulatory women. Also, assessment of endometrial development and cervical mucus are both important in determining the best regimen for letrozole use in future cycles as explained above, and to decide on HCG (human chorionic gonadotropin) ovulation trigger, as well as fertilisation timing as explained next.

2. The second reason is to decide on when to trigger ovulation with HCG injection. It is important to mention here that we found [1] LH levels during letrozole treatment to have bimodal rises, one early during the first few days of letrozole treatment (LH levels rise in response to decreased negative feedback effect of oestrogen, when oestrogen levels are low) then high LH levels later in the cycle in association with LH surge (LH levels rise due to positive oestrogen feedback associated with rising oestrogen levels close to ovulation). We also found LH levels around the peak of LH surge to be significantly higher with letrozole treatment compared to other ovarian stimulation protocols [5]. Such a unique LH pattern (bimodal rise) associated with letrozole treatment may result in confusion when LH ovulation detection kits are used to monitor letrozole treatment. LH kits may show false-positive ovulation early in treatment and a too early true positive response when LH surge has not reached a true peak yet, as the peak of LH surge associated with letrozole treatment is much higher as explained earlier. Again, in this situation, ultrasound examination should help alleviate any confusion regarding best timing of ovulation trigger and fertility treatment, e.g. IUI (intrauterine insemination).

3. The third reason is to determine fertility treatment timing including timing intercourse and IUI. As explained above, a coordinated timing of ovulation based on assessment of follicular size, endometrial development and cervical mucus are necessary because timing seems to play a significant role in fertility treatment success.

4. The fourth reason is to assess the risk of multiple pregnancy if any. Ultrasound is necessary to determine the number of mature follicles, an important predictor for multiple pregnancy risk. However, the literature has suggested a much lower risk of multiple pregnancy associated with letrozole treatment when compared to other ovarian stimulation treatments [3].

To conclude: ultrasound during letrozole treatment may be highly recommended, advisable and required in the following situations:

- Highly recommended for safety when ruling out possible underlying pregnancy and ovarian cysts.
- Advisable to determine stimulation protocol, and response to letrozole treatment, as well as timing HCG administration and fertility treatment including timing intercourse and IUI.
- At least required to determine the risk of multiple pregnancy which is pretty low with letrozole treatment.

References

1. Mitwally MF, Casper RF. Aromatase inhibition: a novel method of ovulation induction in women with polycystic ovary syndrome. *Reprod. Technol.* 2000;10 (5):244–7.

2. Mitwally MFM, Casper RF. Reprint of: use of an aromatase inhibitor for induction of ovulation in patients with an inadequate response to clomiphene citrate. *Fertil Steril.* 2019 Oct;112(4S1):e178–82. doi: 10.1016/j .fertnstert.2019.08.087.

3. Diamond MP, Mitwally M, Casper R, et al. Estimating rates of multiple gestation pregnancies: sample size calculation from the assessment of multiple intrauterine gestations from ovarian stimulation (AMIGOS) trial. *Contemp Clin Trials.* 2011 Nov;32(6):902–8. doi: 10.1016/j.cct.2011.07 .009.

4. Mitwally MF, Casper RF. Single-dose administration of an aromatase inhibitor for ovarian stimulation. *Fertil Steril.* 2005 Jan;83(1):229–31.

5. Mitwally MF, Casper RF. LH surge is associated with higher LH levels and more physiologic estradiol levels in aromatase inhibitor ovarian stimulation cycles. *Fertil Steril.* Sept 2004;82(Suppl 2):S144.

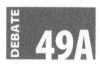

Progesterone Levels Should Be Measured on the Day of hCG Administration

For

Ernesto Bosch

Introduction

The possible impact of serum progesterone (P) levels on the day of human chorionic gonadotropin (hCG) administration in IVF outcome has been a matter of debate for the last 30 years. To date, there is sufficient scientific evidence available to prove that high P levels on the day of triggering negatively impact pregnancy rates. Therefore, measuring it becomes necessary in order to detect these cases and take clinical decisions to minimise its impact.

However, serum P determination is not fully extended, and still some detractors consider that this simple low-cost practice is not justified. In order to demonstrate the clinical value of measuring P the day of triggering, I hereby purpose the most objective and evidence-based approach to analyse the cause-effect association between two clinical events.

The Bradford-Hill Criteria

In 1965, Sir Austin Bradford-Hill, an epidemiologist Professor of Statistics in the University of London, defined the nine criteria that differentiate the causation from the association between an environmental factor and a disease [1]. In this text, we will filter the relationship between high serum P levels the day of triggering and IVF cycle outcome through each of the nine Bradford-Hill criteria.

1. Temporality: Does the Cause Precede the Effect? -- The cause, elevated P the day of trigger, precedes embryo implantation, that occurs after 6 to 9 days after fertilisation. This means that P elevation happens 8-11 days before its effect.

2. Plausibility: Is the Association Consistent with Existing Knowledge? -- It is well-known that P elevation after ovulation induces secretory changes in the endometrium to turn it receptive. A proper synchronisation between P elevation and endometrial maturation is mandatory to allow embryo implantation. Classic studies show the importance of an in-phase endometrium for embryo implantation.

3. Consistency: Have Similar Results Been Shown in Other Studies? -- One of the largest meta-analyses ever published in *Reproductive Medicine*, which includes 63 studies and more than 55,000 subjects, shows that high P is associated with poorer outcome, even with a wide range of thresholds [2].

4. Strength: What Is the Strength of Association Between the Cause and the Effect? -- In a prospective cohort study including more than 4,000 patients, our group demonstrated that high serum P had a strong impact of ongoing pregnancy rate, almost halving it (OR: 0.53; 95% CI 0.38–0.72) in both GnRH agonist and antagonist cycles [3].

5. Dose Response: Does Increased Exposure Equal Increased Effect? -- The study mentioned above [3], showed that patients with higher P levels had lower ongoing pregnancy

rates. Also, it has been reported that the more days of elevated P before triggering, the lower the cycle outcome.

6. Reversibility: Does Removal of a Cause Decrease the Risk of the Effect? -- It has been shown that freezing all the embryos when P levels are high, and transferring them in a subsequent endometrial preparation cycles, under normal P values, restores pregnancy rates. Therefore, removal of the cause, eliminates the effect [3].

7. Is the Evidence Based on a Robust Study Design? -- If we assume that meta-analysis is the cusp of the pyramid of scientific evidence, the one mentioned above [2] proves this query. Moreover, many of the studies included in this meta-analysis are large prospective cohort studies, which also provide high quality scientific evidence.

8. Evidence: How Many Lines of Evidence Lead to the Conclusion? -- Essential protection against flawed ideas is triangulation. This is the strategic use of multiple approaches to address one question. Each approach has its own unrelated assumptions, strengths and weaknesses. Results that agree across different methodologies are less likely to be artefacts. A different way to prove the impact of elevated P on endometrial receptivity is to analyse this effect directly on endometrial samples. Two studies have shown a dramatic variation on the gene expression profile of the endometrium when it has been exposed to high P levels, affecting to genes involved in cell adhesion and structural proteins of the endometrium.

9. Similar Agents Cause Similar Results -- The cause–effect relationship between serum P levels on the day of triggering and cycle outcome has a direct analogy with the more recently observed impact of serum P levels the day of embryo transfer after artificial endometrium preparation cycles and ongoing pregnancy rates. In this case, insufficient exposure to P during the luteal phase leads to a lower outcome [4]. This proves from a different perspective the importance of and adequate exposure of the endometrium to P for an optimal receptivity.

Conclusion

The analysis presented here proves in a very systematic and objective way the cause–effect relationship between serum P levels on the day of triggering and cycle outcome. The nine Bradford-Hill criteria to demonstrate a cause–effect relationship are fulfilled. Moreover, it is demonstrated that there is a strong dose-dependent relation, with elevated P shown to almost halve the ongoing pregnancy rate.

Previous studies show that when serum P is monitored, the proportion of patients that may have an elevation is under control (8–10%); however, when serum P is not controlled, the number of patients than can have an increase can be as high as 38% [5].

Determining serum P is a simple, low-cost practice, that involves very little investment and change in daily practice. Most IVF units perform in-house steroid analysis (mainly for estradiol determination), in platforms that can also determine serum P. While the cost of a serum P is low, the benefit for patients is very high, as clear clinical decisions can be taken to avoid its impact when high levels are detected. Therefore, P levels should always be determined on the day of hCG administration if a fresh embryo transfer is planned.

References

1. Hill AB. The environment and disease: association or causation? *Proc Royal Soc Med.* 1965;58:295–300.

2. Venetis CA, Kolibianakis EM, Bosdou JK, Tarlatzis BC. Progesterone elevation and probability of pregnancy after IVF: a systematic review and meta-analysis of over 60,000 cycles. *Hum Reprod Update.* 2013;19:433–57.

3. Bosch E, Labarta E, Crespo J, et al. Circulating progesterone levels and ongoing pregnancy rates in controlled ovarian stimulation cycles for in vitro fertilization: analysis of over 4000 cycles. *Hum Reprod.* 2010;5:2092–100.

4. Labarta E, Mariani G, Holtmann N, Celada P, Remohí J, Bosch E. Low serum progesterone on the day of embryo transfer is associated with a diminished ongoing pregnancy rate in oocyte donation cycles after artificial endometrial preparation: a prospective study. *Hum Reprod.* 2017;32:2437–42.

5. Bosch E, Valencia I, Escudero E, et al. Premature luteinization during gonadotropin-releasing hormone antagonist cycles and its relationship with in vitro fertilization outcome. *Fertil Steril.* 2003;80:1444–9.

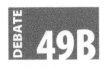
49B Progesterone Levels Should Be Measured on the Day of hCG Administration

Against

Alan Penzias

The foundational base upon which all reproductive care rests is the physiology and endocrinology of the normal menstrual cycle. To decrypt and treat abnormalities in menstrual and reproductive function, we must understand normal first. Few hormonal changes in the human body are as dramatic as the rise in progesterone in the luteal phase. Levels rise by a factor of 20–40× however, almost no other hormone value is as misunderstood or misinterpreted as the simple serum progesterone level.

There isn't universal agreement on the serum level above which ovulation – egg release – has clearly occurred. To the contrary, since the inception of fertility treatment, the assumption that a rising or elevated progesterone level means that ovulation has occurred has been proven false. Further muddying the waters are the variations in hormone levels by different assays [1]. Whether through coincidence or merely poor luck, the variation in readout between commercial platforms seems most pronounced at the level where many fertility specialists make a clinical decision to proceed with fresh embryo transfer in an IVF cycle or cryopreserve all embryos for transfer in a subsequent treatment cycle.

Beyond mere confusion at a critical decision threshold, the odds of premature ovulation, a term indicating the release of eggs from the ovary prior to planned oocyte retrieval, is miniscule. Use of gonadotropin-releasing hormone (GnRH) antagonists or agonists have changed the face of IVF by reliably preventing premature ovulation [2]. The ordinary time sequence in IVF is a course of patient self-administered gonadotropins accompanied by the co-administration or addition of GnRH analogue. At a time point determined by measurement of growing ovarian follicles and rise in serum estradiol, human chorionic gonadotropin (hCG) is self-administered and surgical egg retrieval is scheduled to occur approximately 36 hours later.

With very rare exception the follicles seen at the last ultrasound scan are almost always present at egg collection. The serum progesterone level is nearly entirely unrelated to the presence or absence of oocytes. A progesterone elevation at the time of hCG administration is rarely due to premature ovulation as evidenced by the almost invariant presence of eggs at retrieval. The elevation is also unrelated to the physiologic rise in luteinising hormone (LH) that precedes ovulation in the course of a normal menstrual cycle. In our pharmacologically managed IVF cycles the LH rise is thoroughly prevented by the GnRH analogues. Too many IVF cycles in days gone by were cancelled unnecessarily due to the presumption of premature ovulation. Now there is a clearer understanding that rising progesterone is not an indicator or premature egg release.

Where then does the rising progesterone level come from? It seems that in some patients but not all each developing follicle begins producing a small amount of progesterone during gonadotropin stimulation. The aggregate total production from a large field of follicles can be detected in serum assay. In fact, the number of oocytes retrieved appears to correlate with follicular phase progesterone level with more eggs being retrieved at higher progesterone levels [3]. It does appear to be true that a very elevated progesterone level prior to oocyte retrieval decreases the odds of pregnancy with fresh embryo transfer. Various thresholds have been proposed above which the pregnancy rates with fresh embryo transfer decline because the progesterone has influenced the endometrial lining unfavourably causing it to mature out of synchrony with egg and embryo development [4]. If the serum progesterone measurements are performed in different laboratories during an IVF cycle or on different platforms within a large reference laboratory, the clinical value of the serum progesterone level declines because of potential differences in assay norms.

What about oocyte function after pre-retrieval progesterone exposure? The good news here is that eggs seem entirely unphased by pre-ovulatory exposure to progesterone and function no differently than eggs not exposed to progesterone [5].

In summary, progesterone is an essential component of the natural menstrual cycle and its timely production and decline is necessary to normal function. IVF treatment evolved to its present state by applying knowledge of fundamental principles and creating medications that essentially allow physicians to apply levels of control to individual cycle elements to the benefit of the patient. Interpreting data gathered in an IVF cycle through the lens of a spontaneous menstrual cycle should be done with caution because pharmacologically managed treatment is notably different. Measuring serum progesterone levels on the day of hCG administration risks misunderstanding its origin and impact and could lead to clinical intervention where none is needed.

References

1. Maas KAK, Nguyen K-H, Spratt DI, Penzias AS. Inter-assay variability of progesterone in patients undergoing assisted reproductive technology (ART). *Fertil Steril.* 2011; 96:S122–3.

2. Kolibianakis EM, Collins JC, Tarlatzis BC, Devroey P, Diedrich K, Griesinger G. Among patients treated for IVF with gonadotrophins and GnRH analogues, is the probability of live birth dependent on the type of analogue used? A systematic review and meta-analysis. *Hum Reprod Update.* 2006;12:651–71.

3. Racca A, Santos-Ribeiro S, De Munch N, et al. Impact of late-follicular phase elevated serum progesterone on cumulative live birth rates: is there a deleterious effect on embryo quality? *Hum Reprod.* 2018;33:860–68.

4 Humm KC, Ibrahim Y, Dodge LE, et al. Does elevated serum progesterone on the day of human chorionic gonadotropin administration decrease live birth rates? *J Reprod Med.* 2012;57:9–12.

5. Ubaldi F, Smitz J, Wisanto A, et al. Oocyte and embryo quality as well as pregnancy rate in intracytoplasmic sperm injection are not affected by high follicular phase serum progesterone. *Hum Reprod.* 1995;10:3091–6.

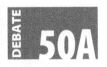
50A Progesterone Treatment Does Not Help Recurrent Miscarriage Patients

For

Raj Rai

Recurrent miscarriage, defined as the loss of three or more consecutive early pregnancies, affects 1–2% of the population. In at least 50% of cases this is due to recurrent fetal aneuploidy. Despite numerous proposed aetiologies (endocrine; immune and anatomical), only obstetric antiphospholid syndrome has withstood critical evaluation over an extended period – 30 years.

Progesterone, secreted by the corpus luteum, is recognised to play a cardinal role in early pregnancy. Its actions are mediated through both genomic (via nuclear and membrane bound receptors) and non-genomic mechanisms which include modulation of the maternal immune response; promotion of a TH2 cytokine response and up-regulation of tissue factor and PAI-1 activity. A murine knockout model of progesterone receptor A demonstrates impaired endometrial decidualisation and implantation failure.

Seminal work by Robert Casper reported that progesterone secretion by the corpus luteum is an absolute requirement for a successful pregnancy. Lutectomy before 8 weeks of pregnancy results in a decrease in progesterone levels and miscarriage. Pregnancy is rescued by the administration of exogenous progesterone. Administration of an anti-progesterone, mifepristone, leads to pregnancy loss. Progesterone levels are lower in pregnancies that miscarry compared to those that are on-going.

Hence, both in vitro and in vivo data has led to the expectation that progesterone supplementation can prevent miscarriage. Until recently, this belief was supported by the results of small individual studies, all of which were of poor quality, often non-randomised/non-blinded and with a low Jadad score. In addition, these early studies used different forms of progestogens (dydrogestone or 17 hydroxyprogesterone) with different routes of administration (oral, vaginal, intramuscular) and differing doses.

To address limitations of existing data, a large prospective randomised double-blinded placebo controlled study (PROMISE) was conducted between 2010 and 2013 to answer the question of whether micronised vaginal progesterone commencing between a positive pregnancy test and 6 weeks gestation and continued until 12 completed weeks or miscarriage led to an increased live birth rate amongst women with 'unexplained' recurrent pregnancy loss [1]. A total of 836 women from 36 UK centres and nine centres from the Netherlands were randomised. The rate of live births after 24 weeks of gestation was 65.8% (262 of 398 pregnancies) in the progesterone group, compared with 63.3% (271 of 428 pregnancies) in the placebo group (relative rate, 1.04; 95% CI 0.94–1.15; absolute rate difference, 2.5 percentage points; 95% CI −4.0 to 9.0). In addition, a further post-hoc sub-group analysis reported *no* difference in the live birth rates in micronised progesterone versus placebo amongst those with a history of three, four, five, and six or more miscarriages.

The largest and most recent meta-analysis of 10 studies (including PROMISE) reported a marginal benefit of progesterone supplementation in early pregnancy in reducing the risk of first trimester pregnancy loss (RR 0.72; 95% CI 0.53–0.97) and increasing the live birth rate (RR 1.07; 95% CI 1.02–1.15) [2]. This analysis however, included studies spanning 60 years with 7 of 10 included trials pre-dating 1990; it used different progesterone/progestins and allowed randomisation as late as 16 weeks gestation. The authors themselves acknowledge that this raises serious concerns about the quality of the included data and hence the conclusions.

The most recent international guidance on the use of progesterone supplementation as a treatment for recurrent miscarriage was published by ESHRE (The ESHRE Guideline Group on RPL et al. 2018). It concluded that vaginal progesterone does not improve live birth rates in women with unexplained recurrent pregnancy loss and that there is insufficient evidence to recommend the use of progesterone to improve live birth rate in women with recurrent pregnancy loss and luteal phase insufficiency [3].

Following on from the PROMISE study, the PRISM trial examined the use of micronised progesterone amongst women *with bleeding* in early pregnancy [4]. There was a small non-significant effect of progesterone on the live birth rate (RR 1.03; 95% CI 1.0–1.07). A subsequent post hoc analysis reported that amongst those with a history of three or more miscarriages and experiencing bleeding in early pregnancy, progesterone was of benefit. However, the validity of this, has to be questioned as the number of previous miscarriages was not identified in the randomisation and stratification variables of the PRISM study. Furthermore, a meta-analysis combining the results of PROMISE and PRISM, reporting a benefit of progesterone amongst those with three or more miscarriages, combines the results of two studies addressing two different questions, with different start times for progesterone. Is the publicity – 'Progesterone could prevent 8450 miscarriages/year in the UK' – and 'marketing' of progesterone justified by the data? Perhaps not.

In conclusion, whilst progesterone is essential for the maintenance of early pregnancy and low serum progesterone is associated with an increased risk for miscarriage – vaginal progesterone supplementation does *not* increase the livebirth rate. Whether different progestogens, starting treatment after ovulation, and in those with a high number of miscarriages, is of benefit remains to be tested in randomised studies meeting contemporary trial criteria.

References

1   Coomarasamy, A, Williams H, Truchanowicz E, et al. A randomized trial of progesterone in women with recurrent miscarriages. *New Engl J Med.* 2015;373 (22):2141–8.

2   Saccone G, Schoen C, Franasiak JM, et al. Supplementation with progestogens in the first trimester of pregnancy to prevent miscarriage in women with unexplained recurrent miscarriage: a systematic review and meta-analysis of randomized, controlled trials. *Fertil Steril.* 2017;107 (2):430–38.e3.

3   The ESHRE Guideline Group on RPL. Atik RB, Christiansen OB, Elson J, et al. ESHRE guideline: recurrent pregnancy loss. *Hum Reprod Open.* 2018;2018(2):hoy004.

4   Coomarasamy A, Devall AJ, Cheed V, et al. A randomized trial of progesterone in women with bleeding in early pregnancy. *New Engl J Med.* 2019;380(19):1815–24.

5   Coomarasamy A, Devall AJ, Brosens JJ, et al. Micronized vaginal progesterone to prevent miscarriage: a critical evaluation of randomized evidence. *Am J Obstet Gynecol.* 2020;223(2):167–76.

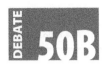

50B Progesterone Treatment Does Not Help Recurrent Miscarriage Patients

Against

Arri Coomarasamy

Introduction

Progesterone is critical for the maintenance of a pregnancy. The central role of progesterone in early pregnancy led clinicians and researchers to speculate that progesterone deficiency could be a cause of miscarriages. This idea resulted in several clinical trials of progesterone treatment in women at high risk of miscarriage. The two important groups of women at particular risk of miscarriage are those with a history of recurrent miscarriage and those with early pregnancy bleeding. This article focuses on women with recurrent miscarriage. The first randomised trial in women with recurrent miscarriage was published in 1953, and several trials followed in the subsequent decades [1]. However, these trials used different progestogens, were small and methodologically weak, producing heterogenous and unreliable results. Policy makers have therefore been unable to make evidence-based recommendations on the use of progestogen supplementation to improve outcomes in these cohorts of women. The PROMISE Trial was conducted to provide robust evidence [2].

The PROMISE Trial

The PROMISE trial is a well-powered randomised trial in women with unexplained recurrent miscarriages [2]. The intervention was 400 mg micronised progesterone taken vaginally twice daily from no later than 6 weeks until 12 weeks of gestation. The comparator was placebo. The primary outcome was live birth beyond 24 weeks of gestation. It is a high quality trial, with computer-generated third party randomisation, allocation concealment, double-blinding, placebo-control, excellent follow-up rate, and a pre-specified statistical analysis plan that was meticulously implemented. The trial recruited 836 women from 36 hospitals in the UK and nine hospitals in the Netherlands.

The primary analysis of the PROMISE trial found the live birth rate was 66% (262/398) in the progesterone group, versus 63% (271/428) in the placebo group (1.04, 95% CI 0.94–1.15, P value = 0.45) [2]. There was a 3% higher live birth rate with progesterone, but the trial finding was reported as not statistically significant due to the large P value (P = 0.45) and the consequent statistical uncertainty. We then performed a pre-specified subgroup analysis by the number of previous miscarriages; the findings (Figure 50B.1) suggested a trend for greater benefit with increasing number of previous miscarriages [3]. A biological gradient related to increasing number of previous miscarriages appeared to be present. We have since confirmed this subgroup effect, and biological gradient, according to increasing number of previous miscarriages in another large trial of 4153 women with threatened miscarriage (the PRISM trial) (Figure 50B.2) [3, 4].

Synthesis of the Totality of Evidence

Practitioners and policy makers need to know the totality of evidence before a recommendation can be made. A systematic review of randomised trials is the gold standard to

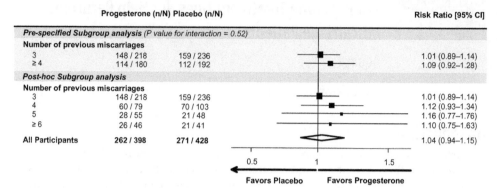

Figure 50B.1 PROMISE Trial subgroup analysis by number of previous miscarriages on the outcome of live birth >24 weeks.
(Reproduced from AJOG, 2020 [3])

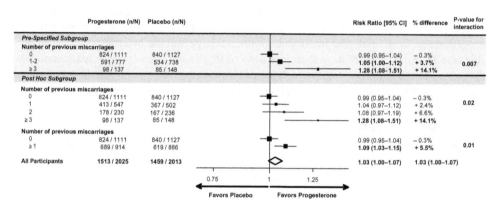

Figure 50B.2 PRISM Trial subgroup analysis by number of previous miscarriages on the outcome of live birth ≥34 weeks.
(Reproduced from AJOG, 2020 [3])

synthesise the effectiveness data. An updated systematic review of all trials of progesterone or progestogens in women with threatened miscarriages and recurrent miscarriages is given in Figure 50B.3 [3]. Eight studies, including a total of 1574, evaluated the effects of progesterone or progestogen in women with a history of recurrent miscarriage. The totality of effectiveness evidence showed an increase in livebirth or ongoing pregnancy with progesterone or progestogen treatment (RR = 1.08, 95% CI 1.03–1.14). There was high level of consistency in the findings, as demonstrated by an I [2] of 0% (Figure 50B.3) [3].

Type of Progestogen

We used vaginal, micronised progesterone in the PROMISE and PRISM trials. The results from these trials are not necessarily generalisable to *progestogens* such as dydrogestone or 17-hydroxyprogesterone. The natural progesterone used in the PROMISE and PRISM trials has an identical chemical structure to physiological progesterone synthesised in the human body. Synthetic progestogens, which include dydrogesterone and 17-hydroxyprogesterone have a different molecular structure, pharmacodynamics and pharmacokinetics, as well as a

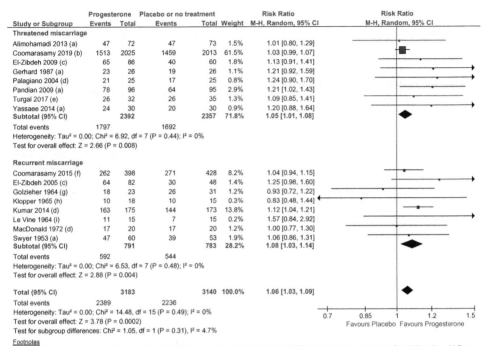

Figure 50B.3 Meta-analysis of all progesterone and progestogen studies for the outcome of live birth or ongoing pregnancy.
(Reproduced from AJOG, 2020 [3])

different safety profile. For example, there is evidence of potential harm from dydrogesterone, particularly an increase in congenital heart disease [5].

Discussion

The role of first trimester progesterone supplementation in the treatment of pregnancies at high risk of miscarriage is a long-standing research question that has been debated in the medical literature for over 60 years. The PROMISE and PRISM trials are two very high quality trials that have addressed the effects of first trimester use of vaginal micronised progesterone treatment in women at risk of a miscarriage.

A history of previous miscarriage identifies women at risk of a future miscarriage, and the risk of a future miscarriage increases with the increasing number of previous miscarriages. Specifically, it is the risk of euploid miscarriages that increases with increasing number of previous miscarriages, meanwhile the risk of miscarriage from sporadic aneuploidies remains broadly constant regardless of the number of previous miscarriages. If one of the causes of euploid miscarriage is luteal phase defect, and progesterone is effective in treating at least some women with luteal phase defect, then we should see an increase in the level of benefit with progesterone treatment in women with increasing numbers of previous miscarriages. This subgroup effect, along with a biological gradient in effect, was observed in both PROMISE and PRISM trials [2–4]. Policy makers and guideline developers will need to consider the evidence carefully to make a balanced recommendation.

References

1. Haas DM, Hathaway TJ, Ramsey PS. Progestogen for preventing miscarriage in women with recurrent miscarriage of unclear etiology. *Cochrane Database Syst Rev.* 2018;10:CD003511.

2. Coomarasamy A, Williams H, Truchanowicz E, et al. A randomized trial of progesterone in women with recurrent miscarriages. *N Engl J Med.* 2015;373:2141–8.

3. Coomarasamy A, Devall AJ, Brosens JJ, et al. Micronized vaginal progesterone to prevent miscarriage: a critical evaluation of randomized evidence. *Am J Obstet Gynecol.* 2020;223(2):167–76.

4. Coomarasamy A, Devall AJ, Cheed V, et al. A randomized trial of progesterone in women with bleeding in early pregnancy. *N Engl J Med.* 2019;380:1815–24.

5. Zaqout M, Aslem E, Abuqamar M, Abughazza O, Panzer J, De Wolf D. The impact of oral intake of dydrogesterone on fetal heart development during early pregnancy. *Pediatr Cardiol.* 2015;36 (7):1483–8.

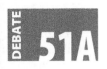

51A The Microbiome Environment Influences IVF Results

For

Sam Schoenmakers and Joop Laven

Introduction

In 2016, the cumulative outcome per egg retrieval cycle lingered around 45%, decreasing to about 4% in women aged older than 42 years, despite introduction of new stimulation schedules and novel methods of optimal embryo selection. To improve IVF outcome, the local microbiome environment has increasingly been sampled, analysed and is being interpreted to understand and predict IVF outcome. The last decade has shown that the human microbiome environment is an essential, integrated and part of normal human physiology and homeostasis. The environment of the gut microbiome directs metabolic and epigenetic processes, regulates the immune system and forms a first line of defence against pathogens. When the balance between host and microbes is disturbed, a dysbiotic state occurs, which is associated with disease and negative health outcome. Since the different, local environments of the female reproductive tract also harbour a unique microbiome, including bacteria and viruses (reviewed in [1]), the balance between host and microbes also affects reproductive health and outcome. Several studies into the relationship between the reproductive microbiome environment and IVF have reported associations with either IVF outcome, pregnancy outcome and embryo quality.

When interpreting microbiome results, the sampling technique, and most important, the possibility of false-positive results based on cross-contamination from other adjacent anatomical regions, should be considered. Only the vaginal environment can easily be collected and even self-sampled without risking cross-contamination by microbes of surrounding anatomical regions. The cervical region can be accessed by speculum investigation, but when sampling the local microbiome, one needs to be extremely cautious not to come into contact with the vaginal walls and environment. Endometrial, fallopian tubes, follicular fluid or peritoneal fluid sampling all involve invasive procedures with high contamination risk, and thus ensure cautious interpretation of the results.

Vaginal Microbiome Environment

In a recent prospective cohort of women eligible for IVF/IVF-ICSI, the vaginal microbiome was sampled prior to the start of hormonal treatment. Retrospective analyses after fresh embryo transfer (ET) within 2 months of sampling and IVF outcome, showed that as well the absence, the presence as the relative abundance of certain specific bacterial species were strongly associated with reproductive outcome. Especially, the combination of a relative abundance of *Lactobacillus* <20%, a relative detection of *Lactobacillus jensenii* >35%, the presence of *Gardnerella vaginalis* or *Proteobacteria* >28% of the total vaginal bacterial biomass was predictive of a chance of less than 6% of achieving a pregnancy after fresh ET, and was defined as an unfavourable microbiome composition. However, predictive outcome was more favourable when balanced with a relative abundance of >60% of *Lactobacillus crispatus* or >60% *Lactobacillus iners* (>60%), which resulted in higher chances to achieve a pregnancy after IVF/ICSI with a fresh ET, respectively of 24% and >50%. These analyses of the combined results of the vaginal microbiome profile and IVF/ICSI outcome resulted in a clinical applicable predictive algorithm for pregnancy change.

Recent research has identified a specific composition of bacterial microbiome environment in the vagina prior to start of hormonal treatment for IVF and hence the transfer of fresh embryonic transfer, which is predictive of IVF outcome [2]. More importantly, it proved to be highly predictive of a failure to achieve within 2 months after the moment of sampling of the vaginal microbial environment.

Intra-uterine Microbiome Environment

Ascending in the female reproductive tract, it was recently reported that the endometrial bacterial environment, sampled via a transcervical approach, and just prior to the transfer of a fresh embryo after an IVF cycle, was predictive of the implantation success of the transferred embryo [3]. Regarding the dynamics of the vaginal microbiome [4], the composition of the endometrial microbes was relatively stable within the same cycle [3]. Due to differences between the community of the endometrial microbiome and the composition of simultaneously collected paired vaginal samples, the endometrium and vaginal microbiome are unique, but can still be a continuum. In line with the findings of the vaginal microbiome, the presence of high numbers of *Lactobacillus* spp. are associated with successful implantation, while the presence of fewer *Lactobacillus* spp. and a high percentage of *Gardnerella vaginalis* are linked to negative reproductive outcome, as is the presence of *Streptococcus*. In line with these findings is a recent study in infertile Japanese women, which showed their endometrial environment is mostly non-*Lactobacillus*-dominant [5].

Follicular Fluid Microbiome Environment

Even high up in the female reproductive tract, within the follicular fluid itself, microbes have been identified [6]. Initial research showed that with culture-dependent and independent techniques after simultaneously sampling of both follicular fluid and the vaginal environment, in order to correct for contamination during the procedure of oocyte pickup, specific microbes were detected within the collected follicular fluid. Important for IVF procedures, was the fact that detection of the presence of *Lactobacillus* species within the follicular fluid was positively associated with better embryo quality and pregnancy outcome. Recently, the same group used scanning electron microscopy to detect and reveal the presence of microbes within fallopian tube samples collected after surgery. However, it is unknown if the detected microbes within the fallopian tube environment are associated with the outcome of IVF techniques.

Conclusion

The microbial environment of different parts of the female reproductive tract, especially both the presence and absence of certain microbes, are to some extent related to the success of IFV-treatment. As in the human gut environment, the local reproductive tract microbes could actively be involved in the local immune responses and as such could influence the initial process of successful implantation. Interpretation of microbial analyses of samples invasively collected higher up the reproductive tract should take possible cross-contamination into account. The non-invasive and self-collectable vaginal microbiome can be interpreted without these limitations and due to the continuum of the reproductive tract microbiome could serve as a biomarker for implantation possibilities and thus fertility outcome after IVF.

References

1. Koedooder R, Mackens S, Budding A, et al. Identification and evaluation of the microbiome in the female and male reproductive tracts. *Hum Reprod Update.* 2019;25(3):298–325.

2. Koedooder R, Singer M, Schoenmakers S, et al. The vaginal microbiome as a predictor for outcome of in vitro fertilization with or without intracytoplasmic sperm injection: a prospective study. *Hum Reprod.* 2019;34 (6):1042–54.

3. Moreno I, Codoner FM, Vilella F, et al. Evidence that the endometrial microbiota has an effect on implantation success or failure. *Am J Obstet Gynecol.* 2016;215 (6):684–703.

4. Gajer P, Brotman RM, Bai G, et al. Temporal dynamics of the human vaginal microbiota. *Sci Transl Med.* 2012;4 (132):132ra52.

5. Kyono K, Hashimoto T, Nagai Y, Sakuraba Y. Analysis of endometrial microbiota by 16S ribosomal RNA gene sequencing among infertile patients: a single-center pilot study. *Reprod Med Biol.* 2018;17 (3):297–306.

6. Pelzer ES, Allan JA, Waterhouse MA, Ross T, Beagley KW, Knox CL. Microorganisms within human follicular fluid: effects on IVF. *PLoS ONE.* 2013;8(3):e59062.

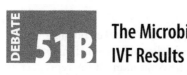

51B The Microbiome Environment Influences IVF Results

Against

Peter Humaidan

The human microbiota is one of the most intriguing areas of biomedical research today. The key is to understand possible associations between dysbiosis/eubiosis and disease or health, and if proven ultimately to investigate how to modulate the microbiota to improve health. In assisted reproductive technology (ART), the microbiota has been studied in recent years, potentially offering new pathophysiological insights – and possibly treatments – for polycystic ovary syndrome (PCOS), endometriosis and infection-related infertility. This opinion paper critically assesses the alleged correlation between genital tract dysbiosis and infertility.

How Is the Endometrial Microbiota Assessed?

To avoid cervico-vaginal bacterial contamination, the most optimal design to study the existence of a specific endometrial microbiota is the use of endometrial samples from hysterectomised women [1, 2]. The limited evidence available until now points towards the existence of a low-biomass endometrial microbiota in some, but importantly not all women; thus, a recent study showed that a substantial number of pre-menopausal women had an endometrial bacterial biomass no different from negative controls [1]. One study showed a strong correlation between the vaginal microbiota and the upper genital tract microbiota [2], whereas another study did not [1]. Moreover, bacterial ascension could be related to different pathophysiological states, as patients with vaginal dysbiosis e.g. in terms of bacterial vaginosis (BV) have an increased risk of the presence of typical BV-type bacteria (e.g. *Gardnerella vaginalis*) in the endometrium [2]. In contrast, common eubiotic vaginal lactobacilli are not necessarily found in the endometrium [1]. Thus, the presence or not of a specific endometrial microbiota has far from been scientifically proven.

Vaginal Microbiota and IVF Results

It was recently hypothesised that if a critical amount of dysbiotic bacteria were present in the vagina these bacteria (e.g. *Gardnerella vaginalis*) might ascend to the endometrium, causing a subclinical endometrial infection which in turn hampered embryo implantation [3]. Indeed, the clinical pregnancy rates per transfer of that study were intriguing, 44% (27/62) versus 9% (2/22) in patients with normal and abnormal vaginal microbiota, respectively [3]. Moreover, a Dutch study recently used another method to determine an 'unfavourable' and 'favourable' vaginal microbiome showing similar results [4], 41% (65/158) versus 6% (2/34) in eubiotic versus dysbiotic samples. Although tempting to draw immediate conclusions, the sample sizes of both studies are relatively small and, importantly, other studies did not corroborate these striking results [5]. In this aspect, the most critical point is the fact that a clear definition of abnormal/unfavourable/dysbiotic vaginal microbiota does not exist – so how can results be compared? For all medical interventions prior to diagnosing, consensual definitions are mandatory and we have to await these definitions to draw any conclusions.

Endometrial Microbiota and IVF Results

Following the idea of a dysbiotic endometrial microbiota which would hamper embryo implantation, the ideal diagnostic samples would be endometrial samples. However, by necessity these samples can only be made trans-cervically with the risk of contamination from the endocervical microbiota, resulting in huge similarities between vaginal and endometrial samples. Nevertheless, these samples could provide some insight into which bacteria ascend to the endometrium. In one study, a live birth rate of 59% was reported (10/17) in patients with a lactobacillus dominated endometrial microbiome (>90%) whereas patients with a lower concentration of lactobacilli had a 7% (1/15) live birth rate per transfer. In contrast, a recent Japanese study investigating blastocyst transfers only, did not find any positive effect of a lactobacillus dominant microbiota on the ongoing pregnancy rate, 38% (26/68) versus 45% (14/31) for the dysbiosis group. Again, the number of patients is extremely small to draw any conclusions whatsoever, and the difference in results between the two studies most certainly could be caused by different methods and assays, exposing the uncertainty as regards the correlation between genital tract microbiota and IVF outcomes.

Next Steps: Cause or Association – Will Modulation of an Unfavourable Microbiota Improve Live Birth Rates?

The future next step should be to investigate causation by treating genital tract microbiota to explore whether this improves the live birth rate in patients undergoing IVF treatment. Until now the only reports on modulation of the genital tract microbiota to improve IVF outcome are casuistic. Most evidence builds on established treatments of BV, i.e. metronidazole and clindamycin. However, some definitions of 'unfavourable microbiome' for IVF outcomes may not be the same as for BV and, thus, the subsequent medical treatment strategy might differ. Another possible future treatment option is to use bacteria therapeutically, either as probiotics or in the form of the new developing drugs, so-called live biotherapeutic products which are well-characterised bacteria undergoing regulatory drug approval prior to clinical usage. Probiotics are not drugs, and to the knowledge of this author no probiotic has been successful in obtaining a health claim. Hence, the current clinical usage of probiotics is problematic. Currently studies are ongoing using different treatment strategies, but until we have the results of those studies, we should be cautious when trying to apply the until now very poor evidence into daily clinical practice.

Conclusions

Taken together, although there is clearly much controversy within the area of vaginal and endometrial microbiota, as usual within the field of reproductive medicine, diagnostics have already been commercialised, suggesting definition of an unfavourable genital microbiota – disregarding the poor evidence. Importantly, until now there is no consensus on the definition of an unfavourable genital tract microbiota, whether the unfavourable genital tract microbiota negatively impacts IVF outcomes, and which treatment the patient with an unfavourable genital tract microbiota should be offered. Thus, as for all research, clinicians and patients should be cautious and refrain from commercialisation and clinical usage until the scientific evidence is present. Until now we just scratched the surface of the possible correlation between genital tract microbiota and IVF outcomes. The results are interesting – but contradictory. Further research should be awaited before any conclusions are drawn.

References

1. Winters AD, Romero R, Gervasi MT, et al. Does the endometrial cavity have a molecular microbial signature? *Sci Rep.* 2019;9(1):9905.

2. Mitchell CM, Haick A, Nkwopara E, et al. Colonization of the upper genital tract by vaginal bacterial species in nonpregnant women. *Am J Obstet Gynecol.* 2015;212 (5):611.e1–9.

3. Haahr T, Jensen JS, Thomsen L, Duus L, Rygaard K, Humaidan P. Abnormal vaginal microbiota may be associated with poor reproductive outcomes: a prospective study in IVF patients. *Hum Reprod.* 2016;31(4):795–803.

4. Koedooder R, Singer M, Schoenmakers S, et al. The vaginal microbiome as a predictor for outcome of in vitro fertilization with or without intracytoplasmic sperm injection: a prospective study. *Hum Reprod.* 2019;34 (6):1042–54.

5. Haahr T, Zacho J, Bräuner M, Shathmigha K, Skov Jensen J, Humaidan P. Reproductive outcome of patients undergoing in vitro fertilisation treatment and diagnosed with bacterial vaginosis or abnormal vaginal microbiota: a systematic PRISMA review and meta-analysis. *BJOG.* 2018;223(2):167–76.

Index